THE COMPLEXITY OF CONNECTION

The Complexity of Connection

Writings from the Stone Center's
Jean Baker Miller Training Institute

Edited by

JUDITH V. JORDAN
MAUREEN WALKER
LINDA M. HARTLING

THE GUILFORD PRESS
New York   London

© 2004 The Guilford Press
A Division of Guilford Publications, Inc.
72 Spring Street, New York, NY 10012
www.guilford.com

Printed in the United States of America

This book is printed on acid-free paper.

Last digit is print number: 9 8 7 6 5 4 3 2 1

Library of Congress Cataloging-in-Publication Data

The complexity of connection : writings from the Stone Center's Jean
Baker Miller Training Institute / edited by Judith V. Jordan, Maureen Walker,
Linda M. Hartling.
        p. cm.
Includes bibliographical references and index.
    ISBN 1-59385-025-5 (pbk. : alk. paper) — ISBN 1-59385-026-3 (hc. alk.
paper)
    1. Feminist therapy. 2. Group psychotherapy. 3.
Psychotherapy—Social aspects. 4. Interpersonal relations. 5.
Women—Psychology. 6. Interpersonal relations and culture. I. Jordan,
Judith V. II. Walker, Maureen. III. Hartling, Linda M.
    RC489.F45C66 2004
    616.89'14—dc22

                                                        2003025344

In memory of Irene P. Stiver and
Alexandra Kaplan
with love and gratitude
for their essential contributions to our work

About the Editors

Judith V. Jordan, PhD, is the codirector and a founding scholar of the Jean Baker Miller Training Institute of the Stone Center at Wellesley College. She is an assistant professor at Harvard Medical School and works as a therapist, supervisor, and consultant, offering hundreds of workshops and conferences on the psychology of connection throughout the United States and Europe. Dr. Jordan is a coauthor of *Women's Growth in Connection* (1991, Guilford Press) and the editor of *Women's Growth in Diversity* (1997, Guilford Press).

Maureen Walker, PhD, is a licensed psychologist with an independent practice in psychotherapy and multicultural consultation in Cambridge, Massachusetts. She is a member of the faculty and the director of program development at the Jean Baker Miller Training Institute. Dr. Walker is the coeditor of *How Connections Heal* (2004, Guilford Press) and has authored several papers in the Stone Center's Works in Progress Series. She is also the associate director of MBA Support Services at Harvard Business School.

Linda M. Hartling, PhD, is the associate director of the Jean Baker Miller Training Institute. She is also a member of an international team establishing the first Center for Human Dignity and Humiliation Studies.

Contributors

Margarita Alvarez, PhD, Department of Psychiatry, Harvard Medical School, Cambridge, Massachusetts.

Andrea Ayvazian, PhD, School for Social Work, Smith College, and Communitas, Inc., Northampton, Massachusetts

Stephen J. Bergman, MD, PhD, Gender Relations Project, Stone Center at Wellesley College, Wellesley, Massachusetts, and Department of Psychiatry, Harvard Medical School, Boston, Massachusetts

Robin Cook-Nobles, EdD, Counseling Service, Stone Center at Wellesley College, Wellesley, Massachusetts, and Antioch New England Graduate School, Keene, New Hampshire

Cate Dooley, MS, Jean Baker Miller Training Institute, Stone Center at Wellesley College, Wellesley, Massachusetts, and private practice, Newton, Massachusetts

Natalie S. Eldridge, PhD, Boston University Counseling Center, Boston, Massachusetts, and Jean Baker Miller Training Institute, Stone Center at Wellesley College, Wellesley, Massachusetts

Nikki M. Fedele, PhD, Jean Baker Miller Training Institute, Stone Center at Wellesley College, Wellesley, Massachusetts, and private practice, Wayland, Massachusetts

Joyce K. Fletcher, DBA, Graduate School of Management, Simmons College, Boston, Massachusetts

Maryellen Handel, PhD, Tufts University School of Medicine, Boston, Massachusetts, and Behavior Health Network, Concord, New York

Linda M. Hartling, PhD, Jean Baker Miller Training Institute, Stone Center at Wellesley College, Wellesley, Massachusetts

Judith V. Jordan, PhD, Jean Baker Miller Training Institute, Stone Center at Wellesley College, Wellesley, Massachusetts, and Department of Psychology, Harvard Medical School, Boston, Massachusetts

Jean Baker Miller, MD, Jean Baker Miller Training Institute, Stone Center at Wellesley College, Wellesley, Massachusetts, and Department of Psychiatry, Boston University School of Medicine, Boston, Massachusetts

Wendy B. Rosen, PhD, McLean Hospital, Belmont, Massachusetts, and private practice, Cambridge, Massachusetts

Irene P. Stiver, PhD (deceased), Jean Baker Miller Training Institute, Stone Center at Wellesley College, Wellesley, Massachusetts; McLean Hospital, Belmont, Massachusetts; and Harvard Medical School, Boston, Massachusetts

Janet L. Surrey, PhD, Jean Baker Miller Training Institute, Stone Center at Wellesley College, Wellesley, Massachusetts, and McLean Hospital, Belmont, Massachusetts

Beverly Daniel Tatum, PhD, President, Spelman College, Atlanta, Georgia

Maureen Walker, PhD, Jean Baker Miller Training Institute, Stone Center at Wellesley College, Wellesley, Massachusetts, and private practice, Cambridge, Massachusetts

Contents

Part II. Applying the Power of Connection

THE COMPLEXITY OF CONNECTION

Introduction

JUDITH V. JORDAN *and* MAUREEN WALKER

*T*he primacy of connection in women's lives is not a new idea. The initial Stone Center model, which was called "self-in-relation," began with that idea but has been evolving ever since. That evolution has been a movement from a psychology of separation to one of connection, and it represents a profound change in our approach to understanding people. Putting connection at the center challenges core beliefs of Western social, psychological, and economic systems. Connection is not a simple, cozy, or easy concept; viewed as the primary organizer and source of motivation in people's lives, it is powerful, complex, and revolutionary, challenging some of the basic tenets and values of 21st-century Western culture.

In 1991 five women (J. V. Jordan, A. G. Kaplan, J. B. Miller, I. P. Stiver, & J. L. Surrey) published *Women's Growth in Connection*. Four of us had been meeting since 1978, trying to learn together, to break free of some of what we felt were the damaging effects for women of traditional therapy. We began cautiously, some of us not quite taking our own ideas seriously. But by 1981 we were writing papers to be presented at conferences, and we had found an institutional home at the Stone Center at Wellesley College where Jean Baker Miller served as the first director; we were literally coming into voice. *Women's Growth in Connection* contained the essential early papers that were an effort to better understand and represent women's lives. We questioned the usefulness of a psychology that elevates and celebrates the separate self. Self is a metaphor, a highly valued concept in Western culture, particularly in the culture of the 21st-century United States. The dominant (white, male, middle-class, heterosexual) culture valorizes separation. To the extent that relationships are emphasized, they are viewed as primarily utilitarian, as aids to the achievement of a separate self. Our Western psychologies focus on individual personality traits, movement toward autonomy, independence, success accomplished through competitive achievement. They underemphasize the importance of connection, growth-fostering relationship, and the need to participate in the growth of relationship and community. The clinical practices that derive from these traditional developmental and clinical models typically overemphasize internal traits, intrapsychic conflict, and striving for independence. Therapeutic practices reflect the dominant culture of separation and power over others.

By the time our second volume of papers, *Women's Growth in Diversity*, was published (Jordan, 1997), we were referring to the Stone Center relational model. Connection, not self or even self-in-relation, was now (and still is) at the center of the model. The Stone Center model posits that connection is at the core of human growth and development. Isolation is seen as the primary source of human suffering. We believe that human beings grow through and toward connection. The path of human development is through movement to increasingly differentiated and growth-fostering connection; chronic disconnections result from the unresponsiveness of important people in our lives. When we are hurt, misunderstood, or violated in some way, when we attempt to represent our experience to the injuring person and we are not responded to, we learn to suppress our experience and disconnect from both our own feelings and the other person. If, on the other hand, we are able to express our feelings and the other person responds with care, showing that we have had an effect, then we feel that we are effective in relationship with others, that we matter, that we can participate in creating growth-fostering and healthy relationships. Ultimately we feel anchored in community and we experience relational competence.

Women's Growth in Diversity emphasized the importance of connection as it also sought to move the model away from the biases of white, middle-class, heterosexual experience, from woman's voice to women's voices. Since publication of that book we have continued to explore connection, especially connection across difference. We are concerned about the suffering incurred at an individual level when people experience a sense of personal isolation, immobilization, and not "mattering" in the world. But we also care deeply about the effects of disconnection at a societal level, the ways that power differentials, forces of stratification, privilege, and marginalization can disconnect and disempower individuals and groups of people. The exercise of power over others (dominance), unilateral influence, and/or coercive control is a prime deterrent to mutuality.

Mutuality involves profound mutual respect and mutual openness to change and responsiveness. It does not mean equality. When it comes to the therapeutic relationship, it does not mean blurring of the roles of therapist and client. As Jean Baker Miller once said, "In order for one person to grow in a relationship, both people must grow." This involves intersubjective, cognitive–emotional change; there is a certain, although different, vulnerability for both participants. Although we ultimately believe safety lies in building good, growth-fostering relationships and not in establishing separation from and power over others, building authentic connection is predicated on tolerating uncertainty, complexity, and the inevitable vulnerability involved in real change. It is far from easy or being perpetually "nice."

Women's Growth in Diversity brought a phenomenological focus to the experience of women whose voices had been historically marginalized from the mainstream writing about women's development. The inclusion of these voices was intended to challenge our assumptions of a powerful mythic norm that would define "woman" as a white, economically privileged, able-bodied, and heterosexual female. Unchallenged, this norm becomes a standard against which all women's experience is interpreted and evaluated. Therefore, the extent to which any individual woman conforms to this norm becomes almost by default the measure by which she is deemed worthy of notice or fit for connection. The publication of *Women's Growth in Diversity* was therefore a critical step in the evolution of the model, one that emphasized the significance of cultural context to human development.

In this third volume of Stone Center papers, readers will see a further shift from the relational model to relational–cultural theory (RCT). This represents our growing awareness of the impact of culture. It follows from increased recognition that relationships do not exist as atomized units—separate and distinct from the larger culture. Indeed, relationships may both represent and reproduce the cultures in which they are embedded. Accordingly, theories about human development must answer the question: What purpose and whose interests does the theory serve? The history of psychological theory is replete with evidence of complicity with cultural arrangements and power practices that divide people into groups of dominants and subordinates. One example of this complicity was the proliferation of psychiatric diagnoses in the 19th century ascribing certain "personality traits" to African slaves that supposedly made them susceptible to "rascality, episodes of running away and disregard for owner's property" (Thomas & Sillen, 1972). More recently, feminist theorists (Broverman, Broverman, Clarkson, Rosenkranz, & Vogel, 1970; Gilligan, 1982; Jordan et al., 1991; Miller, 1976, 1987; Miller & Stiver, 1997) have noted how the traditional theories of psychological maturity tended to overpathologize women as inherently needy, overly emotional, and dependent. Rarely was there any attention to the social structures and power arrangements that circumscribed the relational roles designated for women in a gender-stratified culture. When "personality traits" are attributed to a subordinate group and pathologized, psychological theories help to justify and preserve the culture's power stratifications. In sum, the shift from self-in-relation to RCT signifies an intentional focus on the social implications of theory development.

Through exploring connection and disconnection at both the individual and social levels, we begin to understand how the political becomes psychological/personal and vice versa. Connections form or fail to form within a web of other social and cultural relationships. As we more deeply understood the central role of culture and power differentials on relationships, we felt the model's name needed to signal this.

To place culture, alongside connection, at the center of the theory is to break a critical silence. First, it acknowledges that social and political values inform theories of human psychology, including those that valorize separation and autonomy. Relational–cultural theory does not pretend to be value neutral. RTC recognizes that to feign value neutrality is to perpetuate the distortions of the stratified culture in rather predictable ways. First, theory itself becomes exempt from social scrutiny and takes on an aura of truth. Second, such hierarchical "power over" theories control how all members of the culture are defined and known. Third, it does this by tending to degrade or pathologize the experiences of marginalized people. Fourth, it tends to overvalue and privilege the perspectives of people who are culturally dominant. Miller (1976) and others have pointed out that as one gains dominance in a culture of stratified power, enabling supports and connections are rendered invisible. By placing culture at the center of the model, RCT strives to make visible the multilayered connections that belie the myth of separation (Miller & Stiver, 1997).

In a culture that valorizes separation and autonomy, persons with cultural privilege can falsely appear more self-sufficient and so will be judged as healthier, more mature, more worthy of the privilege the society affords. Those who enjoy less cultural privilege (whether by virtue of race, ethnicity, sexual orientation, or economic status) will more likely be viewed as deficient and needy. They are more likely to be subject to systematic disadvantage and culture shaming.

By bringing a phenomenological focus to cultural context, a more complete and accurate picture of human experience and possibility emerges. Without such a focus, the experiences of both the socially privileged and the socially disadvantaged are subject to distortion. A brief example might illustrate this point.

"Sarah" was a late-middle-aged white woman who had just completed her graduate degree in history. As she spoke with her counselor about her career prospects, she began to bemoan the fact that she lacked a "spirit of adventure." As if to prove her point, she recounted a media story she had heard about a young woman who was described as having dropped everything to travel to another continent to study and write about tribal naming practices. As the conversation progressed, Sarah's counselor encouraged her to consider the contextual factors that informed her career path and to speculate as to whether there might be meaningful differences between her own situation and that of the "adventurous" younger woman. Sarah had started graduate school following an economically devastating divorce. Although she did not bear economic responsibility for her grown children, she did assist in providing resources and caretaking for her aging father. Sarah began to see that she did not suffer from lack of ambition or adventurous spirit, but rather that her relational context—including the changing nature of her relationship with her father and her socioeconomic status—required exquisite attunement to contingencies and complexities of life. She also began to see the irony in a story that would applaud individual pluck and ambition, when an intricate web of relational supports must be in place before someone could "drop everything."

The illusion of separation and the mistaken belief in autonomy contribute to the denial of the basic human need to participate in the growth of others and to being open to being moved by others. And yet the power to move others, to find responsiveness, to effect change, to create movement together is a vital part of good connection. How power is defined and expressed is crucial. For instance there is the power to name, to shame, and to define another's value or lack thereof, the power to distribute resources. If this power is expressed unilaterally, it reduces the strength and power of the other person or group of people who do not hold this power. As it is held onto and denied to others, it creates disconnections and disempowerment. Inequalities in power distribution occur in families, in therapy relationships, in work relationships. At a societal level, unequal distribution of power among groups—those largely defined as marginal by dominant center groups—

is rampant and the source of pain and disconnection among the members of the marginalized groups.

The complexity of connection and of relationships arises from unequal power, from working with difference, or from trying to manage conflict creatively. RCT recognizes that all relationships are punctuated by disconnections, misunderstandings, and conflict. Connecting in a real, growthful way with others is not always harmonious or comfortable; we all experience fear, anger, and shame. We move away to protect ourselves, particularly if we are not met with empathic responsiveness or if we feel we do not matter to the other person. But when we can renegotiate these inevitable disconnections, the relationship is enhanced and personal feelings of well-being, creativity, and clarity increase.

The path of connection is filled with disconnections, the vulnerability of seeking reconnection, and the tension around needing to move away, possibly to hide in protective inauthenticity. But we believe there is a powerful force behind the movement toward connection, a yearning for connection, a desire to contribute to others, to serve something larger than "the self."

In this volume we turn toward the complexity of connection. These papers ask: How can we create a radical new language of connection and fully appreciate the fundamental contribution of relationship to human development? How can we appreciate the power of "controlling images?" Described so powerfully by Patricia Hill Collins (1990), these images are often about race, class, gender, and sexual orientation, and are imposed by the dominant culture to disempower and marginalize subordinate groups. This volume seeks to examine how cultural stratification along multiple social identities shapes developmental experiences and relational possibilities. Specifically, many of the authors explore how experiences of race, ethnicity, sexual orientation, class, and gender affect the development of authenticity and mutual empathy in relationship. In previous volumes, we have elucidated the relational consequences of interpersonal disconnection, describing it as a primary source of human suffering. As we further examine the complexities of connection, we will explore the thesis that a "power over" culture is itself an agent of disconnection that, left unchallenged, effectively diminishes the relational capacities and confidence of all its members. For example, because unilateral power breeds fear, it also diminishes the relational capacities of those who hold power over others. When the purpose of a relationship is to protect the power differential (maintain the gap between those who hold privilege and those who do not), it is highly unlikely that authentic responsiveness can unfold. Indeed, authentic engagement and openness to mutual influence may be viewed as dangerous practices.

True to Jean Baker Miller's original conception, the writings emanating from RCT are still referred to as "works in progress." These ideas have evolved in a relational context characterized by responsiveness and mutual creation. As a group we revisit, rethink, and question our own formulations with the same curiosity and, at times, uneasiness with which we address other models

We have published more than 100 works in progress and many books. Our group has been changed by time and sadly the deaths of one of our founding members, Irene P. Stiver, and of our very early important contributor, Alexandra G. Kaplan, Both of these colleagues were crucial to the growth of our ideas and practices. Despite our personal and professional grief at these losses, we continue with new core contributors, new directions, and new energy. The coeditors of this volume, Maureen Walker and Linda M. Hartling, are two of these very treasured and core voices.

Part I of this volume, "Deepening Our Understanding of Relationship," begins with new theoretical contributions that seek to apply a relational rather than a separation model to competence (Chapter 1), resilience (Chapter 2), and relational awareness (Chapter 3). These chapters challenge the notion that resilience and other characteristics attributed to individuals are really internal, individual traits. Chapter 4 examines therapists' authenticity. Chapters 5, 7, and 8 specifically address an RCT theoretical understanding of race and racism. In a culture where race is a central stratifier, those on both the dominant and the subjugated sides of the racial divide are likely to experience significantly distorted relational expectancies and possibilities. Chapter 6 examines how shame and humiliation can disrupt connection and lead to isolation; the privilege–power dimension is always at the core of this inquiry, whether it be about race, gender, or sexual orientation. How does a group with less power, given less respect by the dominant groups, maintain a sense of dignity? How do marginalized people resist the forces of shame that are directed at them to disempower and silence them? Moreover, as with other social stratifiers, the experience of race and racism also affects how one interprets other aspects of a complex cultural environment.

Part II of the book, "Applying the Power of Connection," RCT is applied in Chapter 9 to couple therapy, work that depends on establishing a "we" relationship and addressing the relationship itself. Our more recent work with groups and time-limited therapy is included in Chapters 10 and 12, respectively. In Chapter 11 we also look at the ways in which this model helps us better understand boys and men. The book ends in Chapter 13 with our most recent application of RCT to the workplace and organizations. How can we rethink the place of relationship in the workplace, making the invisible strengths of connection visible and validated?

We hope that readers who know our earlier work will find a deepening of understanding in this volume. For those of you new to this work, we hope you find resonance and a sense of possibility. We also hope that questions will arise for all who join us in this journey: How is RCT different from other models of therapy? What are the implications for organizing social institutions differently around a core belief in connection rather than separation? We also continue to live with these recurring questions: What makes for change in therapy? How can we use what we learn in psychological practice and theory to facilitate social change? Psychological theory and feminist practice in no way have all the answers. The path of connection is filled with complexity, contradiction, and uncertainty. In the face of the unknowns and the humbling blindspots, we are dedicated to learning, to being responsive. In a world that is increasingly disconnected, violent, and filled with fear, where community needs are obscured by individual greed and competition, we feel a commitment to connection. And in turning to connection, we feel hope.

REFERENCES

Broverman, I. K., Broverman, D. M., Clarkson, F. E., Rosenkranz, P. S., & Vogel, S. (1970). Sex-role stereotypes and clinical judgements of mental health. *Journal of Consulting and Clinical Psychology, 34*(1), 1–7.

Collins, P. H. (1990). *Black feminist thought: Knowledge, consciousness, and the politics of empowerment.* Boston: Unwin Hyman.

Gilligan, C. (1982). *In a different voice: Psychological theory and women's development.* Cambridge, MA: Harvard University Press.

Jordan, J. V. (Ed.). (1997). *Women's growth in diversity: More writings from the Stone Center.* New York: Guilford Press.

Jordan, J. V., Kaplan, A. G., Miller, J. B., Stiver, I. P., & Surrey, J. L. (1991). *Women's growth in connection: Writings from the Stone Center.* New York: Guilford Press.

Miller, J. B. (1976). *Toward a new psychology of women.* Boston: Beacon Press.

Miller, J. B. (1987). *Toward a new psychology of women* (2nd ed.). Boston: Beacon Press.

Miller, J. B., & Stiver, I. P. (1997). *The healing connection: How women form relationships in therapy and in life.* Boston: Beacon Press.

Thomas, A., & Sillen, S. (1972). *Racism and psychiatry.* New York: Brunner-Routledge.

Part I

Deepening Our Understanding of Relationship

1

Toward Competence and Connection

JUDITH V. JORDAN

In the Stone Center model, the yearning for and movement toward connection are seen as central organizing factors in people's lives and the experience of chronic disconnection or isolation is seen as a primary source of suffering (Jordan, Kaplan, Miller, Stiver, & Surrey, 1991; Miller & Stiver, 1997). When we cannot represent ourselves authentically in relationships, when our real experience is not heard or responded to by the other person, then we must falsify, detach from, or suppress our response. Under such circumstances we learn that we cannot have an impact on other people in the relationships that matter to us. A sense of isolation, immobilization, self-blame, and relational incompetence develops. These meaning systems and relational images of incompetence and depletion interfere with our capacity to be productive, as well as to be in a creative relationship. They inhibit our engagement with life and our capacity to love and to move with a sense of awareness to meet others, to contribute to their growth, and to grow ourselves. The need to connect and the need to contribute in a meaningful way, to be competent, productive, and creative, optimally flow together. Yet, in a system that overvalues competition and highly individualistic goals, a system that pits the individual against society and other individuals, the pursuit of competence and connection can be at odds. Further, in a system characterized by competitive individualism, the people who are more invested in relationship and community typically will feel this conflict more acutely.

The word "competence" has its roots in two Latin words: *com,* meaning "together," and *petere,* to aim at, go toward, try to reach, seek (*Oxford English Dictionary,* 1971). It shares these roots with the word "compete." In fact, competition used to mean "to strive after [something] in company or together." Much later did competition come to mean "to be in rivalry with" or "the action of endeavoring to gain what another endeavors to gain at the same time" (*Oxford English Dictionary,* 1971). Current notions of competence are saturated with images of "mastery over" and competition. The verb "to master" suggests "to reduce to subjection, to get the better of, to break, to tame" (*Oxford English Dictionary,* 1971). Evelyn Fox Keller (1985) notes that Western models of science are based on a "Baconian" model of mastery over nature. The competition and mastery implicit in most models of competence create enormous conflict for many people, especially women and other marginalized groups, people who have not traditionally been "the masters." Rather than focus on the problem of these groups for being unable to fully participate in "the psychology of being a master," perhaps we need to focus on the problems of a system that replaces ability, confidence, creativity, and participation in growth-fostering relationships with being the lone star at the top, dominance, being a master, and ultimately participating in oppression of those who are not fully invested in the power that this model confers (Walker, 1998). Today I would like to begin a reexamination of this system of competitively defined competence and begin to suggest what Carol Gilligan (1990) calls some strategies of resistance and transformation.

Most of the original work done on competence and competence motivation was undertaken by Robert White (1959), who suggested that there is an intrinsic motivation to be in effective interaction with the environment and that all people experience a need to feel effective, able to move or change things. The extent to which the environment responds to the efforts and actions of the individual determines the extent to which the individual feels competent or effective. When one is not able to effect a change in one's environment, one might experience a sense of incompetence, or what Seligman (1972) has called "learned helplessness." The signs of learned helplessness are close to what would be the opposite of Jean Baker Miller's "Five Good Things": a drop in zest, decreasing clarity, withdrawal from connection, less self-knowledge, and a decrease in sense of self-worth (Miller & Stiver, 1997; see also Miller, 1987).

Competence, as traditionally defined, usually refers to mastery of a task, the capacity to be instrumentally effective and competitively successful. Taking the individualistic road and "beating" others comes to be seen as interpersonally strong, good, and competent. The irony is that one's sense of self-worth is rarely buttressed in any long-term way in such a competitive system. As Morton Deutsch notes, "self-esteem is more negative in a competitive system than in a cooperative grading system. Winning doesn't satisfy in an ongoing way and losing makes us feel like losers. King of the Mountain doesn't work" (1985, p. 399). Furthermore, competition can damage relationships. Karen Horney (1936/1973) noted such a system creates "envy toward the stronger ones, contempt for the weaker, distrust towards everyone" (p. 161).

As Alfie Kohn (1986) points out, myths supporting the importance of competition suggest it is an unavoidable fact of life and that it motivates us to do our best. A distortion of Darwin's work on evolution would have us believe that we are engaged in a competitive struggle toward the "survival of the fittest." On the contrary, Stephen Jay Gould states that "there is no necessary relationship between natural selection and competitive struggle . . . [and] that success defined as leaving more offspring can be attained by a large variety of strategies including mutualism and symbiosis . . . that we could call cooperative" (Kohn, 1986, p. 21). Yet, our education systems and our systems of assessment actively encourage this emphasis on winning, on being the best, and on competence defined by competitiveness. Assessing a child in a play setting, Jean Piaget asked, "Who has won?" When the child responded, "We both won," Piaget continued, "But who has won most?" (1965, p. 37). What are we teaching? Separate-self models in traditional psychology suggest that we are self-centered, self-gratifying at heart, and that competition is inevitable. The model of separate self, of autonomous self, of self disconnected from others, contributes to a self that is free to compete. Psychology's elevation of separation and autonomy thus contributes to the ascendance of a competitive, individualistic, sociopolitical agenda. A psychology of connection, on the other hand, poses challenges to the larger competitive system.

The dominant myths of instrumental competence, which largely coincide with the myths of masculinity, include:

1. The myth that competition enhances performance
2. The myth of invulnerability
3. The myth of certainty, what I call the cultivation of pathological certainty
4. The myth of self-sufficiency ("I did it alone, so can you.")
5. The myth of mastery ("I mastered it, I *am* the master.")
6. The myth of objectivity

7. The myth of the expert
8. The myth of unilateral change (in an interaction, the less powerful person is changed)
9. The myth that hierarchy and ranking produces incentives and that people assume their places in the hierarchy by virtue of merit
10. The myth that power over others creates safety
11. The myth that rational engagement is superior to and at odds with emotional responsiveness

Since women have typically performed differently from men in areas of achievement, defined largely by masculine standards, women have often been viewed as having "problems with competence and achievement." A whole theory of women's fear of success was developed to explain this problem (Horner, 1970). When women opt out of positions of leadership, leave positions as CEOs, the question is asked: "What's wrong with these women? Can't they hack it in the real world of competition?" How long will it be before we will say, instead, "What's wrong with our construction of competence and success?" There has been one reigning definition that has emphasized competition, mastery, control, having an impact on the physical world, and it has notably omitted the world of relationships and connection.

One of the reasons that the competitive ethic is aversive for so many girls is that girls have learned a "double voice discourse," representing what they want and paying attention to the needs of others at the same time (Tannen, 1998). Girls and women typically care about the impact of their feelings and actions on the other person. I have called this *relational awareness*, being attentive to self, the other, and the relationship. Boys tend to use "single voice discourse," pursuing their own self-interest without orienting to the perspective of the other (Tannen, 1998). Women practice not only empathic listening, but also empathic speaking. They use what I have called *anticipatory empathy*, speaking and moving with an awareness of and concern for the possible consequences of their feelings and actions for other people while also remaining aware of their own needs and the needs of the other person(s) (i.e., relational awareness). I believe this to be one of the greatest human capacities, involving significant skill; it can potentially avert much harm and suffering. It contributes to building relationships where neither person is at the center—relatedness is. Conversely, the individualistic way is to put *the self* at the center and in opposition to society.

What I am proposing is that we need more than one way to conceptualize competence and we need to be very aware of the power of context to shape a person's sense of competence. We also need to question a value system that pits connection against competence, that dichotomizes the two and does not see the possibilities and strengths in the development of relational competence.

RELATIONAL COMPETENCE

The capacity to move another person, to effect a change in a relationship, or effect the well-being of all participants in the relationship might be called *relational competence*. This capacity does not mean simply influencing another person or having an impact on another person, which might produce a sense of power. From a relational point of view, we look at the quality of the impact on the other person and on the relationship. Does this change have value for both (or more) people and the relationship? Does the relationship expand, grow, and become more mutually empowering as well as contribute to the movement and growth of others beyond this immediate relationship?

Another way of framing relational competence is to speak of the ability to participate in growth-fostering relationships. This is the ability to "move" someone or a relationship in the emotional, cognitive, and behavioral realm. The Latin root for "emotion" is the verb "*motere* . . . to move" (*Oxford English Dictionary*, 1971). It is in being in touch with our own feelings—and with our own hearts—that we touch the hearts of others and both people grow.

Relational competence involves:

1. Movement toward mutuality and mutual empathy (caring and learning flows both ways), where empathy expands for both self and other
2. The development of anticipatory empathy, noticing and caring about our impact on others
3. Being open to being influenced
4. Enjoying relational curiosity
5. Experiencing vulnerability as inevitable and a place of potential growth rather than danger
6. Creating good connection rather than exercising power over others as the path of growth

Relational competence occurs within a context of wishing to empower others and appreciating the life-giving nature of community building, of creating strength with others rather than in isolation.

OBSTACLES TO RELATIONAL COMPETENCE

There are several obstacles to the development of a sense of relational competence and many routes to the silencing of women's relational voices (Gilligan, 1982) and the disappearing of women's relational ways of being (Fletcher, 1996). As Beverly Tatum notes, "dominant groups . . . by definition set the parameters within which the subordinants operate. They define a mythical norm" (1997, p. 23). Dominant groups ensure their power advantage by directly and indirectly subverting the competence and limiting the power of connection among the subordinate groups. Karen Laing (1998) noted, "Isolation functions as the glue that holds oppression in place." This is a profound truth. Undermining the sense of competence and courage of a person or a group also serves to keep oppression in place. Thus, to increase connection and a sense of competence, particularly among marginalized or disenfranchised groups, threatens prevailing norms and power dynamics. It is a revolutionary act.

The development of relational competence depends on being in a context that is responsive to one's voice and actions. Resistance to interpersonal influence is a major impediment to relational competence. Nonresponsiveness is also a major component of the exercise of "power over"; those in power are taught to resist the influence of others. Maccoby (1990) has noted this resistance to influence in 3½-year-old boys, and this resistance increases as boys grow older. In fact, a defining characteristic of boyhood and manhood in this culture is the capacity to resist influence, particularly from females. Studies have indicated that between the ages of 3½ and 5½ all children show a dramatic increase in their efforts to influence other people (Maccoby, 1990). This may be a time when children are particularly focused on exploring the world of interpersonal competence. However, the ways girls and boys attempt to influence others differ. Girls tend to make suggestions, whereas boys make more direct demands. Furthermore and more important, in the two years before school, boys appear to actively develop strategies to resist being influenced by others. While, in part, these may be strategies of disconnection, I would suggest that they are invoked largely because of the competitive ethos that pervades the socialization of boys.

In a Western European system, in order to compete successfully (hence, to be a competent male), one must not be vulnerable; one must be armored. I believe denial of vulnerability is one of the greatest costs of male socialization. It also places significant strain on relationships. While girls are still effective in influencing other girls and adults, they progressively fail to have an impact on boys. Eleanor Maccoby, in her classic review of these patterns, suggests that "girls find it aversive to try to interact with someone who is unresponsive and . . . they begin to avoid such partners" (1990, p. 343). Gender-segregated play groups become powerful socializing environments, with boys and girls learning very different styles of interaction and play. Boys are more likely to interrupt one another, refuse to comply with others' demands, and threaten others. All-girl groups are more likely to express agreement and pause to give another girl a chance to speak.

But in adolescence girls and boys move into mixed-sex pairings and groups. The boys, armored to resist influence from others, meet the girls who are organized around relationships and mutual responsiveness. Because the competitive, influence-resistant style is the socially privileged and dominant style, the girls' more mutual and relational approach is seen as deficient, with very serious results for the girls and for our total society, as Gilligan (1990) suggests.

OBSTACLES TO RELATIONAL COMPETENCE/ GENDER ISSUES

In primary heterosexual pairings women complain often of being "stonewalled," not listened to, not taken in, not having impact. A recent study by Gottman, Coon, Carrere, and Swanson (1998) of married couples suggests that divorce is predicted most accurately in marriage by a husband's refusal to accept influence from his wife. Very succinctly Gottman and colleagues note, "husbands do not want to share power with their wives" (p. 12). The issue of avoiding influence is clearly a power dynamic. To be denied the ability to influence another person is to be disempowered and to have one's relational competence undermined.

It worries me that the nonresponsive neutrality of traditional therapies is similarly disempowering and undermining of the development of a sense of relational competence for both clients and therapists. Many therapists get caught in needing to appear to be the expert or needing to appear to be perfectly warm, loving people. When they are inevitably thrown off balance or feel vulnerable during some of the therapy work, they sometimes attribute it to the "manipulativeness" of the client or the client's use of "projective identification."

The traditional culture of therapy supports the following myths of competence: therapists are the experts; change is unilateral; and the person with power, the therapist, should be invulnerable or should not be too emotionally responsive. In such a professional context, the therapist who believes in mutual empathy, the importance of being moved and being emotionally present, may inevitably feel she is "doing it wrong." Furthermore, if she believes she has to be an expert, she will often feel incompetent and fraudulent, particularly when she experiences uncertainty or needs to ask for consultation (which I consider to be a clear sign of relational competence rather than incompetence). In fact, serious difficulty occurs in therapy when therapists deny their vulnerability and refuse to reach out for help from colleagues.

I have written about shame in the therapist, and I think much of this is anchored in unrealistic expectations about how we should be able to help our clients (Jordan, 1989). Managed care and increasing expectations for quick, clear fix-ups only add to the burden that many therapists already feel. I think many of us spend much time struggling with a sense of incompetence or that recurring feeling that "surely someone else would be better at this than I am" (or maybe I should just speak for myself).

Therapists' sense of incompetence can become a major source of disconnection. When I feel helpless and unable to bring something useful to a therapy session, I often feel incompetent. I *believe* in the mystery of therapy, and I *believe* in staying open in vulnerability. Unfortunately, in therapy sessions that are particularly challenging or unclear, the old voices of supervisors in my head, or what I call the rules of "the general internalized psychotherapy culture," demand I have more clarity and certainty than I do. In the face of my own internal critics, I begin to pull out of connection with myself and with my client. As I withdraw, I sink into a deeper sense of incompetence. The irony, of course, is that in therapy the more I can move into being present in a relationship, the more effective the therapy is. Healing is about *staying with*, providing an opportunity for connection, and bringing awareness to patterns of disconnection. Stephen Levine noted, "Healing is to enter with mercy and awareness that which has been withdrawn from in judgment and hatred" (1997, p. 17). While this sounds so seamless and easy, in practice it is challenging and confounding at times! We struggle to bring this attitude of compassion to both our clients and ourselves.

Further, unrealistic expectations of ourselves as human beings are epidemic among therapists. A seasoned, exceptionally talented therapist I am treating noted recently that she spends most of her time feeling fraudulent with her clients. She stated, "If they knew all of the confusion and personal struggles that exist in my life, they would never listen to me." Struggling with these feelings myself, I said something muted or stiff like, "I'm not sure we have to be relational experts in our own lives to be decent therapists." She, being quite attuned, scanned my face and said, "Oh, I'm not the only one!" and we shared a moment of ironic laughter.

I know that when I am caught up in trying to preserve some image of myself as "the good therapist" or "the psychologically healthy adult," I am likely, in fact, to be less present and less relationally competent. Preoccupations with images of who we are or who we *should* be take us out of authentic connection and close us down. This happens in and out of therapy.

RELATIONAL COMPETENCE IN ORGANIZATIONS

Pressure to be the expert, the authority at the top dispensing wisdom, is widespread. I would like to share another vignette about the pressure to be "the expert" from the world of business. Laura is a woman in the Stone Center's study group that is exploring relational practice in organizations and institutions. This vignette exemplifies another way in which relational competence can be completely congruent with and contribute to effective work practices—competence and connection do not have to be at odds.

Laura, who is a senior corporate vice president, noted that she took a job managing a large engineering group whose technology she knew only superficially. In her first week, the project team, many consisting of 10-year veterans with this product, was holding a meeting to determine if the new product was ready to ship. She attended the meeting expecting to take a back seat. When she entered the room, the meeting fell silent. All eyes turned to her. With a sinking feeling, she reports, she realized the decision would be hers—not because she had the information to make the decision but because she had the positional responsibility to do so! To avoid that responsibility would be to let the group feel leaderless. To make the decision independently would have been foolhardy if not impossible (although that's what the situation pulled for). So she outlined the process they would use. She would make the decision and take responsibility if it turned out badly. But first, she'd do some research. She went around the room asking each person, "If you were in my shoes, what would you decide and why?" By the end of the meeting she was able to make a decision, informed by all the real decision makers, the project team (Woodburn, 1998).

In this example, Laura demonstrates the ability to move aside from the expectations for expert, top–down leadership and the unrealistic expectations for an expertise she couldn't possibly hold, and she makes beautiful use of relational competence. She turns to the other workers, the people with the relevant experience, and invites them to take part in the process at the same time that she accepts her defined task as the one who holds the responsibility.

Expanding our notions of competence, then, involves moving away from the dissociated manipulation of objects or from an abstract intellectual exercise to an appreciation of relational competence and the capacity to make things happen for the good of the relationship and the community. A part of this expansion is bringing into clear articulation and focus that which gets devalued and "disappeared," a term Joyce Fletcher (1996) has used.

Relational competence, as shown by Laura, is not a function of some intuitive, biologically given instinct that women possess. It involves vision, philosophy, emotional and cognitive skills, and the development of relational practice. There is relational problem solving in which the power of dialogue, of asking for help, and of sharing uncertainty is openly acknowledged. Cooperative efforts, rather than competitive one-upmanship are encouraged. There is value placed on competence that is in service of the community. When we build relational competence in organizations, we work to empower others and the project, the work, or the community, not just to assert self-dominance or elevate individual needs (Fletcher, 1996).

RESISTANCE AND TRANSFORMATION

Operating within a system that overemphasizes certainty, competitive success, and tough adversarial standards of conduct disempowers people who value connection and community; bell hooks (1991) speaks of the power of the black women's "oppositional gaze." Tracy Robinson and Janie Ward (1991), writing about African American girls, speak about transforming the "resistance of survival" to the "resistance for liberation." They point to the importance of African American women acknowledging the problems of, and demanding change in, an environment that oppresses them, thus transforming self-directed anger into striving for justice. One approach to helping women and other marginalized groups is to foster awareness of the specific expectations and standards of the dominant group and to explicitly critique and name alternative values or ways of constructing reality. The shaming and silencing strategies of the dominant group can be countered with this consciousness along with the support of others who share this awareness.

When I was helping to organize a women's treatment program at a psychiatric hospital, one of the early tasks given to us by the administration was to make an organizational chart of our program. All of us in the leadership group knew what an organizational chart looked like, but we felt that the usual box at the top, followed by two boxes down, and so on, did not fit the way we were trying to operate. So we put together an organizational chart made up of intersecting circles. At the top of the page we placed the patient council and advisers. We placed what we thought of as the leadership coordinating committee at the bottom.

When we showed the chart to the chief administrator of the hospital, his first response was "Didn't anyone teach you how to make an organizational chart?" When we responded that we were well aware of what many people's organizational charts looked like and that we felt our chart did in fact represent our program, his next question was "But who do we go to when we need a decision made?" We noted that we had a committee that made decisions, in consultation with the other groups. This was met with an exasperated, "Oh, *ladies*! . . . Who do we go to when we want a *final* decision?" We persisted. Hence, we were persistently treated as if we were quite incompetent leaders and quite irritating people. Together we held our ground. But when we were dealt with alone (and that was a definite strategy of disempowerment by the administration), each of us often felt more anxious and we would rush back to the others to shore ourselves up.

At a recent conference on relational leadership, a woman in the audience noted she had been chided by a boss for being too interested in "the soft stuff," the emotional, relational aspects in her company. Initially she felt ashamed that she was not thinking about the really important stuff—the hard stuff—the *real* stuff. Then, when she thought about it she realized "the soft stuff *is* the real stuff." However, it is often the unacknowledged, invisible, dismissed and demeaned stuff. It is the stuff of relational competence.

AM I THE PROBLEM?

We need to develop critical relational consciousness and question social norms that devalue and undermine relational values. We need to question situations that leave girls and women feeling much too frequently that "I am the problem." Perhaps just asking the simple question "Am I really the problem?" would begin to free girls and women from blaming ourselves and accepting the shame that the culture puts on us for functioning in a way different from the dominant patterns. bell hooks (1984) enjoins us to see the social world critically and to oppose ideas that disempower us and all women. We need to be critical or resistant, not to disempower other people but to disempower the disempowering ideas and values (hooks, 1989). We must be careful not to focus only on changing the girls to increase their sense of connection and competence but, more important, to focus on changing the

systems within which the girls lose their voices, their sense of competence, and their real sense of connection with themselves and others.

I want to suggest several beginning strategies for resistance and
transformation. These might also be seen as antishaming strategies: (1)
naming the problem, (2) complaining, (3) claiming/reframing strengths,
and (4) developing communities of resilience and courage.

NAMING THE PROBLEM AND NOTICING WHO MAKES THE RULES

Naming what is valued and privileged in any situation is essential.
Pointing to the fact that these standards and values are created by a
particular community removes their absolute power. Developing critical awareness of existing norms and practices is the first step to dismantling them. Alternate values and practices then need to be named
and encouraged. Whenever "outsiders," however, are critical of the
prevailing way of doing things and suggest changes, they are often met
with the disempowering response of "you will be *lowering* (not *changing*) the standards."

There could be nothing more transformative for the dominant
American culture than shifting from the myth of "rugged individualism" to embracing the centrality of connection. We need to develop an
ethic of empowering people who will in turn empower others to develop expanding circles of care and competence, a kind of "relational
ripple." We need to exercise competence in the service of community,
to "uplift the community rather than assert individual rights" (Belenky,
Boyd, & Weinstock, 1997), to develop womankind and mankind (women
don't object too vigorously to being lumped as a part of mankind, but
what man would stand for being called a part of womankind?). We
need multiple perspectives on competence; we particularly need to listen to people on the margin, the greatest social critics and sources of
new strength available to us. In the year 2000, 65% of entrants into the
workplace will be women and minorities. The margin will be the center.

COMPLAINING

In transforming the knee-jerk question "What's wrong with women?"
whenever women don't fit in, we need to listen carefully to women's
complaints. Complaining is one of the most important human capacities we can exercise to name injustice and seek change—if someone is

listening (Jordan, 1997). Women's complaints about many social systems, including the workplace, schools, and therapy, are not signs of women's weakness. Women and other marginalized people (e.g., people of color, gays and lesbians, the physically challenged) are the potential leaders for transformation of the existing disconnected and nonrelational social systems. But we are silenced when we complain ("Don't you women ever do anything but whine and complain?"). We are criticized if we speak with a clear, firm voice (I was called "strident" three times on a panel by a male scholar who professes to be a friend of feminism). You're damned if you do and damned if you don't. As Beverly Tatum notes, writing primarily about racism, "racism is a system of advantage based on race. Someone benefits from racism or sexism. . . . The targeted group is labeled as defective or substandard in significant ways" (1997, p. 23). In other words, oppression is a way of making people feel incompetent. We *need* to complain. With encouragement from others, complaints become protest. When protest is supported by community, it becomes social action. When communities join together to protest and take social action, social revolution is born.

MOVING OUT OF SILENCE

Mary Belenky and colleagues (1997) asked why do so many smart women feel so dumb? How are smart women led to believe they have nothing important to say? A very bright and articulate colleague was commenting on her usual stance in a rather adversarial academic seminar with peers. She noted that whenever she starts to think about saying anything contradictory, she goes blank. Later, driving away from the meeting, she recovers what it is she had hoped to say. I remember sitting in agonizing silence in adversarial seminar after seminar in graduate school, unable to speak, fearful I had nothing to say. My silence increased after the only other two women in this nine-person program dropped out at the end of the first year. I was told by a professor and two fellow students that I was "wasting space" in the program because as a woman I would never fully use this education. I was reminded of my mother's story when she bravely traveled across the country to apply in person for admission to medical school 50 years earlier. She was told, "Why don't you go home, find a nice husband, and raise a family?" (She didn't take this advice.)

One well-meaning professor of mine suggested I had a phobia about speaking in public and lent me a relaxation tape and cognitive behavioral workbook. I felt stupid and embarrassed, and tried hard to improve myself. I, like my professor, felt I was the problem. I remember another occasion when each person in our Stone Center theory group, began to share our fears that we weren't really smart, that our ideas weren't that new. As I listened to each of my colleagues, I could barely believe my ears that these intelligent women had any doubts about their competence, but as I uttered my own doubts and fears, spoke my own conviction of incompetence, I felt as though I was speaking the deep, dark truth.

CLAIMING STRENGTH

In an interdependent world, we need cooperation more than competition. Those who buy into the competitive, individualistic model often believe that those who urge cooperation do so because they do not have the strength or the resources to "go it alone." Naming the strengths involved in relational competence, making these strengths explicit and clear, is a first step. The skills of mutual empathy, connection building, empowering others, anticipatory empathy, and contributing to the community can be detailed and celebrated. We also have to find ways to stay connected to our internal resources as well as the resources in the world around us. This involves connecting with external allies who can validate and support our truths as well as push us to grow, as we encourage them to build their authentic strength as well.

COMMUNITY

We should always remember that strength and competence grow in context with ongoing encouragement and support. We generate resilience and courage in community. African American women speak of "community othermothers" who help nurture community by listening and encouraging others into voice. Given the right context, the right listening, I can be smarter than I am smart and in other circumstances I am dumber than I am dumb. Bernice Johnston Reagon of Sweet Honey in the Rock notes, "Black women have had to have the standing power of rocks and of mountains—cold and hard, strong and stationary. That quality has often obscured the fact that inside the strength, partnering the sturdiness, we are as honey. If our world is warm, honey flows and so do we. If it is cold, stiff and stay put, so do we" (1993, p. 24).

Morrie Schwartz, quoted as he was dying, suggested, "The way you get meaning into your life is to devote yourself to loving others, devote yourself to your community around you and devote yourself to creating something that gives you purpose and meaning" (Albom, 1997, p. 43). Stephen Levine noted, "Love is the only rational act" (Levine, 1997, p. 52). In order to transform a culture of disconnection into a culture of connection we need to develop new images of strength, in which vulnerability, connection building, serving others, seeking justice, and being encouraged and emboldened *by community* as *we build community* are at the core. The existing privileged models of success and competence, which are characterized by defensive armoring and disconnection, are not working. A woman at a meeting recently asked me if I knew what gave the giant sequoia trees their strength. When I admitted I didn't know, she said they actually have very shallow roots but the roots of nearby trees intertwine and support one another. These biggest and oldest of trees, these images of power and strength, literally hold each other up. (A follow-up call to Muir woods confirmed this.) We need to move beyond models of resistance to models of transformation.

We need to shift the dominant images away from war making and elevation of individual specialness to the creation and sustenance of connection and community. There is nothing wrong with someone who wants to give and serve and contribute to the growth of others. There *is* something wrong with a culture that cannot appreciate and validate the centrality of connection in the world.

CONCLUDING COMMENTS

Finally, I want to leave you with two playful images, two points, and two questions, mostly borrowed from others.

The two playful images:

1. The expansive movement of relational ripples
2. A global singing group called the Resister Sisters

The two points:

1. Isolation is the glue that holds oppression in place (Laing, 1998).
2. The soft stuff *is* the real stuff.

The two questions:

1. Why do so many smart women feel so dumb?
2. Am I *really* the problem?

REFERENCES

Albom, M. (1997). *Tuesdays with Morrie*. New York: Doubleday.

Belenky, M., Bond, L., & Weinstock, J. (1997). *A tradition that has no name: Nurturing the development of people, families, and communities*. New York: Basic Books.

Deutsch, M. (1985). *Distributive justice: A social psychological perspective*. New Haven, CT: Yale University Press.

Fletcher, J. (1996). Relational theory in the workplace. *Work in Progress, No. 77*. Wellesley, MA: Stone Center Working Paper Series.

Gilligan, C. (1982). *In a different voice: Psychology theory and women's development*. Cambridge, MA: Harvard University Press.

Gilligan, C. (1990). Joining the resistance: Psychology, politics, girls, and women. *Michigan Quarterly Review, 29*, 501–536.

Gottman, J., Coan, J., Carrere, S., & Swanson, C. (1998). Predicting marital happiness and stability from newlywed interactions. *Journal of Marriage and Family, 60*, 5–22.

hooks, b. (1984). *Feminist theory: From margin to center*. Boston: South End Press.

hooks, b. (1989). *Talking back*. Boston: South End Press.

hooks, b. (1991). The oppositional gaze: Black female spectators. In M. Diawara (Ed.), *Black cinema* (pp. 151–170). New York: Routledge Press.

Horner, M. (1970). Femininity and successful achievement: A basic inconsistency. In J. M. Bardwick, *Feminine personality and conflict* (pp. 24–49). Belmont, CA: Brooks/Cole.

Horney, K. (1973). Culture and neurosis. In T. Millon (Ed.), *Theories of psychopathology and personality* (2nd ed., pp. 37–54). Philadelphia: Saunders.

Jordan, J. V. (1989). Relational development: Therapeutic implications of empathy and shame. *Work in Progress, No. 39*. Wellesley, MA: Stone Center Working Paper Series.

Jordan, J. V. (1997). Relational therapy in a nonrelational world. *Work in Progress, No. 79*. Wellesley, MA: Stone Center Working Paper Series.

Jordan, J. V., Kaplan, A. G., Miller, J. B., Stiver, I. P., & Surrey, J. L. (1991). *Women's growth in connection: Writings from the Stone Center* New York: Guilford Press.

Keller, E. F. (1985). *Reflections on gender and science*. New Haven, CT: Yale University Press.

Kohn, A. (1986). *No contest: The case against competition*. Boston: Houghton Mifflin.

Laing, K. (1998). Katalyst Leadership Workshop "In Pursuit of Parity: Teachers as Liberators," held at the World Trade Center, Boston.

Levine, S. (1997). *A year to live: How to live this year as if it were your last*. New York: Bell Tower.

Oxford English Dictionary (Compact ed.). (1971). Oxford, UK: Clarendon Press.

Maccoby, E. (1990). Gender and relationships: A developmental account. *American Psychologist, 45*, 513–520.

Miller, J. B. (1986). *Toward a new psychology of women* (2nd ed.). Boston: Beacon Press.

Miller, J. B., & Stiver, I. R. (1997). *The healing connection.* Boston: Beacon Press.

Piaget, J. (1965). *The moral judgment of the child* (M. Gabain, Trans.). New York: Free Press.

Reagon, B. J. (1993). *We who believe in freedom: Sweet honey . . . still on the journey.* New York: Doubleday.

Robinson, T., & Ward, J. (1991). A belief in self far greater than anyone's disbelief: Cultivating resistance among African American female adolescents. In C. Gilligan, A. Rogers, & D. Tolman (Eds.), *Women, girls, and psychotherapy: Reframing resistance* (pp. 87–103). Binghamton, NY: Harrington Park Press.

Tannen, D. (1998). *The argument culture: Moving from debate to dialogue.* New York: Random House.

Tatum, B. (1997). *Why are all the black kids sitting together in the cafeteria?* New York: Basic Books.

Seligman, M. (1972). Learned helplessness. *Annual Review of Medicine, 23,* 407–412.

Walker, M. (1998). Race, self, and society: Relational challenges in a culture of disconnection. *Work in Progress, No. 85.* Wellesley, MA: Stone Center Working Paper Series.

White, R. (1959). Motivation reconsidered: The concept of competence. *Psychological Review, 66,* 297–333.

Woodburn, L. (1998). *Beyond "how-to's": A relational reframing of workplace leadership* [Individual presentation during workshop]. Workshop presented by J. V. Jordan, J. K. Fletcher, L. Woodburn, S. Eaton, & M. Harvey, sponsored by the Jean Baker Miller Training Institute, Wellesley College, Wellesley, MA.

This chapter was originally presented at the Learning from Women Conference sponsored by the Jean Baker Miller Training Institute and Harvard Medical School/Cambridge Hospital on May 1, 1998. © 1999 by Judith V. Jordan.

2

Relational Resilience

JUDITH V. JORDAN

Given that life subjects all of us to tensions and suffering and that relationships as well as individuals are buffeted by forces that create pain, disconnection, and the threat of dissolution, the capacity for relational resilience, or transformation, is essential. Movement toward empathic mutuality is at the core of relational resilience. When individuals move from mutually empowering and mutually empathic relationships (Miller, 1986; Surrey, 1985) into disconnection, they are often beset by a damaging sense of immobilization and isolation. They lose the sense of a life-giving empathic bridge. In describing this loss, one client spoke movingly of her identification with the elderly Alzheimer's patient who was abandoned, without identification, by relatives at a race track in Idaho—utterly alone, utterly helpless, unable to even name or speak the horror.

When people are unable to move from disconnection to connection, the resulting combination of immobilization and isolation may become a prison, (not unlike Jean Baker Miller's notion of "condemned isolation" [1988]) and may contribute to psychological anguish, physical deterioration, and sometimes even death. Thus, we can no longer look only at factors within the individual that facilitate adjustment; we must examine the relational dynamics that encourage the capacity for connection. Reframing our understanding of resilience in terms of a relational model has implications for both psychotherapy and social change. Therapy, then, can be understood as largely an effort to explore and enhance the capacity for relational resilience. And in moving beyond personal resilience to personal transformation and social change, the relational context is central.

TRADITIONAL VIEWS OF RESILIENCE

Rutter, who has written extensively on resilience, views it as evident in an "individual who overcomes adversity, who survives stress, and who rises above disadvantages" (1979, p. 3). Block and Block (1980) refer to "ego resilience" in contrast to a condition they call "ego brittle." "Ego resilience refers to the ability to adapt flexibly and with 'elasticity' to changing circumstances" (Dugan & Coles, 1989, p. 112).

Some researchers in the field of resilience have focused on factors within the person, like temperament or personality. Suzanne C. Kobasa has developed the notion of "hardiness," which is thought to protect one from the harmful effects of stress: "Persons high in hardiness easily commit themselves to what they are doing, . . . generally believe that they at least partially control events, . . . and regard change to be a normal challenge or impetus to development" (Kobasa & Puccetti, 1983, p. 840). On the other hand, "learned helplessness," a condition studied by Seligman (1975) that "results when people believe or expect their responses will not influence the future probability of environmental outcomes," is seen as rendering people vulnerable to stress and depression (McCann & Pearlman, 1990, p. 53).

Along these lines, some have suggested that girls develop "pessimistic coping strategies" that interfere with persistent problem-solving efforts. This suggestion is based on studies indicating that girls' expectations of future performance are affected more by past or present failures than by successes, a kind of reflexive pessimism. Girls attribute failure to internal factors, whereas boys tend to attribute failure to external factors and success to internal factors (Dweck, Goetz, & Strauss, 1980; Dweck & Reppucci, 1973); girls blame themselves more than do boys and also take less credit for success; and studies indicate that college women are more self-critical than men in response to failure (Carver & Ganellen, 1983).

In several studies of resilience, freedom from self-denigration emerged as the most powerful protector against stress-related debilitation; mastery and self-esteem were also seen as important (Pearlin & Schooler, 1978). In general, women have been found to be "lower on self-esteem and higher on self-denigration than are men" (Barnett, Biener, & Baruch, 1987, p. 319). Some have gone so far as to conclude that much of psychological literature "depicts women as having been socialized in a way that keeps them from developing resilient personalities" (Barnett et al., 1987, p. 319). But, as Carol Gilligan and colleagues note, girls show an advantage in dealing with stress until they reach adolescence when they become more depressed, more self-critical and begin to move into silence (Gilligan, Lyons, & Hanmer, 1990). As they write, "For girls to remain responsive to *themselves*, they must resist the convention of female goodness; to remain responsive to *others*, they must resist the values placed on self-sufficiency and independence in North American cultures" (Gilligan et al., 1990, p. 11; their emphases). We might well question how women's sense of worth can remain intact when the dominant culture denigrates the relational values that are at the core of our sense of aliveness and worth.

The Role of Control

In addition to the importance of hardiness and self-esteem, some have noted that stress is most clearly buffered by the sense of control, a personality attribute (Cohen & Edwards, 1986). Although there has been little observation of gender differences in the need to control one's environment, it might be argued that a generalized need to be in control may be more pertinent for men than for women (Pearlin & Schooler, 1978). A model of development that suggests there is a power/control mode into which males in this culture are socialized and an empathy/love mode into which girls are acculturated (Jordan, 1987) would imply that different coping strategies would develop as part of these general gender-related modes of being.

Indeed, studies have indicated that women's coping styles are more emotion focused (talking about personal distress with friends, sharing sadness) and men's styles are more problem focused or instrumental (taking action to solve the problem, seeking new strategies) (Lazarus & Folkman, 1984). In line with a research bias that generally overlooks complex context–person interactions, however, early studies on this dimension did not actually assess the degree to which control was possible in various situations. More recently, researchers have noted that emotion-focused coping is adaptive in situations where one actually has little control, and problem-focused coping is useful where one can effect change. In general, it may be that women inhabit worlds where, due to a lack of power, the possibility of changing things is unrealistic; hence emotion-based coping strategies may often make the most sense (Lazarus & Folkman, 1984). We have seen in the early 1990s (in the Anita Hill case and in the public shaming of rape victims) that awful forces can be brought to bear against women who begin to feel they might actually have an effect on the system—particularly if the patriarchal power system is threatened.

The "control hypothesis," furthermore, takes as a given, it seems to me, the notion that women really *do* control vast areas of our lives and that this control protects us from an intolerable sense of vulnerability. It further supports the "just world theory" (Lerner, 1980), that is, that people get what they deserve and deserve what they get. This notion contributes to victim blaming (the rape victim must have provoked it) and preserves the myth that misfortune will not happen to me if I behave according to certain rules. The overemphasis on control also reinforces the blaming of those in the system whose sphere of influence is severely limited by established patterns of power.

Action arising out of emotionally focused coping is possibly more characteristic of a relational model than a power model. Women's consciousness-raising groups in the 1960s and 1970s have much to teach us about this, as do the earlier suffragists, birth-control pioneers, and more recently incest and rape survivors. As one survivor of therapist abuse put it, "When I felt I was the only one and it was my fault, I fell into a black pit. I felt isolated, self-blaming and utterly unable to do anything to make it better. When I can just remember to reach out and talk to someone, both the isolation and sense of immobilization change. And then actually, when I feel less alone and self-blaming, I find new ways to act. It isn't just talk *or* do, connect *or* solve . . . talking about feelings *is* doing and it helps me move into other action."

Separate-Self Biases

In addition to an interest in intrapsychic or personality variables, such as control, many researchers have pointed to the beneficial and protective function of social support in minimizing the destructive consequences of stressful life problems (Cobb, 1976; Dean & Lin, 1977; Kaplan, Cassel, & Gore, 1977; Suls, 1982). In a study done in Georgia, House, Robbins, and Metzner (1982) found that men *with* multiple social ties were two to three times *less* likely to die than men without them. Recent literature on stress and resilience indicates that social support can prevent low birth weights and premature deaths, and protect people from arthritis, tuberculosis, depression, alcoholism, and other psychiatric illnesses brought on by disconnection and isolation (Cobb, 1976). Beardslee and Podorefsky (1988) summarized the literature on stress and resilience, noting that relationships are protective in a wide variety of risk situations. The approaches that emphasize control, self-esteem, and social support, however, are all characterized by the bias of a separate-self model; that is, they look either only within the individual for sources of resilience or, in a one-directional way, only from the point of view of one stressed individual looking for support from some other or others.

Few studies have delineated the complex factors involved in those relationships that not only protect us from stress but promote positive and creative growth. Thus many of the studies have simply counted the number of "social supports" that exist for an individual undergoing adversity but have ignored the *quality* of connectedness; more especially, few have looked at what interferes with movement into mutually enhancing relationships, or what hampers our capacity to transform potentially disconnecting experiences into movement toward greater connection and mutual growth.

A RELATIONAL VIEW OF RESILIENCE

From a relational point of view, the focus of the inquiry might be: What makes for relational resilience and mutuality and ultimately encourages the transformation from isolation and pain to relatedness and growth? In exploring this, I suggest we need new models. I believe we must make the following moves:

1. From *individual "control over"* dynamics to a model of *supported vulnerability*
2. From a one-directional *need for support from others* to *mutual empathic involvement* in the well-being of each person and of the relationship itself
3. From separate *self-esteem* to *relational confidence*
4. From the exercise of *"power over"* dynamics to *empowerment*, by encouraging mutual growth and constructive conflict
5. From *finding meaning* in self-centered *self-consciousness* to *creating meaning* in a more expansive *relational awareness*

I will now turn to these five ways of reframing our understanding of resilience.

From a Model of Individual "Control Over" Dynamics to Supported Vulnerability

In the personal domain, one must be willing to risk the vulnerability of emotional responsiveness. Since we do not want to open ourselves to unnecessary risk, we must learn how to judge when our trust and confidence in the other person is warranted and when it is not. If our experience has taught us to doubt other peoples' trustworthiness, we will have difficulty at the very first step of engagement.

The capacity to ask for and give support is an essential aspect of most relationships, not just those defined as "helping relationships." In a state of stress, personal vulnerability increases, as does the need to enter a more supportive relationship.

Women in particular are asked to "hold" vulnerability and then are often scorned for it. Women are constantly told that we are more vulnerable in every way in a world that takes advantage of, rather than respects, vulnerability: "Both females and elderly individuals report feeling much more vulnerable to criminal victimization than do their male and younger counterparts, respectively" (Perloff, 1983, p. 46). We are bombarded by media evidence that women are endangered; the statistics and lurid details on rapes, wife battering, and sexual harassment are daily reminders of women's vulnerability to greater physical strength and violence. Faludi (1992) suggests that currently we are all being battered by the backlash against feminism. In this year of setbacks for women, I personally have alternated between feeling demoralized and completely inadequate to the task at hand, on the one hand, and outraged at the injustices that have been allowed to occur, on the other.

But vulnerability per se is not the problem. Awareness of vulnerability, in fact, suggests to me good reality testing. It is the *disowned* vulnerability that becomes problematic. An openness to being affected is essential to intimacy and a growth-enhancing relationship; without it, people relate inauthentically, adopting roles and coming from distanced and protected places. Open sharing of our need for support or acceptance may be an essential factor in developing a sense of close connection. Therefore, part of what we are trying to transform is the illusory sense of self-sufficiency and the tendency to deny vulnerability. We need a model that encourages supported vulnerability.

From the Need for Social Support to Mutual Involvement

Social support has been studied largely in the context of buffering stress or contributing to resilience following some particularly pernicious stress: "Having a confidant is one of the best buffers against the negative health outcomes, including cardiovascular disease, often associated with occupation-based stress and negative life events" (Barnett et al., 1987, p. 358; Belle, 1982). A 1989 study at Stanford University of 86 women with advanced breast cancer found that those in support groups not only experienced less anxiety, depression, and pain than those who did not participate, but they also lived twice as long: 37 months compared to 19 months (Spiegel, 1991). While the researchers focused on the support *received*, it is likely that *both* the giving *and* receiving of support, a sense of *mutual involvement*, led to these remarkable outcomes. Women are more likely to turn to others for social support than are men, but women are also more likely to be expected to provide social support (Fischer, 1982). There are more reports of husbands being affirmed and better understood by spouses than of wives. Among college seniors, loneliness is negatively correlated with time spent with women but not with men (Wheeler, Reis, & Nezlek, 1983); that is, for both men and women, spending time with a man is less likely to alleviate the sense of loneliness than spending time with a woman.

One of the dimensions of support that researchers have examined is whether or not people ask for help directly or indirectly. Asking for support directly, which ostensibly is the most effective, is also seen as putting the person doing the asking most at risk—we feel most vulnerable when we let people directly know about our need. Studies have shown that people tend to be the most direct in seeking assistance in those relationships which are the most committed, such as marriage, and tend to be more indirect (e.g., stating a problem without explicitly asking for help) in relationships that are less established and reliable. People also sometimes wish that another person would know what is wanted without their having to state it directly; the care is considered better when another person is tuned in to our unstated needs (Duck, 1990). Men, in particular, see having to make direct requests for help as a threat to their notions of masculine self-sufficiency. In many ways women, socialized to be empathic caregivers, are trained to pick up the unspoken needs of others, particularly male partners. This makes men's dependency and need for support much less visible. Ironically, however, when women need support in mixed-sex situations, they are often with men who have not been socialized toward caring and attuning to unspoken needs. Given that the open expression of needs is seen as weak, if women do express their needs more directly, they are often belittled for their "neediness" or seen as demanding.

While empathic sensitivity to the unspoken needs of others is an exceptionally important skill, it works for the good of both partners only if it is mutual. In close relationships, we have the opportunity to learn one another's distress signals and intervene more effectively when support is needed; but we can hope to make the direct expression of vulnerability less toxic and threatening for all people. A portion of the difficulty arises because we live in a cultural milieu that does not respect helpseeking and that tends to scorn the vulnerability implicit in our inevitable need for support. The ethic of individuality and self-sufficiency still takes precedence over an ethic of mutuality.

From Self-Sufficiency to Relational Confidence

Acknowledging vulnerability is possible only if we feel we *can* reach out for support. To do so we must feel some *confidence in the relationship.* We must also have some confidence in our ability to create growth-enhancing relationships as well as trust that others will join us in that creation. A personal sense of worth or confidence ideally is not just feeling good about oneself but also involves a sense that one has some-thing to contribute to others and that one is part of a meaningful rela-tionship. Self-confidence, as an expression of independent, detached feelings of well-being, does not seem to fit women's experience, just as self-sufficiency does not seem a reasonable goal of human develop-ment. Rather, confidence in the other person (trust) and confidence in the relationship, if it is mutual, serve to support a personal sense of confidence and contribute more fully to a sense of well-being and pos-sibility. Confidence in a relationship depends on mutual trust in the empathic response of the other and commitment to one another and to the relationship; it also grows from reliability, a shared purpose of mak-ing the relationship mutually enhancing for both people, and a deter-mination to honor and respect each other. A history of successful reso-lution of injuries and hurts helps build this sense of confidence.

From "Power Over" Dynamics to Empowerment and Mutuality

We must also learn to discriminate mutual from nonmutual relation-ships and discern which are the relationships that warrant our trust and confidence and which are not. Such distinction involves finding ways to evaluate when an interaction is mutually empathic and mutu-ally empowering versus when it is imbalanced or governed by destruc-tive "power over" dynamics. Commitment to an ethic of mutuality is es-sential. In a relationship we must learn to notice both when we are "reaching" or "touching" another person and when movement stops.

When one person is in a position of "power over" another, there can be little room for the kind of movement in mutuality that I am sug-gesting is essential to personal and relational resilience. "Power over" by its very nature dictates the form of relationship; one person has the ability to decide the rules for discourse and the direction that the rela-tionship will take. The more powerful person also has the assumed *right* to receive support from the less powerful, whenever needed and on his/her terms. This system then is by definition rigid, not flexible, and decidedly not mutual.

From Separate Self to Involvement

Very important, the capacity to move beyond the isolation that can both produce and accompany stress involves a movement out of narrow self-consciousness into the awareness of being part of something larger than the separate self, a "resonance with," whether this be a relationship with another person, feeling part of nature, or some aspect of spiritual involvement. It is when we feel most separate from others and from the flow of life that we are at most risk.

Some interpretations of the classic work on the type A personality, which found an association between hostility and coronary heart disease (Friedman & Rosenman, 1974), have suggested that hostility increases one's focus on the self, thus exaggerating one's feeling of isolation and separateness. More self-involved patients tended to have more severe cases of coronary artery disease, as well as a greater likelihood of depression and anxiety (Scherwitz, Graham, & Ornish, 1985). "The type A patient with more good friends had wider, less constricted coronary arteries than did the type A who was more typically alone" (Luks, 1992, p. 95). These data suggest that our emphasis on boundedness, separation, self-sufficiency, and preoccupation with *numero uno* may not only have adverse consequences for us psychologically but may also be physically damaging.

From Self-Consciousness to Relational Awareness

The need to *receive* support, which is cited in most resilience literature, is thus imbalanced if it overlooks the broader need for mutuality and involvement—the capacity to extend one's interest beyond self. What is integral to a notion of relational awareness or relational resilience is moving from the self at the center of motivation and awareness to a broadening experience of "being with," of being part of, of transcending narrow self-interest and self-concern. This does not entail self-denial, but rather it is the movement from a paradigm of egoism versus altruism to one of relational awareness (Jordan, 1987).

TRAUMA: A CHALLENGE TO RELATIONAL RESILIENCE

Traumas, particularly those caused by other humans (e.g., sexual victimization, war, or physical violence), create major disruptions in our experience of relatedness and thus threaten our capacity for resilience. "The role of others' reactions is central to many conceptualizations of victim response"(McCann & Pearlman, 1990, p. 33), whether they be incest survivors not believed by parents or therapists, or Vietnam veterans returning to a devaluing or hostile populace. One definition of trauma suggests that it is a "paralyzed, overwhelmed state, with immobilization, withdrawal, possible depersonalization, evidence of disorganization" (Krystal, 1978, p. 90). The survival skills of the incest survivor—dissociation, hypervigilance, isolation, and lack of trust—all take a person out of connection; they lessen the possibility of successful use of support. Sroufe's (1989) description of the anxious avoidant baby who does not act as if she/he expects to be comforted by contact with the caretaker certainly applies to those who have been violated by a supposed loving and protective caretaker. Where an abusive relationship is defined as a loving relationship, the only outcome can be severe mistrust. As George Eliot wrote in *Middlemarch*, "What loneliness is more lonely than distrust?" (1872/1981, p. 427).

Furthermore, there is complete disruption of self–other–world meaning systems in trauma. Epstein (1985) suggests the world is no longer seen as benign but malevolent, lacking in meaning, and unjust; others are seen as a source of threat, and the self is felt to be unworthy. Janoff-Bulman (1992) observes that our basic assumptions about the world are shattered in trauma. Rieker and Carmen (1986) note: "the child's task is to accommodate to a family in which exploitation, invasiveness, and the betrayal of trust are normal and in which loyalty, secrecy, and self-sacrifice form the core of the family's value system" (p. 364). And Irene Stiver (1990) has written about this dynamic in dysfunctional families where when truth is denied and buried, shame, self-blame, and withdrawal are inevitable. The effort to retrieve some sense of connection through surface accommodation and compliance leads to an increasing sense of isolation and loneliness.

Trauma therefore impedes movement in relationship. When in trauma, we are inflexible, stuck, bound to repetition. Little can be learned interpersonally; we cling to those patterns that are familiar. Withdrawal into mistrust and isolation is rampant. Some have suggested that, ironically, "those individuals who are most vulnerable may be the least effective in eliciting support" (Ganellen & Blaney, 1984). A description of a composite case will illustrate some of these points. A young woman, survivor of repeated sadistic sexual abuse by her father, uncle, and brothers, would typically become enraged when I failed her in treatment (failures included asking a question that felt insensitive, suggesting a consultation, and many other instances that indicated a lack of understanding). These disconnections early in treatment often led to her suicidal phone calls from undisclosed locations, with me feeling anxious and angry because of her refusal to tell me where she was. After some time in therapy, rather than communicating her distress through self-destructive action, she verbally expressed her outrage about our failures to connect. On one such occasion when I tried to convey some apparently inaccurate understanding, she erupted: "Why do you torture me? You act like you know it all." I responded that I had indeed made a mistake, that I did not intend to torture her, that I certainly did not "know it all"—far from it—and that I thought we both had to look at the problem in our relationship created by this misunderstanding. She retorted, "I don't want to hear how *we* have a problem with our relationship . . . this is all your fault and you better own up to it." In her eyes, hurt equaled abuse. If I questioned that equation, I was seen as trying to talk her out of her reality, something that her abusing father did constantly. When these moments occur I have to hold the tension of these differing perceptions: she feels abused and misunderstood, while I feel unskilled in my failure to understand. We experience our interaction differently, although we can now agree that the misunderstanding and possible disconnection is troubling for both of us. Together we have to negotiate how we can "be with" these differences. I have to actively support exploration of this disconnection and encourage the eventual movement back into connection at the same time that I honor her sense of violation and her momentary need to move into protective distancing. Sometimes I have to do this when I may also feel like disconnecting. In this case, I "hold" the possibility for relational resilience, a responsibility that I view as central to my work as a therapist. As we move forward in our work together, this responsibility will be shared more fully by both of us.

While some have stressed the sense of a loss of control and of meaningfulness in victimization (Janoff-Bulman, 1992; Seligman, 1975), I think more particularly that in instances of trauma involving violation by another person, we lose our trust in the goodness of others; we do not see another human being who responds to us in an empathic, responsive, and caring way. With chronic abuse and secrecy, we lose even our hope that there can ever again be a fully empathic, loving relationship with another person. It is not simply that what they do is beyond our control. It violates our most basic need to be cared about and responded to in a valuing, loving way. In abuse, there is a profound disconnection, a violation of human relatedness and meaningfulness in relationship that cuts deep. Finding ways to reestablish the caring connection or the belief in the possibility of love as a response to vulnerability is essential.

Few who have been severely taxed or injured by trauma would choose the path of suffering to accomplish growth. As Harold Kushner, whose book *When Bad Things Happen to Good People* was in part a response to the premature death of his beloved son Aaron, wrote, "If I could choose, I would forego all the spiritual growth and depth which has come my way because of our experience" (1981, p. 133). But working through trauma and severe stress can in fact lead to a deepening appreciation of the preciousness of life, a wisdom that eludes those who maintain illusions about their own invulnerability; it also creates an abiding respect for the power of human connection, accompanied by an increasing awareness of our absolute need for the love and support of others. Further, it can lead to an expansive desire to assist others who are victimized or injured; the movement toward helping others often becomes key to the transformation of private pain and isolation into compassion for the suffering of all human beings.

RELATIONAL RESILIENCE IN THERAPY

In therapy we fundamentally build a relationship in which we can explore and seek to understand patterns of mutuality, resilience, connection, and disconnection. I will briefly point out the ways that the reframing of relational resilience can inform our understanding of therapy.

Supported Vulnerability

Often when people begin therapy the need for safety is paramount. And at such times the movement into a place of supported vulnerability may be the most important work. Dependability, respect, care, and empathic listening contribute to a sense of security.

In therapy, clients learn how to recognize when they need support, what kind of support they need, how they can ask for it and from whom. Clients become aware of those things that interfere with asking for support or bringing themselves more fully into relationship—shame, pride, fear, anger, split off experiences, inability to find trustworthy partners, and so on. Where there has been doubt about the dependability of others, the therapist and client together try to build new relational images and expectations that include a sense of trust, commitment, and respect; we rebuild the broken empathic bridge; we explore the tendency to approach or avoid others in response to problems so that the client can begin to question automatic reactions in either direction. The mutual need to give support, to empathize, also grows as clients move beyond the initial heightened self-concern and painful vulnerability that accompanies the beginning of treatment. Ultimately we need to create meaning and confidence in a caring human community that we are both part of.

Flexibility

After the initial phase in which the client begins to develop a sense of trust in sharing her/his vulnerability, she/he becomes more flexible and increasingly differentiated and self-protective in decisions about whom to trust and in what ways. Demos (1989, p. 5) writes, "Resilience requires the ability to discriminate between situations and people and select only the most appropriate responses from among one's repertoire for each occasion." As therapists, we encourage recognizing those situations where disconnections may be protective versus those where reengagement and growth is possible. When the possibility for mutuality exists, we try to help the client look at the maladaptive ways she/he may avoid engagement. One client became very critical each time she started to feel close to her therapist; as she became more vocal about the therapist's faults, the therapist often became defensive and thus distanced from the client. Attending to the disconnection that was created by these dynamics became crucial to the therapy. It involved the therapist's ability to move out of her own need to be "right" and her willingness to look at how her distancing created more pain for the client. For her part, the client also had to examine her need to move into attack when she felt more open and vulnerable. Together they had to bear and examine the tension that was created in these moments and find new ways of moving beyond these potential impasses and disconnections.

Empowerment and Conflict

Among therapy's central goals is the encouragement and empowerment of individuals to most fully and creatively live their own truths in a way that is respectful of other's lives. Validation of experience, which often includes directly noting the contextual factors that contribute to difficulties, assists in this process.

Learning to trust that we can be ourselves, be different from one another, with the possibility that difference can lead to growth-promoting conflict, is also essential to authentic relating and creative action. We encourage clients to be more comfortable with moving into conflict in relationships by exploring the development of conflict with us (Jordan, 1990).

Mutuality

In therapy the client develops the courage to bring her/himself most fully into relationship and into creative action. Inauthenticity takes us out of real mutuality. People who have learned to manage the image of themselves that they present to others or who have suppressed true responsiveness are often relieved to let another really see them. One client (among many who share a similar feeling), a very competent and intelligent woman, commented that she is very adept at figuring out what people want and gives it to them in order to either get something in return or to be liked. She derives little real pleasure from this dynamic, however, feeling secretly that she is "manipulative" and that the positive feedback she receives is not about her real sense of herself. She thus feels fraudulent. She does not feel either instrumentally or socially competent. (How often have you heard a man worry about being "manipulative" rather than effective and instrumental?)

The moments of disconnection and isolation are not just times of pain but contain possible lessons that both the therapist and the client must be prepared to take in. We learn from empathic failures. As Steiner- Adair (1991) and Miller and Stiver (1991) have noted, we therapists must become sensitive to our own disconnections and try to discern what is happening when we or the other person are moving away from connection. Disconnections must be named and understood.

Relational Confidence

As misunderstandings are renegotiated and empathic failures are reworked, the client slowly develops a sense of relational confidence. The very capacity of the therapy relationship to not only withstand but grow through the shared work on anger, hurt, and pain contributes significantly to the sense of relational confidence. As one client commented, "In the beginning when I'd get mad at you, I expected you to retaliate. I kept looking for the slightest sign that you weren't treating me fairly. Now, I figure, you can take my anger; I know both of us will work to make some sense of the whole thing together. It feels very different, sturdier."

Relational Awareness

While therapists address individual problems and personal change, we also work on developing "relational awareness," which gradually becomes as important as the kind of self-consciousness that is so prevalent, but so paralyzing, for many people when they enter therapy. First, we must shift our focus from one that primarily looks at the intrapsychic, the characterological, to one that focuses on relational elaboration. We engage in articulating, tracing, and getting to know relational movement from connection to disconnection and back into connection in the here and now. We foster an awareness of self, other, and relationship.

While much of the research on resilience has pointed to the importance of instrumental competence, the need to control, or the need to feel in control, as central to personal well-being and growth, a relational point of view would rather emphasize the need for mutual involvement and mutual empathy. As much as we all enjoy the sense of figuring something out, effectively working on something in the external world and seeing ourselves as competent individuals (what many have called mastery or efficacy), the need for a kind of relational competence and belonging is powerful and primary as well.

TRANSFORMATION AND SOCIAL CHANGE

Unlike resilience, transformation suggests not just a return to a previously existing state but movement through and beyond stress or suffering into a new and more comprehensive personal and relational integration. In the case of disconnection, transformation involves awareness of the forces creating the disconnection, discovery of a means for reconnecting, and building a more differentiated and solid connection. The movement into and out of connection becomes a journey of discovery about self, other, and relationship—about "being in relation." The importance of connectedness is affirmed, and one's capacity to move into healthy connection is strengthened. This is indeed transformative.

By speaking of transformation rather than just resilience we move beyond a notion of recovery from individual pain to a sense of greater integrity and integration in the human community as well. Joining others in mutually supporting and meaningful relationships most clearly allows us to move out of isolation and powerlessness. Energy flows back into connection. Joining with others is a powerful antidote to immobilization and fragmentation. It is thus an antidote to trauma. Moreover, the ability to join with others and become mobilized can further efforts towards a more just society.

I would like to suggest that we live in a traumatized and traumatizing society today. Four million children in the United States between the ages of 3 and 17 experience acts of violence, 38% of adult women have experienced at least one incident of incestuous or extrafamilial sexual abuse in childhood, 1,700 women die each year as a result of domestic violence. In 1984, 37 million Americans experienced criminal victimization. Since 1975 more than 700,000 refugees from Southeast Asia have come to this country, many of whom witnessed endless tortures and deaths—2 million deaths in Cambodia alone (McCann & Pearlman, 1990). Each day we are bombarded with details of murders, assaults, tragedies, and global tensions.

As therapists, we must move beyond dealing with individual pain; we must become part of a larger solution by joining with others to transform the social conditions that contribute heavily to individual pain. We can replace an ethic of individualism with an ethic of mutuality. As feminist theorists have been noting, the personal *is* the political. We cannot continue to pathologize individual adaptations to socially destructive patterns. Therapy should not become a part of the problem by suggesting that the pathology is individual and that the solution is individual. We should not become a part of the problem by reinforcing the isolation of women from one another. An African American panelist at a conference recently noted that African American mothers often explicitly teach their daughters how to survive in a racist society; the comparable teaching of *all* girls about how to survive in a *sexist* society rarely occurs in either black or white families.

Patriarchy and existing power structures depend on the isolation and disempowerment of women. Women are pitted against each other in competition for men and in the demeaning of women who choose to be with women. Women of color are separated from white women. Feminists are characterized as "ballbusters" and "angry bitches." Women fighting for reproductive freedom are portrayed as murderers. Those who speak up against rape, harassment, or job discrimination are seen as troublemakers, to be doubted and judged.

Those involved in social change will need to find ways to be resilient and move toward transformation, in much the same way we have suggested individuals need to move. This transformation can be accomplished through extensive use of support networks, finding the places where change is possible, and finding ways to live with those situations that are utterly beyond movement. It may be as simple as heeding Simone Weil's (1983) suggestion that we ask our neighbor, with compassion, "What are you going through?" We might then add, "Is it *necessary* that you go through it? If so, I will stand with you as you go through it. If not, I will help you change it." Much individual suffering could be prevented if as a culture we truly appreciated our essential interdependence and the bankruptcy of "power over" models. We might accept the inevitability of much suffering but apply ourselves strenuously to the elimination of that suffering, which need not be. This is a question that faces us all in our own lives; as therapists we must help people grapple with it daily: "Is this suffering necessary?" If it is, we must support one another, develop compassion, become resilient. If it is not, we must find ways to move through it and thus to transform the conditions creating unnecessary suffering. As Audre Lorde has suggested, "The only pain that is unbearable is wasted pain" (Lorde, 1984, cited in McDaniel, 1989).

REFERENCES

Barnett, R., Biener, L., & Baruch, G. (1987). *Gender and stress.* New York: Free Press.

Beardslee, W., & Podorefsky, D. (1988). Resilient adolescents whose parents have serious affective and other psychiatric disorders: Importance of self-understanding and relationships. *American Journal of Psychiatry, 145*(1), 63–67.

Belle, D. (1982). Social ties and social support. In D. Belle (Ed.), *Lives in stress: Women and depression* (pp. 133–144). Beverly Hills, CA: Sage.

Carver, C. S., & Ganellen, R. J. (1983). Depression and components of self-punitiveness: High standards, self-criticism, and overgeneralization. *Journal of Abnormal Psychology, 92,* 330–337.

Cobb, S. (1976). Social support as a moderator of life stress. *Psychosomatic Medicine, 38,* 300–314.

Cohen, S., & Edwards, J. R. (1986). Personality characteristics as moderators of the relationship between stress and disorder. In R. J. Newfield (Ed.), *Advances in the investigation of psychological stress* (pp. 235–283). New York: Wiley.

Dean, A., & Lin, N. (1977). The stress-buffering role of social support. *Journal of Nervous and Mental Disease, 165,* 403–415.

Demos, V. (1989). Resiliency in infancy. In T. Dugan & R. Coles (Eds.), *The child in our times* (pp. 3–22). New York: Brunner/Mazel.

Duck, S. (1990). *Personal relationships and social support.* Newbury Park, CA: Sage.

Dugan, T., & Coles, R. (Eds.). (1989). *The child in our times: Studies in the development of resiliency.* New York: Brunner/Mazel.

Dweck, C. S., Goetz, T., & Strauss, N. L. (1980). Sex differences in learned helplessness: IV. An experimental and naturalistic study of failure generalization and its mediators. *Journal of Personality and Social Psychology, 38,* 441–452.

Dweck, C. S., & Reppucci, N. D. (1973). Learned helplessness and reinforcement responsibility in children. *Journal of Personality and Social Psychology, 25,* 109–116.

Eliot, G. (1981). *Middlemarch.* New York: Signet Classic. (Original work published 1872)

Epstein, S. (1985). The implications of cognitive–experiential self-theory for research in social psychology and personality. *Journal of the Theory of Social Behavior, 15,* 283–310.

Faludi, S. (1992). *Backlash: The undeclared war against American women.* New York: Crown.

Fischer, C. (1982). *To dwell among friends: Personal networks in town and city.* Chicago: University of Chicago Press.

Friedman, M., & Rosenman, R. H. (1974). *Type A behavior and your heart.* New York: Knopf.

Ganellen, R., & Blaney, P. (1984). Hardiness and social support as moderators of the effects of life stress. *Journal of Personality and Social Psychology, 47*(1), 156–163.

Gilligan, C., Lyons, N., & Hanmer, T. (1990). *Making connections: The relational worlds of adolescent girls at Emma Willard School.* Troy, NY: Emma Willard School.

House, J., Robbins, C., & Metzner, H. L. (1982). The association of social relationships and activities with mortality: Prospective evidence from the Tecumseh Community Health Study. *American Journal of Epidemiology, 116*(1), 123–140.

Janoff-Bulman, R. (1992). *Shattered assumptions: Toward a new psychology of trauma.* New York: Free Press.

Jordan, J. V. (1987). Clarity in connection: Empathic knowing, desire and sexuality. *Work in Progress, No 29.* Wellesley, MA: Stone Center Working Paper Series.

Jordan, J. V. (1990). Courage in connection: Conflict, compassion and creativity. *Work in Progress, No. 45.* Wellesley, MA: Stone Center Working Paper Series.

Kaplan, B. H., Cassel, J. C., & Gore, S. (1977). Social support and health. *Medical Care, 15,* 47–58.

Kobasa, S. C., & Puccetti, M. C. (1983). Personality and social resources in stress resistance. *Journal of Personality and Social Psychology, 45,* 839–850.

Krystal, H. (1978). Trauma and affects. *Psychoanalytic Study of the Child, 33,* 81–117.

Kushner, H. (1981). *When bad things happen to good people.* New York: Avon.

Lazarus, R. S., & Folkman, S. (1984). *Stress, appraisal and coping.* New York: Springer.

Lerner, M. (1980). *The belief in a just world.* New York: Plenum Press.

Lorde, A. (1984). *Sister outsider.* Freedom, CA: Crossing Press.

Luks, A. (1992). *The healing power of doing good.* New York: Fawcett Columbine.

McCann, L., & Pearlman, L. (1990). *Psychological trauma and the adult survivor.* New York: Brunner/Mazel.

McDaniel, J. (1989). *Metamorphosis: Reflections on recovery.* Ithaca, NY: Firebrand.

Miller, J. B. (1986). What do we mean by relationships? *Work in Progress, No. 22.* Wellesley, MA: Stone Center Working Paper Series.

Miller, J. B. (1988). Connections, disconnections, and violations. *Work in Progress, No. 33.* Wellesley, MA: Stone Center Working Paper Series.

Miller, J. B., & Stiver, I. P. (1991). A relational reframing of therapy. *Work in Progress, No. 52.* Wellesley, MA: Stone Center Working Paper Series.

Pearlin, L. I., & Schooler, C. (1978). The structure of coping. *Journal of Health and Social Behavior, 19,* 2–21.

Perloff, L. (1983). Perceptions of vulnerability to victimization. *Journal of Social Issues, 39,* 41–61.

Rieker, P., & Carmen, E. (1986). The victim-to-patient process: The disconfirmation and transformation of abuse. *American Journal of Orthopsychiatry, 56*(3), 360–370.

Rutter, M. (1979). Protective factors in children's responses to stress and disadvantage. In M. W. Kent & J. Rolf (Eds.), *Primary prevention of psychopathology: Vol. 3. Social competence in children* (pp. 49–74). Hanover, NH: University Press of New England.

Scherwitz, L., Graham, L., & Ornish, D. (1985). Self-involvement and the risk factors for coronary heart disease. *Advances, 2*(2), 6–18.

Seligman, M. (1975). *Helplessness.* San Francisco: Freeman.

Spiegel, D. (1991). A psychosocial intervention and survival time of patients with metastatic breast cancer. *Advances, 7*(3), 10–19.

Sroufe, L. A. (1989). Relationships, self, and individual adaptation. In A. J. Sameroff & R. N. Emde (Eds.), *Relationship disturbances in early childhood* (pp. 70–94). New York: Basic Books.

Steiner-Adair, C. (1991). New maps of development, new models of therapy: The psychology of women and treatment of eating disorders. In C. L. Johnson (Ed.), *Psychodynamic treatment of anorexia nervosa and bulimia* (pp. 225–244). New York: Guilford Press.

Stiver, I. (1990). Dysfunctional families and wounded relationships: Part I. *Work in Progress, No 41.* Wellesley, MA: Stone Center Working Paper Series.

Suls, J. (1982). Social support, interpersonal relations and health: Benefits and liabilities. In G. Sanders & J. Suls (Eds.), *Social psychology of health and illness* (pp. 255–279). Hillsdale, NJ: Erlbaum.

Surrey, J. L. (1985). The "self-in-relation": A theory of women's development. *Work in Progress, No. 13.* Wellesley, MA: Stone Center Working Paper Series.

Weil, S. (1983). *Gravity and grace.* New York: Octagon.

Wheeler, L., Reis, H., & Nezlek, J. (1983). Loneliness, social interaction, and sex roles. *Journal of Personality and Social Psychology, 45,* 943–953.

This chapter was originally presented at a Stone Center Colloquium on April 1, 1992. © 1992 by Judith V. Jordan.

3

Relational Awareness
Transforming Disconnection

JUDITH V. JORDAN

In a relational model of psychological development, disconnection from others is viewed as one of the primary sources of human suffering. Similarly, disconnection from oneself, from the natural flow of one's responses, needs, and yearnings creates distress, inauthenticity, and ultimately a sense of isolation in the world. We suggest that people gain a central sense of meaning, well-being, and worth through engagement in growth-enhancing relationships; we further suggest that an active interest in being connected and movement toward increasing connection are at the core of human development (Miller, 1988). In speaking about relational being, I am suggesting that there is primary energy that flows toward others, toward joining with others in an expansive sense of interconnectedness. In contrast, the separate-self paradigm would suggest that separation and disconnection is the primary state of affairs ("We are born alone; we die alone"). According to this view, from a place of essential aloneness, we at best reach out to relate to or use "objects" who can meet our needs or provide some passing solace in this lonely journey.

Existing autonomy and self-sufficiency models, then, create a consciousness of separation and a belief that this is at the core of the human condition. Most psychoanalytic or depth psychologies posit that when we peel away the layers of socialization and civilization we find a selfish, aggressive, and isolated individual. Classical Freudians and some object relations theorists see the desire for relatedness as grafted onto other, more primary drives such as aggression, sexuality, or hunger. Connection and love are often seen as illusions, momentarily covering over the more basic condition of isolation and self-interest. Children are then raised to value separation, to feel proud of signs of independence. Normative socialization teaches that we are safer and stronger if we can exist without needing relationships. This concept is at the core of the power/control mode (Jordan, 1987) that informs socialization of the dominant group in most Western cultures but most dramatically in the United States. What we might call "defensive self-sufficiency" is the standard of psychological maturity in this model.

At a personal level when we are injured or violated in important relationships, particularly when this is a chronic state of affairs, we withdraw even more deeply into defensive isolation and fear of connection. There are several forces pushing us toward pervasive experiences of isolation:

1. Normative emphasis on defensive disconnection as a means to feeling strong and self-sufficient (e.g., "becoming your own man"; "standing on your own two feet")
2. Contextually produced disconnections including societal forces that suggest certain "different" or "minority" groups are "lesser than" (e.g., women, people of color, lesbians and gays, older people)
3. Individual pathological disconnections that result from repetitive and ongoing violations in close relationships, particularly those which involve dependency and inability to self-protect, such as between small children and parents

I would like to suggest that the story of our preoccupation with self-sufficiency and autonomy is largely the story of our woundedness, the extent to which the cultural standards of development have warped our natural search for safe and growth-enhancing connection. Pressure toward disconnection is harshly and normatively rendered in the lives of boys and men, with society's insistence on fierce independence, autonomy, and guardedness. Several theorists have spoken about the trauma of the boy's enforced separation from his primary objects: mother and father (Bergman, 1991; Bergman & Surrey, 1993; Pollack, 1995). But I would suggest there is a more pervasive injury in the larger disruption of a sense of connectedness in general, whether with his mother, his father, or all others. The boy is taught to see himself as standing *over* or *against* rather than *with;* in such a stance he is taught to deny basic human engagement and vulnerability. Psychology itself, with its reigning separate-self paradigm, its overemphasis on individualism, and its emphasis on independent "doers" reinforces this sense of separateness. But anyone who has known the experience of "coming home" to connection, whether in the embrace of a loved one, in gazing into the sparkling and responsive eyes of a baby, or in the rapture of a breathtaking sunset, knows there is something basic and beyond doubt about the sense of "being with," being in the flow of relational experience.

Any discussion of disconnections should include the societal factors that push us in the direction of disconnection and do not support the kind of transformation of disconnections into connection that we are suggesting is essential to healthy growth. In addition to the disconnections involved in socializing children toward independence and autonomy, toward an ideal of strength in separation, I would include all the divisive and fragmenting forces in the culture that push people into shame and isolation. Important among these forces are racism, sexism, heterosexism, ageism, and classism; all of the judgments that render groups marginalized, denigrated, or objectified contribute to an experience of disconnection and isolation. Disempowerment and fear usually accompany these disconnections. Furthermore, the suppression of all experience that makes the dominant group uncomfortable or threatened leads to self-protective inauthenticity in many marginalized groups—another source of disconnection.

I would like to add that I think there is a profound antirelational backlash going on at this point in history. This is not just backlash against women but also against relational values and ways of organizing experience that threaten existing patriarchal power systems. In our field of health care this is epitomized by the increasingly dehumanizing delivery of care through managed care systems. A student recently pointed out that a flyer from one managed care program offered a list of dos and don'ts about the efficient delivery of mental health services. On the list was "Don't build relationships with your clients. They lead to regression, increased dependency, and demands for longer-term therapy!"

DISCONNECTIONS

As individuals, we all have particular ways that we disconnect, particular situations that render us most vulnerable to disconnection, and particular patterns for transforming disconnections back into expansive connections; furthermore, ongoing relationships develop their own patterns of disconnection and reconnection. Most of these patterns exist at an unconscious, unexamined level. Questions we might ask when we observe disconnections are: Is it noticed by both people (or all people involved since these observations are not just limited to two-person situations)? Does it *matter* to both people? Will both people try to change it? Will both people work to sustain the connection? And will they work to understand the disconnection? Will both people attempt to understand and look at what is current? Can both people "hold" responsibility for the effect of disconnections on the relationship?

In acute disconnections within primarily growth-enhancing relationships, we have the opportunity to first name the disconnection and explore the interaction pattern, what led up to it; to express our feelings and represent our needs and understandings; and to stay open to the experience of the other person. We can also make an effort to see how our feelings and responses are affecting the relationship.

Often the clue to a disconnection is the drop in energy we feel in the moment. We feel negative affect, sad, angry, or depressed, and the movement in connection either slows down or ceases. There can be fear and immobilization; our sense of investment in the connection diminishes. There is often either heightened self-consciousness or dissociation; both involve a decrease in relational awareness. In acute disconnections, however, the interaction can often be transformed rather quickly. The disconnections to which I am referring are largely in individual interactions, but there are ways these occur in groups as well.

In chronic disconnection, often brought about because the relational context is not mutual or growth-enhancing, there develops a deep sense of immobilization or impasse. In fact, that is what impasse is: a chronic disconnection. The lack of movement and negative feelings that characterize acute disconnection settle in, and one feels depressed, out of touch, stuck. The pattern of immobilization, fear, and self-blame leads to a heightened sense of isolation.

Fear figures importantly in most experiences of disconnection. While a natural, relational response to fear is to turn to another for help, comfort, protection, and love, most of us have a history of being injured in some way when we have sought comfort from another person in times of need or vulnerability. When others have been nonresponsive or, worse yet, abusive in the face of our need and vulnerability, we are left feeling wounded, and we question the wisdom of turning to others in times of need. Trauma reactions are dramatically characterized by this pattern. In trauma a vulnerable person is violated by a powerful other who does not respond with empathy or concern to the injured person. This leaves the victim feeling as if she/he does not mat-

ter and is not respected—a state of disconnection that feels terribly unsafe. The tension between the yearning for connection and the terror
of connection is exquisite and often paralyzing. Jean Baker Miller and
Irene P. Stiver (1994) have written about this as the central paradox of
connections and disconnections:

> In the face of significant and especially repeated experiences of dis-
> connection, we believe that we yearn even more for connections to oth-
> ers. However, we also become so afraid of engaging with others about
> our experience that we keep important parts of ourselves out of con-
> nection; that is, we develop strategies for disconnection. (p. 1)

I would add that the capacity to *hold* the relationship, to be in relational
flow, lessens as we fall into self-protective strategies. Often when we
blame ourselves or others rather than looking at the relational patterns, we are moving out of connection.

Relationships that fail to be mutual or adequately honor both people's realities also push toward disconnection. If one person is continually in the position of accommodating to the other's reality, or if contact with one's inner process is distorted in the process of relating to
another, the relationship becomes illusory. Resentment about the imbalance of mutuality goes underground, and connection begins to fal-
ter.

When we are hurt by those we love and become angry at them for
hurting us but also feel we need them or the relationship and are not
sure we can represent our hurt to them, we often close down or withdraw. When we need them or are dependent on them and feel angry at
them, we may also disconnect or push them away to try to achieve
safety. When mixed emotional states lead us in confusing directions, toward or away from others, it is helpful to begin to disentangle what the
intertwined feelings are. Often simply naming the different feelings as
clearly as possible is helpful. Increased clarity of experience is an important part of moving back into connection.

When we hurt someone we love, we often feel shame and chagrin,
which can also lead us to disconnect. If the suffering in the person we
love is caused by someone else or some other condition, we often feel a
sense of compassion, of bearing the sadness with that person. But
when we actually cause the pain, there is often a conflicting movement
toward and away from the other. We seek to protect ourselves from seeing the hurt that we cause by withdrawing or defending our action at
the same time that we may genuinely feel the pain with the person we
have hurt. In such situations it is essential to witness her/his pain, validate her/his hurt, take responsibility for our part in creating it, and ex-

press sorrow about it. This does not always mean undoing the painful words or actions, as sometimes the pain is inevitable. This is an especially important dynamic for therapists to be aware of, as we often are tempted to disconnect when we fail our clients empathically or hurt them inadvertently (Jordan, 1993).

Shame is another major factor that takes us into isolation. When we feel it is unsafe to bring various aspects of ourselves directly into a relationship, profound disconnection results (Jordan, 1989). The belief that no empathic response will be available from another person leads to deep withdrawal and immobilization.

CLINICAL VIGNETTE OF ACUTE DISCONNECTION

Jane, a 39-year-old teacher, became pregnant in a relationship with her boyfriend, whom she did not want to marry. After much exploration she decided she really wanted to have the baby; she felt quite joyful about this, although she also worried about how she would "manage." When she told her family, who are quite conservative and live in a small midwestern town, they were furious and judging. They wondered, "How could you do this to us? What will people think? Do you think *you* could really be a good mother? If you can't think about our feelings, could you at least think about this poor child who will probably be ruined by your selfish need to have a baby?" Jane felt devastated and moved into significant self-doubt and self-blame about this. She felt all alone, sad, angry, and very needy. Her exaggerated neediness made her feel uncomfortable about turning to anyone for help. She feared she would overwhelm people. Every time she thought of speaking with her friend Cathy about this she felt extreme anxiety. Her attempts to defend against her anxiety led her to become more distanced and closed down. Cathy, sensing this distancing, felt that a "door was slammed" in her face and wondered what she had done to push Jane away or make her angry. She in turn pulled away. Jane noticed Cathy's pain and increasing distance. With difficulty, Jane was able to go to Cathy and tell her she felt lonely and was sad that she had hurt Cathy; she noted she felt disconnected and wanted to try to look at that with Cathy. Cathy responded by saying she had felt hurt by Jane's distancing but that she didn't want to "go away." She wanted to be there for Jane. Jane also acknowledged that she had been feeling what she called "rejection sensitive" and fearful of how "needy" she was. Cathy commented that she too was in a vulnerable place. The two friends began to feel reconnected as Jane began then to tell Cathy about what was behind her original disconnecting. When people feel a need for more care or protection at the same time they feel unsafe, they often develop hypervigilance in order to protect themselves. They look for danger, become supersensitive to rejection, and often defensively distance from the other person in an effort to feel safe or worthy.

While most disconnections are painful, they sometimes serve an important function. That is, we often disconnect in order to keep our truth alive or to maintain a sense of integrity or authenticity. This is akin to Carol Gilligan's (see Brown & Gilligan, 1992) notion of "political resistance" where girls resist letting go of their deep knowledge about relationships when in adolescence the rules change, suggesting they need to suppress their understanding of life. If they do not develop such political resistance, girls then move out of authentic relationship in order to preserve the illusion of relationship or to fit into the only relationships available to them.

Most chronic disconnections, however, lead to a sense of isolation and ultimately interfere with growth as more and more of our experience gets split off from the flow of relationship. Most change occurs by our being able to bring aspects of ourselves into relationships with other persons where we get new responses, build new images, and create new actions. Fixed, chronic disconnections derail our development, particularly if they contribute to a wariness of new connections. Many severe and chronic disconnections do just that. They leave us with an extreme fear of relationships as well as an extreme yearning for connection; Jean Baker Miller and Irene P. Stiver (1994) have beautifully addressed this dynamic.

There are clearly situations when people must move out of nonmutual, hurtful relationships. At such times, disconnecting is healthy. But most often such moves must be made with an awareness of the need for other sustaining connections in a person's life. One of the most important skills a person can develop is to be able to discern those relationships in which one is safe being open or vulnerable and those in which one should be appropriately self-protective. I am not advocating a naive, universal opening to others, although I wish we lived in a world where that could happen. We do not. But as a culture we need a different balance between an attitude of self-protection and self-enhancement, on the one hand, and the ability to be open to being affected, to fostering growth in others, and to caring about the building of relationship, on the other. Our societal imbalance in the promotion of self-interest has been extremely destructive to relationships.

RELATIONAL AWARENESS

Relational awareness involves the development of clarity about the movement of relationship; this importantly includes an awareness of

our patterns and ways of connecting and disconnecting, and transforming the flow from the direction of disconnection to connection. It includes personal awareness, awareness of the other, awareness of the impact of oneself on the other, the effect of other on oneself, and the
quality of energy and flow in the relationship itself. Developing relational awareness is enormously complex. It is different from developing
self-knowledge or analyzing one's past relationship histories. In relational awareness one moves toward greater clarity of what actually exists in the relationship. It is more akin to being "present with" and looking at one's patterns of relating; one has a modicum of distance and
capacity to observe at the same time one is present in the experience.
There is an attunement to self, other, and relational processes. Awareness involves a nonjudgmental stance, an ability to notice and observe
without becoming totally immersed or caught in the experience. One
can learn to see consequences and sequences of behaviors without
moving into paralyzing self-doubt and self-blame.

   We get to know our own state and how we deal with it (e.g., "When
I'm angry I tend to 'go away' so I don't threaten people or the relationship," or "I push people away indirectly so they don't see my vulnerability, leaving others feeling hurt or confused").

   When people increase their capacity for relational awareness, they
dramatically alter their capacity to transform disconnections. They also
enhance their ability to move into growth-enhancing relationships and
to move toward intimacy, closeness, and an awareness of the primacy of
relatedness. Defensive patterns of "turning away" or "against" are transformed into turning "toward" and "moving with."

   Relational awareness is not about "analyzing" relationships. It involves an attitude of openness to learning about our relational patterns.
It often takes place most creatively in active interaction with others; we
also can learn about these patterns in quiet reflection. In order to culti-
vate relational awareness, one must achieve a kind of steadiness and a
sense of the larger perspective. What keeps us out of the relational
present of authentic and close engagement? Obstacles to connection include roles, habit patterns, automatic reactions, dissociation, reactivity
rather than responsiveness, and affective overamplification. Some of
the areas in which we can usefully focus relational awareness are the
following: the difficulty of dealing with mixed feelings; shame; the
need to feel powerful; fear of vulnerability; avoidance of conflict; an
overdeveloped tendency to accommodate to the needs or demands of
another; overreliance on control and will; the need to be admired; and,
importantly, the overdeveloped need to be self-sufficient. Some of
these resonate with Karen Horney's (1942) list of neurotic trends.

   Teasing out what comes from the past and what comes from the present is also helpful. That is, in current relationships, we are often beset by old patterns or relational images that inevitably lead to distortions and unclarity in our current interactions. The capacity for current awareness drops where violation, fear, and trauma patterns dominate.

Not only do old relational images keep us out of connection but what I call "ego strategies" or investment in images of who we are or who we should be take us out of authentic connection and close us down. We become more involved in trying to maintain a certain set of beliefs about ourselves or in wishing to convey certain images of ourselves, and this usually takes us out of connection in a profound way. This striving becomes a straitjacket for the person maintaining the image as well as for the other person who will have to give a certain response in order to support the image being conveyed. Little growth can occur in such relationships. This kind of relating occurs in roles, often in job positions, and in fact is often normative and necessary for such relationships. But it only interferes with the more growth-enhancing or close relationships I am speaking about here. You cannot control another person to make her/him be what you want nor to respond in a particular way and be in authentic connection. You can simply represent your feelings or your own ideas and see whether the other person can respond. Imposition of "power over" another is a forceful and distorting act. One person initiates and directs, and the other person accommodates. Real connection and growth do not happen under such circumstances.

TRANSFORMATION

What helps us stay in the struggle for connection? I believe there is something intrinsically satisfying about being in connection. It feels real; it feels healing; it feels safe. Most of us have proverbial unconscious memories of the sense of closeness and comfort of being held close and feeling at peace. We also have more recent experiences of how good it feels to work through the difficult places in relationships. But it is a struggle, and we need support in our efforts.

Disconnections are inevitable. Empathic failures are inevitable. Hurt feelings and disappointments are inevitable. Acute disconnections can be minor or major; they can hurt a great deal, or they can cause a small loss of energy or decrease in zest. Resilience is the key. Self-empathy and empathy for others can help transform these disconnections and lead to a compassionate attitude in the struggle to stay connected. Essential to the transformation of disconnection is an openness to being moved by the other person. Also essential is an openness

to being seen by the other person. Thus we must be able to open ourselves up to being known, to being moved, and to moving another person. We find ways to avoid getting stuck in disconnection; this is at the
heart of relational resilience. We must move out of more narrow self-
awareness.

Transforming disconnection is not about taking action, doing, fixing, changing, or controlling. It is about dealing with the fear that
largely determines people's movement into separation and isolation.
Safety in separation is part of the model of separate self; I would suggest instead that real safety occurs in the building of growth-fostering
relationships.

The pattern of transformation of disconnection most often involves:

1. Naming the disconnection in a nonaccusatory way. ("I just noticed a shift here. Did you feel it also?")
2. Noticing what was going on when the shift occurred; in therapy
   this is the "Why now?" question
3. Examining one's part in the disconnection and taking responsibility for it ("I think I may have pulled away just then," or "Perhaps I hurt you when I said . . . ")
4. Hearing the other person's sense of what is going on
5. Looking together at the possible relational factors that might
   have contributed to the disconnection ("We've been really out
   of touch recently, and we haven't been taking care of this relationship, have we?")
6. Acknowledging the relational history ("What resources have we
   developed for dealing with these painful times?")
7. Putting the disconnection in a larger context ("This present
   pain is not forever, nor is it the most real aspect of the relationship.")
8. Commitment to the transformation of the disconnection and to
   the ongoing growth-fostering nature of the relationship; commitment to mutual respect and mutual growth is at the core of
   a healthy relationship
9. Reestablishing concern and appreciation for the relationship in
   addition to caring for the individuals in the relationship: the
   willingness to explore what limits relationship is essential; it
   means we must give up our pretensions that we always "do good
   relationships"

We are all wounded, all struggling to be in positive connection. If
we try to maintain the image of being accomplished at relationships,
then we inevitably move out of the real give and take of relatedness.

While idealization is appealing, it is not about growth or about being real. A real relationship is staying with what actually is, trying to be honest, kind, open, and compassionate with the real-life pain that exists everywhere. Instead of judgment, comparison, and distancing in the face of another's pain or in the face of difficulties in relationship, we intend compassion and empathy for ourselves and for the other person. Sharing vulnerability, grief, and suffering is enormously healing in a relationship where we feel trusting and trustworthy. Looking at the things that impede good connection and revealing the blockages that get in our way often opens the way toward reconnection. We cannot always get rid of the blockages to connection, but we can bring awareness to them and bring them into the relationship by communicating about them—and sometimes just doing that does dispel the blockages.

Attention must be paid also to "what holds the relationship." What is the larger context, and how supportive is it of the struggle to stay in connection? Where there is commitment to mutual growth, mutual respect, and the willingness to explore the disconnections and pain in relationship, then there is hope that connection can prevail. When we see someone else as "other"—racially, sexually, or politically—we tend to treat them as an object, as "not I," not someone creating a "we" with "us." This destroys a sense of connection.

Bringing nonjudgmental awareness to ourselves and others is difficult. Often when people point out a problem in us or state that they see something in us we do not like, the response is "Oh, no! Am I like that? I'm terrible." Or we get defensive and look for flaws in the other to explain her/his judgment of us. We need to support one another in hearing descriptive feedback so that we do not automatically move to places of shame or self-blame. Learning how others see us is essential to our growth, and being able to provide that for others is also part of expanding relatedness. By this I do not mean catharsis ("let it all hang out") with each other. I mean responsible empathic attunement to others where we share our reactions and feelings authentically but with concern and attention to their effects on others and on the relationship.

Different emotional states tend to either guide us toward connection or take us away. Depression takes us out of connection, into an unclear state. Sadness can produce powerful connection if we are able to reach toward others to seek support and comfort (Stiver & Miller, 1988). Similarly, anger can lead to connection as an effort to communicate hurt and to get some caring response from the other person who is hurting us (Miller, 1982). Rage, however, usually takes us out of connection because the intensity is too great and is often fed by old, unspoken angers; the preoccupation with self-protection leads to a closing down, and people are frightened by rage. Fear can move us toward or away from others; if we are able to turn to others in fear, we can be comforted and learn new ways to be with our fear. It can be deeply moving, soothing, and trust building. Or, in fear, we can move into hiding and distance. Shame, secrets, and inauthenticity clearly take us out of connection.

Therapists, too, must look at how we disconnect or keep people at a distance in order to create some sense of personal safety. Fear so clearly figures in our movement into separation (Jordan, 1993).

As we build relationships, we need to create a conscious history of relational patterns and specifically relational repair. This helps us learn how we have effectively mended torn places in the relationships before. We might construct a relational resilience inventory as well as an inventory of where we are vulnerable to disconnections.

The ability to reconnect, to be resilient in relationship, to move back into connection to see if mutual growth-enhancing relatedness can be reestablished is one of the most important skills one can develop.

RELATIONAL AWARENESS GROUPS

As part of an effort to facilitate the development of relational skills in recent years, I have been co-leading a group called "a relational awareness practice group." It is run by two co-leaders and is a combined didactic and experiential group in which we seek to help people become aware of their relational patterns. We also try to help people communicate their needs, feelings, and concerns effectively and respectfully at the same time they expand their awareness of self, other, and relationship. This is not a catharsis group, nor is it a group to analyze where the patterns come from in the past, although we notice when feelings that come from the past take over and make staying in the present difficult. We try to help the women identify their relational resources, strengths, and vulnerabilities. Each group begins with a relational "check-in" process. In this check-in, people state in several sentences where they are emotionally or otherwise and what impact they think their current state might have on the other group members. People are encouraged to ask themselves the questions: What do I feel? What do I want? What impact will these have on the other person? What do I need to do to move this relationship in the direction of growth for all of us? What is happening in the relationship right now? What does the relationship need?

We also ask people if they have a relational topic they would like the group to discuss. The co-leaders participate in this check-in, not going into great detail but commenting on their current state insofar as it might impact on the group (e.g., "I'm feeling a bit tired today, so I may seem a little distant," or "I was looking forward to this group a lot, so I may jump in and comment a lot and may possibly crowd people a little"). This particular group is made up largely of trauma survivors.

The kinds of connections we work toward in the group are mutually respectful, empathic, and empowering in which each person notices the effect they have on the others and also notes how they are affected by others. Being mindful or attentive to the relationship is the first step toward becoming aware of what needs work and what people want to happen in the relationship. We do not go into detail about people's histories or even current relationships. Most important, we want people to see their own relational patterns more clearly, particularly how they move into disconnection or might evoke that in others. At the same time we acknowledge that people often feel the need for disconnection, distancing, or establishing a sense of control over their involvement in the interaction. We also honor the longings, resources, and capacity they have to reconnect and try to build on those.

Often the fear of being open, of being affected by another, of taking in something that is offered leaves us feeling disconnected and isolated. A deep and moving discussion occurred in one of our meetings about how much the women wanted to give to one another and wanted to be there for each other. But they then went on to talk about how hard it was to really let someone else have an impact on them or to ask for help from others. They were just too scared about being vulnerable, open, or receptive. As the conversation went on, one of the women suddenly got a look of amazement on her face and said, "Well, what's really going on here then? We're all saying we want to give to one another, but there's no one willing to be open to really take in and be affected by what we're giving! So, is anybody really giving to anyone if no one is there to receive it? Is anything really happening?" For this group of trauma survivors, this became a moment of powerful relational awareness. They saw that reparative, loving connection is what they needed but also saw they were too scared to open themselves to it because their sense of need and vulnerability were so great.

During the check-in at a recent group, several people remarked they felt depressed, anxious, and cut off. One woman spoke for the group: "I'm feeling depressed, immobilized, and withdrawn today. I probably won't be able to participate much in the group: I don't want people to take that personally and think I'm angry at them, 'cuz I'm not." The isolation in the room was palpable. No one had a topic to talk about. After a short but thick and tense silence, one of the co-leaders suggested that it felt like everyone wanted to be out of the room. But we also knew from our history together that if we could begin to name the feelings, then we might experience a shift out of the isolation. There might be good reason for people to feel a heightened self-protectiveness, but we might explore both the disconnection and the reasons for it to see if there were common threads from which we could learn. One woman, Pat, commented, "Well you know, Connie [another woman in the group] and I had a big fight just before the group started, and some people were there. I think it scared people." Another short but painful silence followed. Then Connie responded, "I just gotta say I blew up and lost it. I'm sorry. I'm not angry now. I'm ashamed." The anxiety in the room lessened. Pat responded, "I don't want to keep this going either. It feels better that you said you were quiet 'cuz you feel bad. I thought you were still mad and ready to pounce, so I thought I'm sure as hell not going to open myself up here." Another member then joined in: "I thought you were both mad and I was going to have to fix it all like I used to in my family. Now, instead, I can just say this is making me so tense. And right now I actually feel a little more okay." One of the co-leaders commented on the process of being able to look at how we are affecting each other and how the tension begins to shift when we are able to check things out with each other. All the details of the fight or the past woundings were not necessary to this discussion nor to achieving more clarity together. But being aware of the authentic feelings was. Moving into disconnection was also seen as a necessary self-protective strategy until the safety of the relational context could be evaluated.

In another group meeting, Carol responded to Diane at one point when Diane was describing a painful interaction that had occurred in another setting by saying, "I don't know what you're talking about." Betty heard this as a distancing, critical response, as if Carol were saying to Diane, "It isn't true what you're saying." Betty expressed her anger at Carol. Dottie then said she heard the comment more as curiosity: "Tell me what you're talking about." A discussion ensued, framed in the struggle to stay connected and to learn something about ourselves and others. It did not deteriorate into a standoff, with people venting their anger, distancing, or staying in their isolation and being "right" about what they heard.

Relational awareness allows people to address imbalances, pains, and failures of mutuality before they become too big, before impasses develop. It supports relational resilience. Self-empathy is as important as empathy for the other. To feel competent interpersonally, one must be taken seriously by others. That includes asking for what you want, saying "no" to things you do not want, and learning ways to manage interpersonal conflict. It involves honoring others' needs as well as being respectful of your impact on them. It also involves learning ways to build relationship and honoring the importance of relationship through transforming disconnections. The pattern of opening and closing, transforming disconnections, moving into deeper connection, but then often lapsing into distance is illustrated by some work I have been doing with Beth.

Beth is a successful lawyer who first undertook therapy about 10 years ago to work on anxieties she was experiencing in graduate school and her difficulties getting into a committed relationship with a man. She completed her therapeutic work in 3 years, and she was doing well in a new marriage with a new baby and a career that was extremely successful and gratifying. But about 2 years ago she began to experience disturbing dreams, a sense of isolation, sexual withdrawal from her husband, and a nagging sense that something "big" was wrong. She called to resume therapy. She spoke of feeling very cut off and isolated everywhere in her world. In therapy, she began to recover memories of abuse by an uncle and a general sense of neglect and abandonment in her home. She was indeed profoundly disconnected, often related to people in a distanced inauthentic manner, and felt very unknown and unseen. She said the only exceptions to her cutoff way of being were her three children, with whom she experienced deep connection, warmth, and love. As she contrasted this closeness with the isolation she felt everywhere else in her life for her whole life, she "got how bad it really had been." At this time in therapy she began to feel intense sadness. But she also began to feel increasing hope about the possibility of feeling more love and closeness in her life with others. As she opened more to others she also began to feel more fear; this is part of the paradox of connection and disconnection which Stiver and Miller (1988) describe. It is a common, dramatic pattern in trauma work; as a person begins to heal and open up, she/he is thrown into intense fear, often leading to abrupt, spasmodic closing down. In working with trauma this often leads to a roller coaster (Chu, 1992) or whiplash feeling in the treatment. At best she was able to reach out to me or to her husband and take the risk that this relationship could be different from the violating relationships of her past. At worst she moved back into isolation, fear, and self-blame. In response to her, I validated that it really made sense that she wanted to cut herself off, to withdraw and "numb out," given the context in which she existed as a child and the resulting expectations about relationships with which she was left. In therapy her increasing awareness of how awful, dangerous, and isolated her childhood had been contrasted with her hope of the possibility of something different. She reported, "I feel out of it, under water, hazy. I can't tell what I'm feeling." Then she added, "I feel increasingly scared of being hurt and abandoned." Again, I acknowledged her need to move back into disconnection and isolation, knowing that the larger movement is toward connecting and establishing a different kind of relationship. I said that made sense in the past and empathized with the way things were for her as a child. In therapy, I validated the smaller movement back into disconnection and isolation and knew that the larger movement, even represented by her coming back into therapy and being able to turn to me more frequently in her distress, is toward connecting and establishing a different kind of relationship. This means that we look at the differences in the relational context then and now (as they exist in the therapy and in her relationship with her husband compared to earlier interactions with parents).

Beth's latest crisis of immobility and numbness came after a couples meeting in which she began to reveal more of herself with her husband, a very new and frightening experience for her. She has been increasing her authentic communication in her therapy, in her marriage, and has started doing it with a new friend who is also an abuse survivor. Each time she takes a step forward, she spirals backward into depression, confusion, immobility, and disconnection. In order to move forward she struggles to stay with the sad edge of loss and anger, of what was not there for her, and how sad that is. I empathize with the necessary movement into disconnection and fear, but I do not see it as the whole picture. In moments of fear and trauma, her capacity for relational awareness drops; anger, blaming of self and other, self-destructiveness, and isolation increase. I can help hold the larger picture of hope and connection. I might add that it helps me as a therapist to recognize the spiraling pattern of connection and disconnection in working through the trauma; otherwise I would tend to personalize and blame myself each time Beth goes into major jolting disconnection. That would undoubtedly lead me to disconnect as well.

It is essential that therapists, too, get to know and take responsibility for our disconnections (Jordan, 1993). It is important in therapy as well as in our lives that we not become hemmed in by idealized expectations of how or who we should be; that includes being careful not to set new standards of relational perfection that none of us can live up to. This attempt only contributes to shame, and shame leads to inevitable disconnection and impasse. We are all struggling to stay in growth-enhancing connection; we are all constantly moving into disconnection. If we build impossible expectations of how we should be as therapists or parents or friends or lovers, we will only be building new places for disconnection, as our shame and disappointment in ourselves will lead us away from others. Getting to know our places of disconnection importantly means developing a compassionate attitude toward our needs to disconnect, our yearnings to connect, and our many imperfections in the journey of connection.

REFERENCES

Bergman, S. (1991). Men's psychological development: A relational perspective. *Work in Progress, No. 48.* Wellesley, MA: Stone Center Working Paper Series.

Bergman, S., & Surrey, J. L. (1993). The woman–man relationship: Impasses and possibilities. *Work in Progress, No. 55.* Wellesley, MA: Stone Center Working Paper Series.

Brown, L., & Gilligan, C. (1992). *Meeting at the crossroads: Women's psychology and girls' development.* Cambridge, MA: Harvard University Press.

Chu, J. (1992). The therapeutic roller coaster: Dilemmas in the treatment of childhood abuse survivors. *Journal of Psychotherapy Practice and Research, 1*(4), 351–370.

Horney, K. (1942). *Self-analysis.* New York: Norton.

Jordan, J. V. (1987). Clarity in connection: Empathic knowing, desire, and sexuality. *Work in Progress, No. 29.* Wellesley, MA: Stone Center Working Paper Series.

Jordan, J. V. (1989). Relational development: Therapeutic implications of empathy and shame. *Work In Progress, No. 39.* Wellesley, MA: Stone Center Working Paper Series.

Jordan, J. V. (1993). Challenges to connection. *Work in Progress, No. 60.* Wellesley, MA: Stone Center Working Paper Series.

Miller, J. B. (1982). The construction of anger in women and men. *Work in Progress, No. 4.* Wellesley, MA: Stone Center Working Paper Series.

Miller, J. B. (1988). Connections, disconnections and violations. *Work in Progress, No. 33.* Wellesley, MA: Stone Center Working Paper Series.

Miller, J. B., & Stiver, I. P. (1994). Movement in therapy: Honoring the strategies of disconnection. *Work in Progress, No. 65.* Wellesley, MA: Stone Center Working Paper Series.

Pollack, W. (1995). The trauma of Oedipus: Toward a new psychoanalytic psychology of men. In R. Levant & W. Pollack (Eds.), *A new psychology of men* (pp. 13–35). New York: Basic Books.

Stiver, I. P., & Miller, J. B. (1988). From depression to sadness in women's psychotherapy. *Work in Progress, No. 36.* Wellesley, MA: Stone Center Working Paper Series.

This chapter was originally presented at a Stone Center Colloquium on April 5, 1995. © 1995 by Judith V. Jordan.

4

Therapists' Authenticity

JEAN BAKER MILLER, JUDITH V. JORDAN,
IRENE P. STIVER, MAUREEN WALKER,
JANET L. SURREY, *and* NATALIE S. ELDRIDGE

Relational–cultural theory emphasizes therapist authenticity. In this, it differs from many traditional psychodynamic theories. But what do we mean by therapist authenticity? We will each offer a short answer to that question.

To begin to answer it, we have to set out a few basic notions. Working in a relational way comes out of a wholly different therapeutic approach. It is not a model of the omniscient (and omnipotent) expert *acting on* a person, making interpretations about what's wrong with the "sick," "disturbed" patient. Instead, it is both people—or in group or family therapy, all people—participating in trying to carry out a creative act of countering the destructive effects of a patriarchal, "power over" society and all of its many manifestations, recognizing that these conditions affect us all (Jordan, Kaplan, Miller, Stiver, & Surrey, 1991; Miller & Stiver, 1997).

However, we believe that the therapist should have particular abilities, responsibilities, and knowledge—and the training to acquire these capabilities. What are these abilities? Most important of all, the therapist needs to learn how to participate in the therapy relationship in such a way that she facilitates "movement in relationship." How does she do this? If she is really present and authentic, she will be moved (i.e., feel with the patient's expression of her/his experience). If the therapist can make it known that she is moved, the patient will be moved (i.e., feel with the therapist feeling with her). The patient thus has the very valuable chance to know that her/his thoughts and feelings do reach another person, do matter, and can be part of a mutual experience (Miller & Stiver, 1997). We think that this is the key source of change in therapy. It is so important because the basic trouble has been the disconnections the person has experienced, the disconnections in which the patient had little or no possibility of having an authentic effect on the disconnecting relationship.

This is very different from training someone not to show any response in therapy. However, it requires very good training to express authentic responsiveness in a way that creates movement in relationship.

To be a little more specific, to facilitate movement in relationship, the therapist should know a lot about the strategies of disconnection. They arise out of disconnecting experience. We believe that the central desire of all people is to connect with others. But when people have suffered hurt, danger, humiliation, and many other kinds of disconnection, they continue to try to find whatever connections they can. Now, however, they feel they can do so only if they keep significant amounts of their experience and responses out of connection. This is what we call the *central relational paradox*. The methods people develop to keep parts of themselves out of connection are called the *strategies of disconnection* (Miller & Stiver, 1997).

Seemingly paradoxically also, we believe that one of the most important ways to facilitate movement in relationship is to truly honor the strategies of disconnection. We must realize the deep reasons for these strategies and the fear or terror that people feel at the threat of losing them—even as we believe that they create the problems (i.e., they are the very obstacles to connection) (Miller & Stiver, 1997).

We assume that the therapist knows how to work with the strategies of disconnection. That is her job. Authenticity, then, means that the therapist tries to be with the thoughts and feelings occurring in the relationship. It also means that the therapist tries to be with the movement toward connection, the fears of that movement, and the strategies of disconnection. She should be "in" this moment-to-moment interplay. She should try to convey that she has felt with the patient and raise questions when she hasn't, questions that will help them both move toward the mutuality we've described (Jordan et al., 1991). This moment-to-moment responsiveness is the most important part of authenticity.

What about the question of the therapist "disclosing" facts about her own life—or even her feelings? If such "disclosures" do not advance the movement in relationship, there is no place for them in psychotherapy. If they will advance the movement or will help to convey that the therapist is honoring the strategies of disconnection, they may be important. If not bringing them in will interfere with the movement in relationship, then they may need to be brought in. This is where training and judgment—and often discussion with colleagues and supervisors—come in.

One brief example may illustrate these points. The question of my physical disability from polio comes into therapy with everyone with whom I've worked, although in many different ways and sometimes very indirectly. One example of this occurred early in therapy with a woman I'll call Constance. She never expressed any negative feelings. She said things like "I hate complainers. What have I got to complain about? Some people have it so much harder."

On the one hand, I like and admire Constance's awareness of hardships in the world. But this can also be a person's way of avoiding deep feelings of hurt, disappointment, anger, and other important feelings that she hasn't yet shared; that is, it can be a strategy of disconnection. I didn't know if Constance was trying to stay away from certain feelings, so I asked, "When you say that are you thinking about my disability? Do you wonder if I've had a hard time?" This may not have been what she was thinking. I, however, believed it was important to explore this possibility since it may have been a part of her strategies of disconnection.

As I have become more relational in my approach to therapy, I've become more open about my experience. Specifically, I have become more open whenever it is required to facilitate movement in the therapeutic relationship. Of course, this always depends upon where the relationship is during the course of therapy.

So my openness varies with every patient. In this instance with Constance, I said, "I had polio when I was very young and there were some hard times. I, too, know that people endure much worse hardships in life. But I don't think we can compare these things. What hurts you, hurts you. And you have the right to experience that and explore how it affects you. So my polio and more extreme hardships don't negate anything you feel. Also, it's important that you feel able to bring this up whenever you want to."

The subject of my disability comes up repeatedly in different forms with patients. I watch for it, among watching for lots of other things. It comes up in the words people use, in their dream images, and the like. When I suspect that something personal, like my polio, is interfering with the movement in the relationship, I try to offer the patient an open, authentic response that may facilitate movement toward better connection.

To summarize, I want to emphasize that relational authenticity never means that the therapist uses therapy to meet her own needs. If I had a need to talk about my polio, I certainly shouldn't impose that on anyone's therapy. But if I suspect that my polio may be getting in the way of movement in therapeutic relationship, then the therapy needs me to talk about it.

We'll now move into more complex aspects of this topic.

JUDITH V. JORDAN

Relational authenticity in therapy is not the same thing as total honesty on the part of the therapist; it is about a *quality of presence* that contributes powerfully to healing in connection. The therapist's emotional presence is *an important source of information* for clients and *a resource for growth* in the therapy relationship. It's important for clients to develop an awareness of the impact of their actions and words on other people and on relationships. The therapist's authentic responsiveness contributes to a sense of relational competence as the client begins to experience her/himself as effective in moving or affecting the therapist. It also leads to the development of anticipatory empathy in the client; this involves learning how to anticipate how she/he affects and moves others. The therapist, in being engaged and authentic, gives important information about what impact the client has on her. Clients need to develop relational awareness, looking at interactions and learning what they contribute or how they affect the flow of the relationship. They need to ask questions like "Where is this feeling coming from—is this about me or is this about you?"; "Are you bringing this into the session or have I affected you in some way?"; "Am I stimulating something in you in some way that I may not even be aware of?"; and "What am I contributing and what are you contributing to this interaction?" This leads to the growth of mutual empathy and relational awareness.

Mutual empathy, an essential component of authenticity, is the core relational dynamic that leads to growth in therapy. It depends on the client seeing that she/he *has an impact* on the therapist. In order for the person to know that she/he matters, that she/he influences or moves us, she/he needs to see and feel the therapist's response. This clearly goes against rules about neutrality, nondisclosure, or nonresponsiveness held by many traditional therapists. Also, in order to grow we all need the sense of connection that arises in this flow of mutual empathy. I would suggest that this process changes over time in therapy and my authenticity as a therapist changes over time in working with somebody. We're building a relationship in which trust is growing both ways. Both therapist and client develop increasing trust based on our shared history of movement through connection and disconnection. This opens the way for more relational authenticity.

In discussing therapist authenticity, I want also to make the distinction between relational responsiveness and reactivity. Reactivity is impulsive, entirely spontaneous, and based only on the internal experience of one person (e.g., I feel angry, I just have to express it regardless of the context and the responses of the other person). Relational responsiveness involves a consideration of context and concern about the possible impact of our actions or words on the other person and the relationship. Therapeutic responsiveness also includes the intention to be of help to the client. Therapist authenticity is always informed by that intention.

In the course of therapy the therapist also develops a kind of anticipatory empathy that allows an informed, considered responsiveness quite different from "knee-jerk reactivity." Anticipatory empathy is based on the history of the relationship, a knowledge of the client, and working hypotheses about what the client and the relationship need at this time. It is practiced with the aim of empowering the person and the relationship. It involves a great deal of clinical judgment and sensitive attunement to the client's responses. Anticipatory empathy moves the relationship and increases the sense of connection. It contributes to and arises within an atmosphere of care.

If the therapist is responsive to the client, the inevitable disconnections that occur all the time in therapy will lead on to new connection. In fact, in the reworking of disconnections, connections are strengthened and transformed (not merely repaired) and the relationship develops a stability and trustworthiness that allows further growth to occur. This is where the real work of therapy happens, in navigating and transforming the inevitable disconnections.

In our model, the source of pathology is *chronic disconnection*, not just disconnection; and chronic disconnection results from the nonresponsiveness of one person (particularly the more powerful person) when disconnections occur within the relationship. Consequently, nonresponsiveness of a therapist is not only not helpful to most clients but it is actually hurtful to many. Conversely, within a context of relational responsiveness, the client learns that she/he can be effective in relationship, that she/he matters. These empathic moments provide the building blocks for a sense of relational competence. Depriving clients of this information impoverishes the therapeutic work. Moreover, for people who have been particularly wounded by unresponsive others in the past, this nonresponsiveness signals *a kind of danger* that can lead to withdrawal, isolation, and retraumatization.

Boundaries

I also want to address briefly the question of boundaries. When we talk about authenticity, many people say, "Well what about the 'boundary issue.' Isn't it important for therapists to maintain their neutrality, their boundaries and not reveal or disclose too much of themselves or their reactions?" Perhaps we ought to clarify what is meant by "boundaries." The boundary concept is about safety, clarity, and privacy. It potentially includes the capacity to authentically represent one's needs and feelings in a context that holds some promise of mutuality.

It is essential in therapy that the vulnerability of our clients be protected, particularly by making sure the therapist is not using them to meet her own needs. It's also important that we recognize the therapist's legitimate right to maintain her own privacy, and it's essential to clarify the origin of the feelings and thoughts that emerge in a therapeutic encounter—what belongs to the therapist and what belongs to the client. These are all key elements in what is usually covered in the notion of "keeping the boundaries."

By suggesting that therapy involves mutual empathy and the practice of authenticity on the part of the therapist, we are not suggesting that therapists simply engage in an ordinary social relationship with clients. The above discussion of reactivity versus relational responsiveness points to that. The therapy relationship is intentional and professional. Its aim is to help the client. The therapist's energy and thoughts are directed toward helping the client effect a change in her/his life.

The therapist and the client are in particular roles that suggest different kinds of participation. There are power differences. The therapist's role is to facilitate the development of relational awareness and to assist the client in meeting his or her goals. The therapist also belongs to a profession that sets standards of care; protective limits for both people are crucial to this relationship. Respect, clarity, and responsibility on the part of the therapist for the well-being of the client capture for me the values that are often tagged with the word "boundary." Therapist authenticity requires these qualities. It does not involve total self-disclosure and usually it does not even involve disclosure of factual information about the therapist's life, although in the example that Jean just gave that was clearly a very important sharing.

I am reluctant to use the boundary metaphor and language, however, because it connotes a spatial metaphor of "self" experience (in a "separate-self" paradigm) that emphasizes the importance of protection from an impinging context, personal or otherwise, and thus obscures the importance of a *boundary as a place of meeting*. Redefined, boundaries would suggest movement, differentiation, and connection. Perhaps if we could think of boundary as a place of meeting rather than an armored dividing line, protecting against an impinging outside world, this concept would make more sense in a relational model.

For me, the current boundary metaphor partakes of the dominant paradigm of "a self" resisting influence, demarcating spheres of influence or control in order to establish "power over" others as a way of ensuring personal safety. It is important to remember that "self" is a metaphor. There is no such thing as a "self." The bounded self is a metaphor built on a model of separation rather than connection. In contrast, I believe that safety and psychological growth arise in good connection, not in the experience of self-sufficiency, autonomy, and boundedness. Growth-enhancing relatedness depends clearly on respect, clarity, the capacity to represent one's needs and feelings, and an expectation of mutuality. In meeting others authentically, in engaging in growth-fostering relationships, we create a sense of personal meaning and value.

Having said all that, I think it's important to reframe the concept of boundaries and identify specifically what about the concept is useful in therapy. The way it is currently used is too often unexamined and, I think, rather flip. I offer the example of a supervisor saying to a supervisee when she reported she had passed a box of Kleenex to a sobbing client, "Where were your boundaries?!" I've heard many examples like this. There's a "boundary police" mentality that gets going, pushing therapists subtly in the direction of a separation model, which includes therapist nonresponsiveness. This mentality comes from a model in which separation equals safety. Instead, we believe that growth-fostering connection builds safety. This shift from a separate-self paradigm to a relational paradigm makes the current boundary concept problematic.

What do I think is useful about the boundary notion?

1. *Clarity*: It's important that each person's experience is clear and each person knows whose feelings and thoughts belong to whom. It is important to help clients know and express their feelings and needs more clearly. This leads to better connection with one's inner experience and better connection with others. And it is important to develop clarity about which relationships are mutual and growth-fostering and which are not. In the latter case, it is important to assist people in disengaging from destructive or abusive relationships.

2. It's important that the therapist assume appropriate responsibility for the protection of the clients' *safety* and for the relationship.

3. The therapist should *never use* the client to take care of her own needs. This is most clear in the area of sexual exploitation, but it's true in many areas.

4. Both therapist and client have a *right to privacy* and *self-protection*. Learning how to say no to other people and feeling one has a right to say no or to state one's limits is very important for everyone but especially for people who have been violated in relationships. Both the therapist and the client must feel safe enough to stay in the relationship.

I want to underline some language there. As a therapist, I talk about *stating* my limits rather than *setting* limits on the other person. This feels honest and authentic. If I tell a client I cannot handle five phone calls a day from her/him, it's too much for me, that's authentically stating my limits. The need for the calls on the part of my client may be totally legitimate, but I can't meet that need. So, I state that and I say, "You do need to be in contact with me. It is, unfortunately, impossible for me to be there as much as you need. I'm sorry about that. But we need to do some problem solving around this. How are we going to deal with this together?" This is using my *real* response in the relationship to provide some information and to stimulate some collaborative problem solving together.

Both people in a growth-enhancing relationship are moving toward representing their own needs with an expectation of respect from the other. In the therapy relationship it is primarily the needs of the client that are attended to, but the therapist also has needs for safety, self-care, and the right to state certain limits. Both people must have the right to say no, to state their limits, as well as to seek responsiveness in the other person. How this occurs in therapy will depend on certain role constraints and the importance of keeping the client's well-being at the center of all decision making (this is where clinical judgment is crucial). Part of being an adult in a relationship is learning to respect the other person's feelings, limits, sense of privacy, and even flaws. Respect and responsiveness feel like a better route to genuine and mature relatedness than creating a therapeutic relationship with one "powerful," "in charge" person setting limits on, or placing boundaries around, an "out of control" other who must be reined in by force or superior power. Unfortunately, the concept of boundaries is too often laden with power inequity and therefore does not support the client in her/his empowerment or in the development of new relational awareness and patterns.

It is important for the client to learn to grapple with yearnings and needs in the face of another's inability to meet them; and it is important, although difficult, for both the therapist and the client to learn to hold the tension of these encounters. It is important for each person in a relationship to learn to respect the other's vulnerability. In addition, it is important to learn to move into relationships anchored in both self-empathy and empathy for the other. Much can be learned in the course of such struggles and their exploration in therapy. Significant personal growth occurs around the development of relational awareness, which, I believe, is facilitated by the therapist's authentic, relationally responsive presence.

IRENE P. STIVER

Authenticity is ever evolving, not achieved at any one moment—it is a person's ongoing ability to represent her/himself in relationships more fully. Mutual engagement in growth-fostering relationships is the very process that leads to the creation of a relatively safe context in which a person can risk revealing her/his personhood. While we would generally see strategies of disconnection as ways of moving out of authenticity, of not being free to represent oneself, at times these strategies can express a person's truth in some indirect and displaced form.

For example, a patient of mine often rants and rages at members of her family who hurt her and disempower her. Her fury is understandable and legitimate, but her angry outbursts take a form that pushes everyone away (including me). She is seen as "the bitch," yet she is the only one in her family who expresses the rage that all of them must experience. Often this rage spills out to other settings where it is not as legitimate (and in therapy), but it is still a truth about her experience.

I couldn't figure out how to get to these issues without invalidating her feelings. I addressed them by finally saying something like "When you tell me about such-and-such, I really feel how enraging that was for you; yet, I keep wondering if you feel any relief when you get angry—whether you think that you really have expressed how you feel and know it's legitimate?" When she could see she felt worse, not better, after an angry outburst, we could move into more mutual, authentic exploration.

The therapist's efforts to represent herself more authentically facilitate the process of movement toward mutuality. When I feel less authentic, less empathic with my patient, I do not feel connected to her/him and the patient does not feel very connected to me. As a result, I become more inhibited, silenced, and uncertain about how or what I feel and how or what I want to share. When this occurs, I ask myself: What seems to be interfering with my feeling safe enough to be responsive, and what is interfering with our relating in a genuine, authentic way?

In these moments, I have felt least able to authentically represent myself, and least free to express a whole range of feelings and thoughts that I do not think are "good." For example, at that moment I may feel angry, judgmental, anxious, intimidated, as well as ashamed and uncomfortable about my experience. When this has happened, I become afraid that if I speak some truth about my feelings and perspective, without carefully phrasing what I want to say, I might be doing something harmful to my patient. Furthermore, I am very fearful that if I speak my truth about what I am experiencing, my patient may disconnect from me and I would feel cutoff and alone.

During these difficult moments, we therapists often lose faith in the process of how to move from disconnection to new, better connection. This keeps us stuck. I want to suggest that when we feel disconnected we need to exercise greater effort to bring more of ourselves and our experience into the relationship, to feel more present and engaged—even if it means risking a period of disconnection. It may sometimes be a big risk since the patient may feel hurt and/or not understood in response to the therapist's sharing. The work then is to find ways to move from the disconnection to better connection; but we need faith that the process usually works when we create a more mutually empathic, authentic context while we are trying to transform the rupture.

When I am in that nonauthentic space, I need to listen carefully to the ways in which the patient is responding to my lack of "good enough" engagement. I find that if I do listen carefully, the patient will often say something authentic that gives me the opportunity to move into more mutual and authentic connection, as in the example I'll give in a moment.

So both the therapist's taking the risk by moving into authenticity and the patient's taking the risk to convey what she/he is experiencing (and the therapist hearing that message) can move both of them into more connection. However, when I'm in the midst of a major disconnection I forget what I truly believe, which is: when the therapist hangs in there with empathic resonance throughout the worst periods of disconnection, things do begin to move—at least most of the time.

To sum up: Authenticity is a process in movement—we move in and out of more or less authenticity as a consequence of the relational dynamics. Sometimes disconnections in the relationship are an immediate consequence of a therapist taking the risk to express more authentic feelings, but also sometimes they are the consequence of not expressing the truth. When I can appreciate how much a patient's strategies of disconnection contain a truth, I am more able to find something authentic to say which helps move the process into more mutual engagement.

A clinical vignette illustrates some of these issues. I was seeing a woman in her 50s (whom I will call Linda) whose mother was then in her late 80s. Linda had a long history of grievances about her mother—for not ever listening to her, for always lauding how wonderful her brother was who rarely visited or called, for not apparently recognizing what her daughter had accomplished, and especially for past threats to disown her when she married a Jewish man.

I could easily empathize with all these experiences, and I did, but the mother was quite elderly—and living alone in another city. Linda was becoming more gutsy in general, in therapy and life, that is, becoming more authentic, expressing more of what she thought and felt about what was happening in all of her relationships.

In the past Linda and her family had always invited her mother to join them on holidays; someone would pick her up and bring her to their home. Now Linda was refusing to facilitate her mother's visits or to pick her up. She said her mother was perfectly capable of taking a bus. In addition, if she and her mother went out to lunch, she was furious if her mother did not offer to pay (the mother was on a small income and Linda was very well off).

So here is my patient representing herself more fully than ever before. (Prior to this new behavior, Linda would withdraw, drink heavily, and be overly accommodating to her husband, mother, children, and so on.) Now she was speaking more of her truth and was proud of it. I found I could not mutually engage with her perspective; yet, it was clear that she thought I would be pleased at this progress and proud of her speaking up and "expressing herself."

I would listen, not say much, but wanted to say something authentic like "Oh, come on, your mother's 88! And on her own. Of course you're angry with her, but can't you find more generosity of spirit?"—which, of course, I didn't say. After one of these sessions in which I was quite silent, she said, "I guess I got a D in mothers." So maybe I was more authentic than I thought. Her capacity to say that to me allowed me to move and begin to engage more mutually with her and to say at least something more authentic.

I said, "I guess you picked up something about my attitude, and it has been difficult for me to convey it to you. I understand the reasons you're so furious at your mother. I also understand that you want to let her know how much she has hurt you in the past. But I think when you don't seem to take into account that she is old and alone, you end up feeling worse about yourself. It keeps your relationship with her stuck in the past even as you have tried so hard to change it." This opened up her pain about doing what she was doing. We could engage more mutually in trying to understand together why she did not want to give up this behavior; simultaneously, we could engage in understanding how bad this behavior felt. Over time this relationship evolved amazingly well.

In such relatively nonmutual periods in therapy, I feel cut off from my own experience and disconnected from myself and the patient. I was in touch with my age as a contributor to my distress at Linda's treatment of her mother. In addition, images of my own mother at 87 certainly got in my way and silenced me (I would say to myself something like "This is your issue—keep quiet."). Nevertheless, with the help of Linda's response, perhaps to my giving her some authentic message, I finally found one authentic thing to say.

In supervision, when I am not so directly engaged and when this kind of disconnection or an impasse occurs, when the therapist feels unable to say "the right thing" and feels distant and cut off, I always ask, "Can you think of one authentic thing you *can* say?" While this may sometimes cause more disconnection before it moves on to new connection, the therapist feels more real and more mutually engaged and then movement often can occur.

MAUREEN WALKER

About 5 years ago, I had a patient whom I will call John. I was working in a university counseling center, and when John needed a therapist my number came up. We did not choose each other. John came into my office, propped himself in a chair, crossed his legs, and announced that he had come in for some *feedback*, but that he didn't expect very much good to come out of our conversation. He went on to say, and I quote, that he was like any "white, conservative, male Republican. [He wasn't] one of those people who expected somebody else to solve [his] problems." John was quite efficient, economical, and effective in his speech; he had used just four words to let me know what he thought of himself, what he expected of the process and of me. (I must say that I felt totally outclassed in the moment. Because of all of the things I thought about him, no four words would have expressed them.) I think of this particular patient because those first few moments with him typify the impact of a nonrelational culture on relational authenticity. John and I shared the legacy of living in a stratified culture, where people are not just different, but where judgments of "better than" and "less than" are imposed on those differences. Using the coded language of this culture, we were able to traverse the territory of those differences without ever leaving our psychic home. In other words, old relational images could remain intact, and neither John nor I had to risk fuller representation with each other. We were also engulfed in the unnamed shame of an unjust power differential—where people on both sides of the inequality live with a certain amount of mistrust, numbness, and fear.

Disclosure: I did not like John. Had I met him on an airplane, I would have changed my seat. However, in the therapy office different standards apply. The dilemma that I felt in the moment was how to take care of myself, that is, how to hold onto not only my sense of professional competence but also my personal integrity and how to act in his best interest. As an African American women with diverse and extensive clinical experience, I was invested in my image of myself as a culturally competent, politically astute therapist. That image, however, was framed in a cultural context of dominance–subordination, and it left me with two options: fight or flight. To fight might mean that I would level him with some sharp retort or scathing political commentary—rationalizing that anyone who was so politically obtuse was ripe for shaming. At the very least, such a response would have allowed me to turn the tables and reassert my professional dominance. After all, I had been taught that I was *supposed* to be in charge of the session. I knew, however, that that would have been a very harmful response. Adding to the weight of this awareness was my felt sense that anything that I might say in this moment of mutual mistrust could have implications far beyond the therapy room. It had the potential to contribute to either the healing or the further deterioration of the larger culture. Fortunately, we are guided by ethical principles that remind us that our first obligation is to do no harm. If I could not, with any sense of authenticity, offer John warm positive regard, I could at least do no harm. And at that moment, doing no harm translated into one of my favorite strategies of disconnection: when in doubt, get out. I immediately started to think about how I could get John out of my office and preserve my image of myself, if possible in less than the allotted 50 minutes. I was frantically trying to identify one of my colleagues who ideally would be a better "match" for John, or—failing that—somebody who just owed me a favor.

Fortunately, the session did last for 50 minutes, and I was forced to really grapple with my commitment to authenticity—to being honest, caring, and principled. I found myself asking two questions:

1. What would it mean to risk fuller representation of myself with a client whom I did not like and with whom I felt unsafe? Everything in my professional training had taught me that my job was to be less anxious (read: more powerful) than my client. Although my professional culture gave me "power over" John, in the dominant society which provided the larger context for our interaction, John indeed was more valued and had "power over" me. That place of historical and contemporary marginalization is not safe territory for me. It is a place where my competence is questioned. It is a place where the collective relational images of the dominant culture hold sway: where unless I *prove* that I am somehow different (i.e., disconnected from other people who look like me), I could be prejudged of everything from laziness to stupidity to promiscuity. It is very important to own here that adding insult to cultural injury was my own sense of shame at my capacity to be wounded.

2. Under these conditions, what would constitute "good enough" disclosure? What I discovered during those first few moments was that the "power over" model of relationship, whether rooted in my professional culture or the larger dominant culture, left me with an either/or dilemma: being open to John would have felt like erasing myself. Without being able to articulate the specific responsibilities that constitute therapist authenticity in the moment, I knew there had to be a way to communicate more of the truth than either of those options held.

Although the words rang hollow in my ears at the time, I said something to John about how the decision to talk to me must not have been an easy one, and we were able to move on. It wasn't much, but it was good enough. It was enough to allow him to move on and enough for me to feel that I had not abandoned or betrayed myself. In retrospect, it was the "one true thing" that Irene P. Stiver (personal communication, April 20, 1998) described in her reflections on skills for authenticity.

In less than 10 minutes I found myself listening to a man describe his pain as he tried to "balance" his homoerotic fantasies and sexual longings with his attempts to live out a "straight" facade in a corporate context. As we moved deeper into his narrative, I was able to authentically express my sadness at what he had come to see as his personal unworthiness; I could sense his fatigue and feel the burden of inauthenticity in his own life as he had to work harder and harder to keep more and more of himself out of relationship with important people in his life. He was living every day in that place that Jean Baker Miller (1988) refers to as "condemned isolation." There was a lot of movement and mutual growth over the 2 years that we worked together. We laughed and strategized together as he prepared to talk with his girlfriend, whom he described as a religious fundamentalist, about his sexuality. We decided that his wanting to take her to see *My Own Private Idaho* was at least as ineffective as her wanting him to join an evangelical congregation as a "cure." In sum, this relationship became very important to both of us.

Reflections on the Vignette

John came into my office desperately yearning for, but deeply terrified of, connection of any kind, let alone a cross-racial encounter. His strategy of disconnection was to represent himself as a tabloid headline, using emotionally charged language designed to trigger reaction rather than engagement. He knew (probably instinctively rather than consciously) that to initiate our meeting with assertions of race, gender, and political affinity in a culture stratified along those same lines would lessen the possibility that either of us would build or sustain a connection.

My immediate instinct was to feel unsafe, and I found myself floundering in a sea of historical anger and ancient hurt. My strategy of disconnection was to immediately armor myself with old relational images of white, male, conservative Republicans. To protect myself from the wounds of yet another racist encounter, I decided in less than 2 minutes that I knew his story without ever hearing his narrative, thus keeping intact the relational images in which I had previously found safety. In that place of personal and professional vulnerability, it felt safer to respond to John as an abstraction, as a tabloid headline.

Five Critical Learnings about Authenticity

I use this vignette because it illustrates five critical learnings about authenticity.

1. J. D. Frank and J. B. Frank (1991) talked about faith in the process as a nonspecific healing factor. Neither John nor I had much faith in the process during those first few moments. I think for me that loss of faith masked my fear of vulnerability. This fear is especially potent in a nonrelational culture that rewards *invulnerability and power over another* (Jordan, 1997). What I learned from John about how to be a better "therapist-person" was that "good enough" authenticity was not possible without accepting the gift of mutuality. I think

it's important to distinguish between mutuality and sameness. We were not the same, although John and I both knew the pain of being on the "less than" side of a cultural inequality. Mutuality for us meant loosening our hold on the relational images in which we both took refuge. In that way we were both "closeted" and needed to "come out" to relationship with each other and to ourselves in a way that would allow our images to shift.

2. To risk authenticity in a nonrelational culture is to recognize relationship as the bearer of cultural shame. We live in a culture that creates vulnerability through differential valuing and then shames vulnerability by locating the pain within one individual or the other. As Judy Jordan mentioned earlier, projective identification erodes authenticity. In other words, it felt safer to see John as the source of my anxiety and vulnerability rather than to examine the images and meanings that I had internalized as a result of living in a hierarchical culture—to interrogate those with my own shame and anxiety about vulnerability.

3. This differential valuing also means we bring to cross-cultural relationships not only a physical self but also a collective-historical self by means of the relational images that we hold of self and others. Because those images have provided the illusion of safety in a "power over" culture, we may become deeply invested in them. For example, to the extent that my images provided me with a preformed set of expectations and relational possibilities, I can anticipate threats and thus armor myself *against* connection and mutuality. It is important therefore to recognize that relationships across stratification are rife with living and active images that can undermine even the most deeply felt yearnings for connection. It can be as if the actual persons in present time are reduced to spectator roles as the vested relational images spar with each other. As we examine our investment in and our connection to those images (collective-historical self), our capacity for self-empathy grows and allows for expanded knowing of self and other. As I grew in my capacity for self-empathy, I was able to be more fully present with John; I could embrace his impact on my life. As John grew more alive and trusting of himself, he was able to witness his impact on me. He was able to know that I deeply cared about his life. This process of mutuality, by definition, was neither unidirectional nor linear.

4. Self-empathy interrupts denial in a nonrelational culture. One of the signal features of nonrelational culture is that those persons who collectively represent dominance reserve the right to name reality, thus distancing marginalized people from their own experience. Under such conditions it is difficult to embrace and to develop empathy for the totality of one's own experience, irrespective of whether one then chooses to *disclose* it. From my "power over" location in the culture of

therapy, I felt freer to name my anger and indignation at John than to acknowledge the historical pain and vulnerability that our relationship exposed. Movement in the relationship was directly contingent upon my ability to be empathic with my own vulnerability and to remain connected to all facets of the emotional paradox that relationship across stratification holds.

5. What threatened authenticity in my relationship was that my efforts to disconnect signaled my resistance to mutual impact; the resistance was expressed in my need to establish and maintain power over this person while keeping my images intact. The challenge for me to facilitate a relationship that would allow John to come to know and represent himself in his totality and in his particularity: white, male, gay, Republican, perhaps even conservative, not better than nor less than but culturally different from me—and for me to accept him in his fullness: a white, male, gay, conservative Republican could help me *become* and *represent* more fully who I am.

JANET L. SURREY

I would like to look at some particular dilemmas that arise around the therapist representing herself in the therapeutic relationship. Many of these dilemmas are recurrent themes brought up by experienced clinicians working in the relational–cultural model. I describe this aspect of the relational development of therapists as working with the therapist's voice; the "I" voice of the therapist in the therapy relationship.

I, as a therapist, am not here as simply a disembodied presence, a reflecting or projective mirror. I am present as a person with voice, first of all embodied (e.g., I have to miss sessions for illness or surgery; I am tired or I have a headache today).

I am here with a particular social identity (a unique combination of privilege and oppression) and a cultural location (by race, class, gender, ethnicity, sexuality, etc.). All of these get negotiated in every therapy relationship in unique ways.

I am also present with my own particular history, temperament, strengths, weaknesses, vulnerabilities, and my own particular limits and limitations (both personal and professional).

I bring with me my own life context—family, children, professional identity, spirituality, politics, interests, and life commitments. It is interesting and significant that these are often some of the primary reasons particular clients seek me out as a therapist.

I need to represent all these conditions and work with them as they become relevant in the moment in any therapy relationship.

I am also open to growing and changing. Every relationship creates new challenges, questions, and possibilities, with constantly evolving issues of how I (or any therapist) represent myself. Sometimes these flow with very little struggle; sometimes they are very complicated. Some of the ongoing questions I continuously work with moment-to-moment are: How much of my experience do I speak? How? When? Why? What is the impact of not speaking? What about information about me that is not my choice to share, as when a client reads something I've written or when I have to tell something of enormous importance in my life, such as I'm going to China to adopt a baby or I have to cancel a session because my father is seriously ill? How do therapists determine how much to share? How do we deal with major events in *our* lives as they enter therapy? For example, a therapist with metastatic breast cancer came to see me around the process of working with her clients during the last months of her life. Her concern and work to be present but not intrusive in these relationships was incredibly thoughtful and inspiring.

How much do I share responsibly my own experience, life dilemmas, learnings, and stories? How do we make the choices that these will be helpful in fostering the client's growth? How do we assess this?

What about a client who is unusually sensitive to my own level of presence—who deserves to know when (and sometimes why) I am distracted, have low energy, or am stressed? How much do I explain? When does this become intrusive?

When working on impasses in therapy, how much do I share my feelings in the relationship? We know some of our clients already know a lot about us, but how open are we to "owning" and working with our own difficult or complicated feelings?

How much can I risk? Those moments of truth, when the therapist trusts the client and takes the risk to reveal something difficult about herself, often stand out in a client's memory as a key turning point in the relationship. But sometimes these moments can be hurtful to the relationship. How much trust and history is there within the relationship to get through these difficult interactions? And is there really any "safe" place to hide in the end?

We are constantly working with such dilemmas—and often a particularly difficult issue or feeling needs to be talked through with a colleague before one can share responsibly with the client. All of us need ongoing supervision or a peer supervisory relational context in our lives. Sometimes, depending on the history and trust in the relationship and time available (as in longer-term therapy), we can take more risks to be open. In general, I would say that in my own development as a therapist, I am much more likely to try and find a way to bring these dilemmas and my interior musings into the relationship—that is, into the "we."

A significant aspect of our responsibility as therapists is to monitor our self-awareness and to grow in our ability and competency to represent ourselves and to *care for ourselves* in the context of the therapy relationship. Dilemmas around authenticity involve conflicts or tensions between different responsibilities—including to ourselves—all encompassed in the larger, overriding task of fostering the client's growth.

One client, who was struggling with infertility, wrestled for 2 years with whether or not she really wanted to know if I had children. I did not leave that totally up to her but rather tried to look together to see what her knowing, or not, might mean in the relationship to *both* of us. What was authentic and connecting was the struggle to find our way together and not necessarily (in this particular situation) the actual facts of my life. When this client found out a few years later that I was going to adopt my first child, she was truly moved that I had given her the space and time to think through together what had been best for her and our relationship.

The kinds of issues most troubling for me are acknowledging feelings I have in the relationship, which I worry about sharing or about which I feel shame. These raise dilemmas for me of protection verses authenticity, that is, protecting the client (or perhaps myself) versus telling the truth or rather finding a way to be authentic, as Irene has stressed above.

As I describe these dilemmas, I am struck by their resonance with themes I have been writing about regarding the mother's voice in mother–child relationships, as these have been culturally constructed. The mother's "I" voice, her representing herself in the relationship with her children, has historically been seen as dangerous or intrusive but may actually be central in fostering real relational development in her children. Relational dilemmas center around how two voices in dialogue can move toward greater mutuality. Such dilemmas come to the forefront when I feel anger, judgment, fear, hurt, or despair in the relationship and when these are not just fleeting emotions but have some real significance.

To begin with anger: I have grown much more comfortable about receiving a client's anger than I am in responsibly representing my own. I still struggle with old images of anger as destructive rather than as a source of positive energy for change. Furthermore, I do not carry many inspiring relational images of healthy anger in therapists. Sometimes when I need to own my momentary reactive anger, I may say something like "You are right. I do sound irritated, but at the same time I am in touch with a larger understanding about why you may need to push me away." We *are* asking the client to be with us, with our feelings, and to appreciate their impact on us. When I feel judgmental, it usually passes, but if it persists, I believe the client may need this acknowledged. In effect, I am saying that I, too, am human and have a range of feelings and can keep working with them in the service of the relationship.

If a client hits a vulnerable place, either intentionally or unintentionally, I realize that I often feel shame about these feelings. I still hold some image of the therapist as invulnerable or always capable of putting aside her personal reactions. Intellectually, I know that this is not true, but I still feel it is very awkward to work with these reactions when they come up for me in therapy. I am aware that these feelings often arise in the face of the client's strategies of disconnection, and this framework often helps me to find an empathic stance within which I can express my own reactions. However, sometimes it is really just my buttons that are being pushed because of who I am, not simply because of the client's behavior.

A big dilemma for me arises when I am feeling trapped in a therapy relationship. Sometimes it is just a temporary feeling: "I want out; I don't want to be here; this is just too hard; I can't find a way to move." However, sometimes it is really a larger issue of discerning if the therapy is helpful, if I need help with staying in the relationships, or if I need to let go. This is very different from simple countertransference, although countertransference may be a factor. These can be thorny questions. For example, when and how can a therapist decide and negotiate a break or termination of therapy, not simply for the client's welfare but for her own? These questions touch on important issues of our own self-care—questions to be honestly and responsibly negotiated in the therapy relationship.

Part of our responsibility in the therapy relationship is to take care of ourselves so that we can be present and responsive, whether this has to do with taking vacations, time for self-care, personal growth, working to balance our lives, working with vicarious trauma, and the like. This is difficult when our needs or choices are clearly not immediately in the client's interest—although they may well be in the interest of the relationship, which includes the client.

Sometimes self-care in the relationship involves discerning when I feel abused or frightened and need to represent or change something. And sometimes therapists simply need to acknowledge and own their vulnerabilities, limitations, basic values, or concern for the "bottom line" to be able to work productively. For me, the most difficult dilemma arises when my needs really are at odds with what I feel is best or right for the client. For example, when I went away for a 3-month maternity leave, I know this was particularly hurtful to some clients. If the issue is something less than an obvious priority or necessity, how do we negotiate this responsibly? What are the limits and the dimensions of our "promised" availability? Our accountabilities? How do we actually work out such deeply conflicting responsibilities in the relationship?

An experienced clinician consulted me recently to discuss a situation that was very troubling and confusing for her. For a number of years, she had been working intensely with a very fragile client whose mother had died during the client's birth. The client was pregnant with her first child and had expressed to the therapist that, for the first time, she felt she could count on the therapist to be there and not abandon her when she had the baby. The therapist appreciated the meaning of this in terms of the particular event she was facing (giving birth) as well as in terms of the client expressing her need and trust in a very new way.

Closer to the client's due date, the therapist suddenly was offered the opportunity to travel far away to participate in an event with enormous meaning and importance to her. It would mean being away for 3 weeks, including during the client's due date. The therapist felt she needed help to think through what to do. She felt torn and knew she wanted to take this opportunity for herself but could not imagine disappointing the client in this way. In the therapy relationship, she found herself unable to be clear and hold onto her own conviction, she started doubting herself, and she could not speak about the situation.

With a lot of support from me and other colleagues she decided to go and finally told her client that she would be going away. The client felt terribly betrayed, became extremely angry and depressed, and stopped eating. The therapist then wrote her a long letter describing how difficult her decision had been, how terrible she knew the client would feel, and how much she hoped they could hang in together and deal with this. The next 2 months were devastating as the client felt her worst nightmare had been reenacted. She expressed a lot of anger but, over time, also felt that her therapist had really acknowledged her and the importance of the relationship. She also appreciated the therapist sharing the details of her decision and could understand the importance and meaning of the trip to the therapist. This impasse has had a relatively positive outcome so far.

We know, however, that this is not always so. I saw the therapist, the client, and their relationship grow enormously through this time. The therapist sought consultation to gain clarity on her own dilemma.

She was then able to make a clear, honest statement to the client with awareness of the potential impact and with a passionate commitment to stay and grow together through the disconnection.

These dilemmas can be extremely painful and complex—often the stuff of which hard and real relational growth can, but not always does, happen. The call to authenticity is a great challenge. It raises many lively and some painful questions that make it imperative to create opportunities like this to examine together how to move constructively within the relational paradigm.

NATALIE S. ELDRIDGE

Ethical Dilemmas Raised by Conversation on Authenticity

In listening to our conversations about authenticity in the months preceding this conference, I began to consider some of the ethical dilemmas that moving toward authenticity raises in our work:

1. How do we maintain our responsibility for the therapeutic relationship and our responsibility to protect the client; and yet move away from a hierarchical, or paternalistic, stance in the relationship?

2. When our own emotional response takes us out of connection with the client and when acknowledging that response could be experienced as intrusive to the client, how do we decide what to do? Irene's case was a beautiful illustration of this.

3. From an ethical perspective, what is therapeutic safety? When is it "safe enough" to take some risks? Safe for whom? And when is too much safety potentially harmful for the client as well as to the quality of the therapeutic relationship?

4. Finally, new ethical questions emerge from this conversation about what constitutes abuse, negligence, or avoiding harm. If we allow clients to assume that all our feelings and reactions in the therapy room are about them, can we increase the potential for client shame or burden the client with our inauthenticity? Judy has illustrated this well.

Focus on the Context

We cannot answer these questions here; in fact, I do not believe there are universal answers. Rather, faced with these dilemmas, ethical clinical choices must arise from a careful consideration of each therapeutic context. These are some of the questions that might help us consider a specific context:

1. Who are we protecting in a given situation: the client, the relationship, or ourselves? Which is most relevant in this particular therapeutic context?

2. How much risk can we take? Do we have the time within the relational context to "hang in there" and deal with the fallout of a relational risk? Some of the contextual factors to consider include the strengths and vulnerabilities of both the client and the therapist, the stage of the therapy, and the history in the particular therapy relationship of negotiating empathic failures. Sometimes we have little data on the contextual factors, as in Maureen's case, where issues of authenticity arise in the first meeting.

3. What is our relational context as a therapist: do we have a community of colleagues and consultants that can help us to hold these dilemmas and make context-relevant, sound ethical choices? Sometimes there are elements of context we cannot see from inside the therapeutic relationship.

4. For me, ethical dilemmas involving authenticity often arise when I feel particularly inauthentic in a therapy relationship and when I am uncertain how to move back into authentic connection. Disclosure or acknowledgment sometimes is the way to move, but not always. If it is in the service of the relationship with the client and in the service of her healing, then it can be useful, as in the case Jean discussed concerning bringing up her disability in the therapy. However, if disclosure is in the service of reducing the therapist's anxiety only and is done before the client is ready to hear it, then it may be harmful both to the client and to the relationship.

Illustrative Vignette

As a lesbian therapist, I find I must decide with each client how to manage information about my lifestyle. Often, it is not relevant nor an issue, but when it becomes an issue in the midst of a therapy, it can be distracting and it can move me out of connection until I resolve it.

For example, I had worked for a few months with a 20-year-old African American woman who was lonely, shy, and frustrated at her lack of dating experience with men. Our differences in race and in age were self-evident from the beginning of therapy, and she had shared a certain safety she felt in these differences. She was making progress in using the therapy to rehearse how to connect with others, and she was beginning to build an external support system. I was completely unprepared when she arrived in crisis one day because her brother had come out as a gay man to her family and her parents had disowned him. She felt both betrayed by her brother for not telling her earlier and betrayed by her parents for forbidding her to contact him. She was struggling to understand his sexual identity in complete isolation and spoke of how she had never known anyone who was gay.

For her, this revelation changed nothing in the therapy relationship, while for me a dramatic shift occurred. I suddenly felt very inauthentic with her and became distracted by my own anxiety. Was I betraying her by not disclosing my sexual orientation? How likely would it be for her to inadvertently find out this information from someone else in the university community? If she knew I was a lesbian, would she feel compelled to disown me? The shift in the relevance of my sexuality to the therapy relationship created a dilemma for how to move back into healing connection with my client.

What to Do?

First, I held on to the frame of therapy built thus far in our relationship, concentrated on shifting my attention from my anxiety back to what my client was saying, and just plain held on until the end of the session.

Next, I tapped into my professional relational context. Luckily for me, this both included colleagues at the University Counseling Center with whom I frequently discussed cases and included a peer supervision group made up of lesbian therapists from various settings. As I reviewed my dilemma and sorted out whom I was seeking to protect from what, I saw that a disclosure about my sexual orientation might have eased my immediate anxiety about keeping something from her as her brother had done. Yet, it became clearer that disclosure would not relieve her of the sense of betrayal she had concerning her brother and may have distracted her from understanding the meaning of this relationship with him. The major concern for the therapy remained my disconnection from her in the therapy; I had become temporarily less present, less authentic, and I did not want this to persist.

Discussion of the case itself reduced my anxiety, and I was able to shift my focus back to the client's sense of abandonment and disconnection from her brother for whom she felt great affection. My work with her was around supporting her explorations into peer and dating relationships. It also involved exploring her perceived loss of her brother, which was a devastating blow to her growing confidence.

In reviewing the context of this particular therapy relationship, I thought about the brief duration of our work and our anticipated termination in four to five sessions at the end of the semester. I considered our particular relationship history and noted little focus on empathic failures thus far. As I refocused on the client's needs at that time and the power in our relationship to create an environment in which she could move and grow, any consideration of a move to disclose my sexuality to her dissipated. Rather than identifying with the brother, who was disowned and cut off because of being gay, I realigned myself with the client.

I felt sad that, at the moment of the intimacy of learning something significant about her brother, my client had been cut off from the potential of greater connection by her parents who were seeking to protect her from an unknown threat. I felt compassion for the conflicting loyalties she felt, which left her with the perception of an impossible choice of either disconnecting from her parents or disconnecting from her brother. These are things I could share with her—that moved us into greater connection around the relational issues that brought her into therapy. I moved back into an authentic connection with her for our remaining sessions.

CONCLUSION

The ethical processes involved in resolving the kinds of dilemmas raised by our presentation today are complex. Some therapists have oversimplified and vastly misinterpreted the subtle but significant ways we are redefining therapy or, as Jean puts it, our attitudes about therapy. However, it should be clear to all that authenticity does not equal self-disclosure. Mutuality does not mean that the therapist's needs are equal to the client's needs in the therapy relationship.

Rather, ethical clinical choices about how to move toward authenticity emerge only from careful consideration of each therapeutic context, which includes understanding the intentionality or purpose of the therapy, analyzing the power dynamics that influence the specific relationship, and exploring the strategies of disconnection of both the client and the therapist.

REFERENCES

Frank, J. D., & Frank, J. B. (1991). *Persuasion and healing: A comparative study of psychotherapy*. Baltimore: Johns Hopkins University Press.

Jordan, J. V. (1995). Boundaries: A relational perspective. *Psychotherapy Forum, 1*(2), 4–5.

Jordan, J. V. (1997). Relational therapy in a non-relational world. *Work in Progress, No. 79*. Wellesley, MA: Stone Center Working Paper Series.

Jordan, J. V., Kaplan, A., Miller, J. B., Stiver, I. P., & Surrey, J. (1991). *Women's growth in connection: Writings from the Stone Center.* New York: Guilford Press.

Miller, J. B. (1988). Connections, disconnections, and violations. *Work in Progress, No. 33.* Wellesley, MA: Stone Center Working Paper Series.

Miller, J. B., & Stiver, I. P. (1997). *The healing connection: How women form relationships in therapy and life.* Boston: Beacon Press.

This chapter was originally presented as a panel at the Learning from Women Conference sponsored by the Jean Baker Miller Training Institute and Harvard Medical School/ Cambridge Hospital on May 1, 1998. © 1999 by Jean Baker Miller, Judith V. Jordan, Irene P. Stiver, Maureen Walker, Janet L. Surrey, and Natalie S. Eldridge.

5

Race, Self, and Society
Relational Challenges in a Culture of Disconnection

Maureen Walker

*H*istorically, relationships among women of different race in the United States have been filled with disconnection. While individual women have made brave and undeniable efforts to bridge the racial and ethnic differences in pursuit of common goals, there is little evidence of sustained and broad-based movement to overcome the contradictions of living in a patriarchal power structure. The observation has been made that differences of race among women, and the implications of these differences, present the most serious challenge to the mobilization of women's joint power (Lorde, 1984). Comas-Díaz and Greene (1994) assert that skin color is a determinant variable which differentiates the status of women of color from women of European or white extraction. The effects of the differentiation are such that the dynamics of exclusion, marginality, and internecine oppression countermand women's tendencies to strive for good connection. Given the premise that women organize a sense of self around the ability to make and maintain good connections (Miller, 1988), these dynamics are all the more problematic. Lorde (1984) suggests that when there are no models for relating across difference as equals, women may seek to ignore, copy, or destroy difference. In this chapter I examine the historical context of contemporary contradictions and explore the implications of relational–cultural theory (RCT) for developing models of relational competence across racial difference.

SCENARIO 1

A true story was reported to me by a woman (Beverly) who is an American black woman in her mid-30s. One day as she was waiting for service at the perfume counter in Nieman-Marcus, another woman, who seemed to have been browsing in the general area, also came and stood at the counter. This woman was a tall, strawberry blonde, American, white woman who also seemed to be in her mid-30s. She was accompanied by a male whom Beverly presumed to be her husband. After a few moments, the sales clerk, also an American white woman, came up to the counter, turned to Beverly, and very pleasantly asked, "May I help you?" At this, the white woman who was the shopper, also turned to Beverly and said, "You've got to wait your turn. I was over here first." Beverly realized that this was possibly true but felt genuinely affronted by the woman's tone and mannerism. She said to the woman, "I'm not sure what your problem is, but you're yelling at the wrong person." The other woman replied, "Why don't you just take a chill pill?" And she thrust her purchase toward the sales clerk. The discourse became decidedly juvenile at that point, as Beverly replied, "No, you take a chill pill." Without a word, the sales clerk took the other woman's merchandise and quickly disappeared. Beverly then heard the woman mutter to her companion, "This really makes me angry. Who does she think she is? You can't go anywhere now . . . they're everywhere you go." Beverly responded, "What 'they'? Could you possibly be talking about ugly, frizz-dried blondes? You only think that because of all of the mirrors in here." This response was followed by stony glares and hate-filled silence.

The sales clerk returned with the completed transaction, and the other woman was escorted away by her companion. The sales clerk apologized profusely, saying she couldn't understand the woman's rudeness. My friend quickly absolved the sales clerk of any responsibility in the encounter and commented that the woman obviously had problems she wanted to take out on the world. When Beverly reported the incident to me a couple of weeks later, she was still deeply offended. She was more than offended; she was sickened by both the woman's and her own behavior during an encounter that had deteriorated into racially driven nastiness. Beverly, a self-described feminist with experience in successful arbitration, only compounded her despondency by becoming totally de-skilled in the moment, completely incapable of a more self-controlled, self-aware interaction with another woman.

Relational–cultural theory is a worldview that speaks a deep truth about women's relationships; it allows us to make sense out of the seeming contradictions in women's lives without pathologizing women as inadequate, dependent, or counterdependent. By affirming relationality as a central feature in women's development (Miller, 1988), RCT provides a liberating language for conceptions of self—a language that says clearly and powerfully that to grow through action in relationship with others is both necessary and good.

Relational–cultural theory also exposes more sobering and painful realities. Encounters such as the one described by Beverly are not altogether rare. You may, in fact, be thinking now of similar conflictual experiences in which you have been either a witness or a participant. Whenever I am involved in racially charged conflicts, either as a witness or as a "main character," I am compelled to grapple with the complexity of relational challenges in a culture of disconnection.

One of the central tenets of relational–cultural theory is that the ability to make and maintain relationships is central to a woman's sense of self and well-being (Miller, 1988). In the midst of racially charged conflict, however, it is often difficult to see women as the people on this planet more likely to yearn for empathic connection. Certainly it is difficult to see this yearning in Beverly's story. Nonetheless, incidents such as these are instructive because they lead us to ask three questions: (1) How can we use relational–cultural theory to explain the causes of racism in women's lives? (2) How might relational–cultural theory help us to understand the effects of racism on women's lives? (3) What does a relational worldview tell us about possibilities for healing and reconciliation? It is important to recognize that racism manifests not just in the hyperbolic acting out that we are sometimes called to witness (or in which we may sometimes find ourselves entangled). Frequently and also more insidiously, it is present in the inability to represent oneself with authenticity across racial differences and in the resistance to make more of oneself available for growth and change within the context of cross-racial relationships.

Many factors contribute to cross-racial tensions among women, including the following.

"Power Over" Culture/Stratified Difference

People who make the rounds of diversity conferences, as trainers or as participants, are very familiar with the frequently quoted maxim: Race prejudice plus power equals racism. To the extent that this saying is true, I could think of no better place to begin examining the causes of racism among women than in a review of Jean Baker Miller's (1976, 1987) reflections on power. Miller writes that, like all concepts and actions of a dominant group, power may be distorted and skewed. This distortion is manifest in a constant need to maintain an irrational dominance: a dominance built on a foundation that includes restriction of another group. Dominance, then, engenders conflict and simultaneously seeks to suppress it. In speaking to issues of dominance and power, Miller has laid the foundation for a more thorough discussion on race, self, and society. It has become almost a cliché to lament the relational disconnections arising out of racial/cultural *difference* in the United States. It is *not*, however, the differences that plague us. It is rather that the differences are *profoundly stratified*. This stratification is the consequence of systematic miseducation that teaches us that white is superior and black is inferior. The *stratification*, not the *difference*, constrains our capacity for authenticity and undermines our desire for connection. The stratification distorts our answers to the questions: "Who am I? Who is this other person? Who are we together?" These distortions, arising out of stratification, manifest not only in grand political terms but also on the level of more mundane, everyday discourse. In fact, I believe that it is often on this very basic, visceral level that the stratifications have the most destructive impact on women's relationships.

SCENARIO 2

A few years ago, I led a group in which women were discussing culture and race. During the course of the discussion, the women started to talk about aspects of themselves that they particularly enjoyed. One woman, whom I will call Amy, reported that one reason she enjoyed being white was because she didn't have to do "s***loads of stuff to her hair in order to look good." Amy went on to explain that as a college student she had shared a dorm with many black women and had endured the stench that filled the building every time one of them decided to straighten her hair. She expressed some level of sympathy that black women could have such low self-esteem that they would go to extreme and probably painful lengths to look white.

By the time Amy finished her input, a reasonable person might have concluded that the whole U.S. commercial hair products industry was supported entirely by black women. For the most part, Amy was well intentioned and about as relationally skilled as anyone else in the group. Her comments, however, served to illustrate the processes of distortion that can occur in a racially stratified society. She had internalized a stratified cultural aesthetic based on the premise of "better than"/"less than." Therefore, she interpreted what might have been a matter of personal style, taste, convenience, or experimentation as low self-esteem.

What exactly does a discourse on power have to do with hair grooming? It has to do with the *power of naming*: the power to name what's good, what's bad, what's beautiful, what's normal—what is "minority" or "diverse." In Amy's mind, *different* translated into a "better than"/"less than" stratification. Physical appearance and hair grooming practices among women are not simply *different*—one is preferred and the other is demeaned. The important part of this rather ordinary conversation was that one mode of grooming is validated by the dominant cultural aesthetic; the other is subject to being interpreted as an expression of psychological fragility.

We are a multicultural society, and we are also a culture of disconnection. It is not problematic that we are of many different colors and cultures. The problem lies in the fact that the dominant culture has the power to define one group as better than the other. Inevitably, certain relational distortions arise from dominant–subordinate or stratified relationships. The dominant culture distorts images of self, images of other, and necessarily, images of relational possibilities. Unfortunately, there is another, more insidious, consequence of this differential valuing.

In a patriarchal society (in U.S. culture), all women of any race are subject to the oppressive notion that their worth is based largely and sometimes exclusively on physical appearance. From a very early age, young girls receive the message that they must be beautiful in order to enjoy popularity or love or even fresh breath. Added to the devaluing that all women share is a more particularized version of the cultural beauty imperative that says, "How you look is what's most important; and how *you* look can never be good enough. Given your distance from the dominant aesthetic (whether typified by skin color, hair texture, physical features, or some combination of the three), you will always be viewed as comparably less than the purported ideal."

All women are subject to the debilitating effects of white male domination; women of color exist in a culture that devalues blackness as well. On this very primitive, sensate, and often unconscious level, the stratification begins and has the potential to aggravate any of the inevitable conflicts in which women find themselves. If women were to build healthy connections within a multiracial context, issues of color and culture stratification would need to be earnestly addressed. It may be very tempting for women who enjoy educational, class, professional, or political privilege to dismiss these issues as irrelevant and incompatible with a feminist world view. It is important to remember, however, that professional and class privilege (i.e., the ability to attend a conference and be surrounded by colleagues who share similar political values) provide comforts and buffers most women in the United States are denied. Privileged women may therefore be more vulnerable to this cultural imperative.

The following excerpt from Carolyn M. Rodgers's (1968) poem "I Have Been Hungry" illustrates how the dominant aesthetic both reflects and exploits historical stratification among women:

> and you white girl
> shall I call you sister now
> can we share any secrets of sameness,
> any singularity of goals . . .
> you, white girl with the head that
> perpetually tosses over-rated curls
> while I religiously toss my over-rated behind
> you white girl
> I am yet suspicious of . . .

Collective Biography and Relational Images

In addition to illustrating relational consequences of color and culture stratification, Rodgers's poem highlights another significant challenge to women's relational development in multiracial contexts. Because of our specific histories as women in the United States, we bring to each encounter both an individual and a collective biography. Miller (1976, 1987) asserts that each participant in an encounter brings her own state of psychological organization *filled* with conceptions about what she *wants to do* or *could do* or *should do*. Some research suggests, however, that any formulation of personality or any description of psychological organization is *incomplete*—if it does not include the racially informed meanings and images that have developed over time (Helms, 1990). In other words, what I have come to believe about myself as a woman of primarily African descent has a profound impact on my personality formation and, more precisely, on my relational development. Women's shared historical legacy in the United States is that we have been denied access to full participation in the systems and relationships that affect our lives; on a very concrete level, we have been unable to fully participate in setting the terms of how we will relate to the larger world. For women of primarily European descent, this exclusion was traditionally justified by promises of care, protection, and admiration. It is also our historical legacy that the pedestal and the promises, however illusory they may be, have *not* been extended to women of primarily African descent. In fact, the terms of the relationship were such that not only were African women not protected but their very subjugation served to support, on one level, the privilege of European women and, on another level, the degradation of all women. This is called a *setup*. From the inception of this country, women of different race have been set up to wage conflict on terms defined by others. Under these conditions and through this historical conditioning, we develop relational images that hold meaning for us about who we are and who the other is. Such historically conditioned images may constrain our capacity to seriously know what we want, need, and desire in relationships with each other. The historical biography brought to contemporary encounters is one of nonmutuality, one of restricted access to self and to the other.

There are *four* specific consequences of cultural nonmutuality. *First,* under these conditions, American black and American white women become abstractions not only to each other but also to themselves. *Second,* abstracted images become frozen in time, impeding the development of new relational images and new relational possibilities. *Third,* stratification contaminates conflict; under stratified conditions, it becomes very difficult to mutually engage the task of growth through resolution. *Fourth,* with limited opportunities for action in relationship, our capacity for authenticity, and thus for connection is seriously compromised.

Effects of Racism on Women's Relational Development

When we examine the relational consequences of racial stratification on women's lives, it is again helpful to review Jean Baker Miller's reflections on conflict. Miller (1976, 1981) has written that conflict is both inevitable and necessary for human growth. Under conditions of racial/cultural stratification, the basic dominant–subordinate mode of waging conflict—the mode of disconnection—is likely to appear. Furthermore, the conflict may be expressed in extreme forms, as one seeks to hold onto to a sense of well-being and safety either by overwhelming and shaming the *other* or, quite paradoxically, by silencing and shaming oneself.

In speaking about historical or collective biographies, one is inclined to think of a time long past and gone. The time *is* long past but not gone. It is important to recognize the *intergenerational* impact and residual effects of distorted relational images. In fact, ambivalences that remain as a result of old relational images are likely to be exacerbated as opportunities for interaction and expand as cultural norms become more ambiguous. The potential for *dis*connection among women of different race will become more acute. This notion is consistent with Miller's (1976, 1987) hypothesis that people are more aware of conflict precisely because women are trying to act in new ways. To the extent that we are unable to speak with authenticity about conflict, power, and race, we become caught in the grip of shame where historical hurts can override our most genuine yearnings for connection.

SCENARIO 3

A situation between two women, whom I will call Stacy and Sue, illustrates this point. Stacy and Sue were undergraduates who not only worked together in the campus women's association but who had also formed a nice friendship that extended far beyond the obligations of committee work or political activism. Toward the end of the semester, I started to notice that the two women seemed initially to be avoiding each other and later to be actively hostile toward each other. Any comment or inquiry about Stacy would elicit a caustic remark from Sue and vice versa. When I finally commented about the change in their relationship, Sue, first defiantly and later tearfully, told me about the incident that created a rift between the two friends. Sue, who describes herself as a Korean American woman, had darkened her skin and chosen to wear something that she called an "Afro fright wig" for Halloween. Stacy, an African American, felt insulted and betrayed by her friend, whom she perceived to be making fun of African racial features. She retaliated by suggesting that she would go and find a yellow mask with slanted eyes. Sue accused Stacy of being too sensitive and, worse, needing everyone to be politically correct. Stacy accused Sue of being racist and, worse, really wanting to be white. Both women, fearing that their connection had been irreparably ruptured, remained distant from each other for the next several months.

The situation between Stacy and Sue serves as a poignant example of what can happen when two women strive for connection within a context of nonmutuality. In a less stratified society, this minor disconnection could have led to relational movement. In this culture, however, their efforts to be in relationship were sabotaged by a legacy of stratification that probably neither of them understood. This situation also illustrates the pervasiveness of the legacy. Although the template for stratification was originally set in black and white, the effects extend beyond this simple polarity. Relationships among women of any race are vulnerable to the impact of a legacy of culture and color stratification—a system of inequality that has ensconced white on the *top,* black on the *bottom,* and left millions of other not-so-easily classified women on *an ever shifting middle ground* asking the question: Where do *I* fit?

Both Stacy and Sue blamed the other solely for violating the trust between them. They were both unaware of the original violation perpetrated by the dominant culture. As Judith V. Jordan (1993) comments, an abusive society, like an abusive family, effects a pattern of violating vulnerability, actively silencing, and moving people into shame, self-doubt, and isolation. It seems Stacy and Sue were both unaware of their heightened vulnerability as women of color in a society that devalues both their color and their cultures. Neither woman had access to enough of her own internal reality to be appropriately sensitive and intentional in her response to the reality of the other. Their inability to remain active right in the relationship represents yet another relational challenge. That is, as Miller (1988) pointed out, action in relationship enables a stronger thinking/feeling base. As a person develops more clarity about her own thoughts and feelings, she becomes more available to the relationship. In this relationship, she continues to learn about herself and the other person, thereby enhancing her capacity for self-empathy and empathy for the other. I have no doubt that by the end of their first week of estrangement, neither Stacy nor Sue really knew what she was feeling. There was, in fact, a transmutation of feeling as each woman moved farther and farther away from her original feeling/thinking base and started to position herself more and more according to cultural expectations. Stacy became "Angry Black Woman"; Sue became "Aggrieved, Confused Victim." Both became abstractions to themselves and to each other—not daring to represent fully their vulnerabilities, their fears, or their sadness. I can think of no better example of what Miller (1988) has termed *condemned isolation* than the situation in which these two women found themselves. In their efforts to appear invulnerable, each tried in various ways to shame the other, thereby avoiding the cultural shame they both carried as women striving for connection in a stratified society.

Each of the women developed camps of people with whom they would rehash the incident. And in each retelling, the speaker became more and more vociferous in her account of how she had admonished her erstwhile friend. Each speaker became more and more invested in her image of herself as invulnerable and actually having power over the other. In this way, each woman became more and more disconnected from her own experience and less authentic in her presentation to other peers. Within their "camps" each became increasingly strident in expressing her outrage at the other. Each woman became increasingly invested in relational images that helped her to feel safe and protected from impact by the other person.

It is quite likely, in generations past, that this situation would never have developed between Stacy and Sue, precisely because their paths might never have crossed. However, with new opportunities for cross-racial contact, and with increased opportunities to behave in new ways, opportunities for connection and disconnection are potentiated. The paradox is that apparent openings/expansions in the relational arena may lead to a more restricted internal life when one is living in a racially and culturally stratified society.

If Stacy and Sue's experience illustrates the polarization of conflict in a stratified culture, yet another challenge to connection is the tendency to homogenize experience. Because relationship is such a central feature of women's relationships, women in multiracial and cross-cultural contexts will sometimes pretend that real inequalities do not exist. Or, more likely, we may settle for a pretense of connection using a complicated strategy of disconnection. Typical of this strategy is a game called "my inequality is the same as your inequality." Potentially productive discussions about cross-racial relational dilemmas often get derailed with comparisons of oppressions. The comparisons are usually expressed in comments like "sexism is the same as racism" or "classism is worse than racism." Usually these comments are attempts to reduce anxiety about historical racial stratification or, as Carolyn M. Rodgers (1975) said, to express "some singularity of purpose." We are not hard pressed to find a variety of oppressions that plague our society, and more often than not those oppressions are interlinked. However, we do little to promote healing and reconnection when we pit one oppression against the other. In these cases, anxiety about historical and contemporary stratification overrides attempts to stay active in the present relationship. In the attempts to homogenize, precious parts of each person's experience get lost. Some part of each person's experience, perhaps that part that we fear will not be affirmed, is either held out or pushed out of relationship. Experience shows that once those "pushed out/held back" parts can be named and acknowledged, the relationship can move forward with integrity.

Relational Possibilities and Reconnection

It is very clear that women yearn for connection in a cultural context that undermines mutuality. Through acts of omission and commission women have been active participants in sustaining racism, in whatever mutant form, throughout our shared history. Sometimes, women have participated in the development of new strains/variants of racism by exploiting their positioning within the white heterosexist patriarchy. In the United States, this positioning has been used to exclude and oppress both women and men of color. Such shortsighted alliances produce vicarious power, but according to Miller (1976), they also create a fraudulent sense of pride (Collins, 1990). In this regard, power based on race is used to create and maintain *dis*connection. How then, do we face the challenge of moving from cultural disconnection to a place of hope, reconciliation, and reconnection? How does a relational model inform the possibilities for healing and reconciliation? The relational model teaches us to ask: How can I know my "true self"/"healthy self" if it has not been formed in the crucible of relationship with others? Specifically, how can a woman understand herself as a person of whatever racial or ethnic descent—whether white, Mexican American, biracial, Japanese American, or African Caribbean—without such action in relationship?

Action in relationship offers women the gift of conflict, the very process many women have been taught to avoid. In *Toward a New Psychology of Women*, Miller (1976, 1987) wrote that whenever two people interact with each other, each person is presenting something new—something different from what would arise within herself. The ability to engage that "something new" is the source of personal and relational growth (Bergman & Surrey, 1994). When women wage good conflict, old relational images, thin abstractions of self and other, can be replaced by more fully textured images that are authenticated through action in relationship.

SCENARIO 4
(CHANGE TO SOCIAL SERVICE SETTING)

I would like to close by returning to a racial reconciliation for an example of women waging good conflict. Ana, a second generation immigrant from Cuba, engaged another group member, Rhonda, an Afro-Caribbean woman, in a conversation about her experience with a friend and former coworker. Both women were social service providers. Ana reported that in a conversation with this woman, whom she identified as Italian American, they discussed recent changes in Ana's office. The coworker had confided that she was happy that she no longer worked with the agency because the clientele consisted of a new wave of immigrants who were "no longer people like us." Her specific complaint was that people from Haiti were very difficult to work with and were probably best served by people like themselves. Wanting to avoid an emotionally charged disagreement with her friend, Ana responded that "the new people weren't all bad." "Besides," she said, "the government makes us work with them." At this point, Ana very tearfully said to Rhonda, "I feel as if I have betrayed you. I wish I could have been more effective." Rhonda acknowledged that she felt betrayed. She was able to say that she deeply understood Ana's need to protect her relationship with her friend and wished it hadn't been at the expense of herself and other black people. Each woman made herself available to move and be moved by the other. They expressed their ambivalences, disappointments, and desires to stay close to each other even in the midst of grief, guilt, and disappointment. They continued to engage, not only with each other but with the rest of the group as well, as they discussed ways to find and hold onto their own voices in the face of racial disconnections.

Relational–cultural theory tells us that when women learn to make use of conflict, they accomplish two major tasks:

1. They escape the trap of rigged conflict. Rhonda and Ana were able to voice their own desires, to say for themselves what each wanted from the other in relationship. They rejected the archetypal/historical scripts the dominant culture had prepared for them (for Rhonda that may have looked like some variant of "Angry Black Woman"; for Ana, a variation on the theme of "Confused Innocent Caught in the Middle"). Unlike Stacy and Sue in the earlier scenario, they refused to fade into thin abstractions; they remained real and available to themselves and to each other.

2. They understood that conflict is an inevitable part of life, which creates potential for growth. Each woman approached the conflict with a sense of integrity and respect. From this standpoint, they were able to practice both self-empathy and empathy for the other.

The hope in the Rhonda and Ana scenario is that they refused to wage conflict on someone else's terms. They let neither historical stratification nor more contemporary frictions sabotage their desire for connection with each other. Although their conflict involved anger and anguish, each woman left the interaction feeling changed and hopeful, having embraced new possibilities for personal and relational integrity.

Because we live in a culture shaped by a legacy of race-based stratification, *disconnection* often seems the most expedient course as we navigate through our everyday lives. What we learn from RCT is that healing and reconnection are active possibilities only when we make ourselves available to the experience of challenge and the complexities of conflict, as well as the opportunities for resilience and expanded empathy that multicultural connectedness can bring.

REFERENCES

Bergman, S., & Surrey, J. L. (1994). Couples therapy: A relational approach. *Work in Progress, No. 66.* Wellesley, MA: Stone Center Working Paper Series.

Collins, P. H. (1990). *Black feminist thought: Knowledge, consciousness, and the politics of empowerment.* Boston: Unwin Hyman.

Comas-Díaz, L., & Greene, B. (1994). Overview: Connections and disconnections. In L. Comas-Díaz & B. Greene (Eds.), *Women of color: Integrating ethnic and gender identities in psychotherapy* (pp. 341–346). New York: Guilford Press.

Helms, J. E. (Ed.). (1990). *Black and white racial identity: Theory, research, and practice.* Westport, CT: Greenwood Press.

Jordan, J. V. (1993). *Challenges to connection: The traumatizing society.* Paper presented at the Learning from Women Conference, a symposium conducted by Harvard Medical School and the Stone Center, Boston.

Lorde, A. (1984). *Sister outsider.* Freedom, CA: Crossing Press.

Miller, J. B. (1976). *Toward a new psychology of women.* Boston: Beacon Press.

Miller, J. B. (1987). *Toward a new psychology of women* (2nd ed.). Boston: Beacon Press.

Miller, J. B. (1988). Connections, disconnections, and violations. *Work in Progress, No. 33.* Wellesley, MA: Stone Center Working Paper Series.

Rodgers, C. M. (1968). I have been hungry. In C. M. Rodgers, *How I got ovah: New and selected poems* (p. 49). Garden City, NY: Anchor Press/Doubleday.

Rodgers, C. M. (1975). I have been hungry. In C. M. Rodgers, *How I got ovah: New and selected poems* (pp. 49–52). Garden City, NY: Anchor Press.

This chapter was originally presented at the Learning from Women Conference sponsored by the Jean Baker Miller Training Institute and Harvard Medical School/Cambridge Hospital on May 1, 1998. © 1999 by Maureen Walker.

6

Shame and Humiliation
From Isolation to
Relational Transformation

LINDA M. HARTLING, WENDY B. ROSEN,
MAUREEN WALKER, *and* JUDITH V. JORDAN

A RELATIONAL CONCEPTUALIZATION OF SHAME
AND HUMILIATION

Linda M. Hartling

While most of us can think of at least one occasion in which we felt
shamed or humiliated, in many instances these types of experiences are
difficult to identify, difficult to acknowledge, and difficult to express.
To recount experiences of shame or humiliation, we risk revisiting
painful images of being devalued, disempowered, or disgraced, perhaps triggering or reinforcing further feelings of shame. Yet, below our
immediate awareness, these experiences can have a profound and enduring influence over our daily behavior. Jean Baker Miller and Irene
P. Stiver note that "we become so fearful of engaging others because of
past neglects, humiliations, and violations . . . we begin to keep important parts of our experience out of connection. We do not feel safe

enough to more fully represent ourselves in relational encounters" (1995, p. 1). Experiences of shame or humiliation—including experiences of being scorned, ridiculed, belittled, ostracized, or demeaned—can disrupt our ability to initiate and participate in the relationships that help us grow.

To begin examining the painful impact of shame and humiliation, we must call upon our best relational practices to create a context in which clients feel safe enough to represent their experiences. These practices include the following:

1. *Listening and responding.* Experiences of shame or humiliation often alienate and silence individuals, in extreme cases leading them into what Jean Baker Miller (1988) describes as "condemned isolation." To overcome the silence and disconnections induced by these experiences, Judith V. Jordan reminds us that "in real dialogue both speaker and listener create a liveliness together and come into a truth together. Dialogue involves both initiative and responsiveness" (1989, p. 3). Within a context of responsiveness—a context of listening and responding—we offer clients an opportunity to feel safe and to fully represent their experience.

2. *Mutual empathy.* Mutual empathy not only entails empathizing with a client's experience but also encompasses empathizing with the client's *strategies of disconnection* (Miller & Stiver, 1994), the strategies that may have allowed the client to survive sometimes unimaginable dehumanizing encounters with others. Moreover, mutual empathy means identifying and empathizing with *our own* experiences of feeling shamed or humiliated as well as our personal and professional strategies of disconnection, which can interfere with our ability to be fully present and engaged in a relationship.

3. *Authenticity.* The practice of authenticity is about being authentic in a way that facilitates the growth of our clients. It is not about self-disclosure but about being fully present and engaged in the relationship, a point made clear in the Stone Center paper "Therapists' Authenticity" (Miller et al., 1999).

4. *Movement toward mutuality.* Shaming or humiliating interactions can thrive within a context of dominant–subordinate relationships (i.e., nonmutual relationships) in which one person holds the power to degrade another. By moving toward mutuality, we are moving away from the "power over" dynamics that promote and perpetuate shame and humiliation (see Jordan, 1986).

5. *Humor.* One relational practice that many of us use but rarely acknowledge is the practice of humor. Humor can be an effective method of disarming or neutralizing some feelings of shame or humili-

ation, specifically humor in the form of taking ourselves lightly and laughing with each other about vulnerabilities and imperfections that make us unique relational beings.

These are only a few of the relational practices that can potentially bridge the disconnections caused by shame or humiliation. All too often, shaming experiences have taught clients that safety lies in disconnection and separation. Relational practice invites clients back into relationship and offers them the opportunity to find healing through connection.

From a Separate Self to a Relational Perspective

Shame and humiliation, along with guilt and embarrassment, belong to a family of emotions that have been referred to as the *self-conscious emotions* (Tangney & Fischer, 1995). They are called the self-conscious emotions because they cause us to reflect upon ourselves; we become *self-conscious*. However, this view is based on a traditional perspective that emphasizes a separate, independent self as the primary unit of study (Jordan, 1989). If we expand our understanding to incorporate a broader, relational perspective, experiences of shame and humiliation might be described as causing us to reflect upon *ourselves in relationship*. Therefore, it might be more accurate to say that these emotions make us *relationally conscious*, which is most obvious when shame or humiliation serve as precursors to disconnection or rejection.

Relational–cultural theory (RCT) offers us the opportunity to move beyond "separate-self" analyses to an awareness of the relational dynamics of these experiences. Throughout this chapter we describe and expand a relational perspective to achieve a deeper understanding of shame and humiliation.

A Relational Understanding of Shame

The word "shame" comes from a variety of European words that literally mean "to cover, to veil, to hide" (Wurmser, 1981, p. 29). The literal meaning of the word is consistent with the individual responses associated with shame (e.g., feeling exposed, avoiding eye contact, wanting to hide or withdraw). Examinations of shame found in the literature often describe this emotion as an experience of the self, a failure of being, a global sense of deficiency, or a failure to achieve one's ideas (Lewis, 1987). The literature recognizes shame as an intense, enduring experience that affects the whole self.

Applying a relational perspective, Jordan (1989) defines shame as "a felt sense of unworthiness to be in connection, a deep sense of unlovability, with the ongoing awareness of how very much one wants to connect with others." Furthermore, Jordan suggests that shame diminishes the empathic possibility within a relationship, cutting off the opportunity for the individuals engaged in the relationship to progress toward mutuality and authentic connection. All of us can likely recall feeling isolated or cut off from others after experiencing some form of shame. Jordan brings our attention to these relational dynamics. While separate-self analyses acknowledge shame as an intense, enduring experience involving the whole self, a relational perspective significantly enhances our understanding, suggesting that shame is an intense, enduring experience involving one's *whole being in relationship*.

The Relational Dynamics of Humiliation

The word "humiliation" is derived from the Latin root word *humus*, which means earth or soil (Barnhart, 1988). When this root word is combined with the suffix "ate," meaning "cause to be," to humiliate literally means "cause to be soil," or, stated in contemporary terms, to "treat someone like dirt." In other words, humiliation is a form of human interaction that puts an individual—or group—in a degraded or lowly position, inciting feelings of devaluation or disgrace.

Compared to shame, the experience of humiliation has been relatively neglected in the literature (Hartling, 1995; Hartling & Luchetta, 1999). One possible explanation of this oversight is that the characteristics of humiliation do not fit into the individualistic analyses that emphasize experiences of a separate self. Paul Gilbert contends that humiliation is distinguished by a relational dynamic when he suggests that "in shame the focus is on the self, while in humiliation the focus is on the harm done by others" (1997, p. 133). Regardless of this and other possible distinctions, shame and humiliation are frequently used interchangeably in the literature. Perhaps this is because these emotions result in similar behavioral responses (e.g., avoiding eye contact, withdrawing, and hiding). By shifting from an individualistic perspective to a relational view, we may be able to clarify and enhance our insight into both of these emotions.

Judith V. Jordan's relational definition of shame—a felt sense of being unworthy of connection—provides us with a starting point for describing the closely affiliated experience of humiliation. Humiliation might be thought of as a feeling associated with *being made to feel unworthy of connection*. This definition begins to draw attention to the interpersonal characteristics of humiliation: humiliation is inflicted on another person engaged in a relationship. It is a relational violation that causes an individual to feel degraded, devalued, or unworthy of connection. Applying a relational approach, the relational dynamics of humiliation move to the foreground.

Within a broader, relational framework, it may be easier to describe some of the similarities and differences between shame and humiliation, including those characteristics that have important social implications. For example, scholars suggest that these emotions are similar in that they are both more prevalent in relationships characterized by power imbalances, as in hierarchical, dominant–subordinate relationships (Hartling, 1995; Klein, 1991; Miller, 1987). The "power over" conditions that promote shame and humiliation are readily observed in a variety of settings, ranging from playgrounds to battlegrounds.

In describing a difference between shame and humiliation, Donald C. Klein asserts that "*people believe they deserve their shame; they do not believe they deserve their humiliation*" (1991, p. 117; emphasis mine). With shame, we tend to blame ourselves for the damage we have brought upon ourselves (Lewis, 1987). With humiliation, the damage is viewed as unjustly inflicted upon us by others. This distinction helps us understand how shame and humiliation can be used as a form of social control. It is advantageous to the dominant group to persuade the subordinate group that they are deserving of shame, that they are responsible for the damage they have brought upon themselves, that they should blame themselves for some deficiency or supposed inferiority. Convincing subordinates that they are responsible for their humiliation and deserving of shame diverts attention away from the actions of the dominant group. Alternatively, if members of the subordinate group were to clearly identify their experiences as undeserved humiliation, they might begin to focus their attention on the behaviors and practices of the dominant group and challenge those behaviors.

These are only a few of the dynamics illuminated through a relational exploration of shame and humiliation. Continued study may reveal other important characteristics that will enhance our understanding of these emotions.

Shame and Humiliation in Therapy

A relational approach helps us recognize the many types of human interactions that may trigger feelings of shame or humiliation. These interactions can range from interpersonal encounters (e.g., ridicule, scorn, contempt, harassment) to social or institutionalized practices (e.g., racism, sexism, classism, heterosexism). They can even include international events (e.g., ethnic cleansing, armed conflict, genocide; see Figure 6.1). It is important to be aware of the numerous forms of behavior leading to feelings of shame and humiliation as we begin to explore the effects of these experiences in therapeutic settings.

Therapy is a complex relational context. A therapist must navigate the intricacies of the client's culture and experiences (e.g., past neglects, history of abuse, strategies of disconnection, relational strengths), as well as moderate aspects of her/his own culture, experience, education, and training. Furthermore, a therapist must negotiate the influence and impact of the larger culture and the culture of therapy itself, which is largely informed by separate-self models of psychological development (see Figure 6.2). Given these complexities, encounters with the dynamics of shame and humiliation in therapy become almost inevitable.

RCT suggests that relationships naturally move through periods of connection, disconnection, and reconnection. Resolving disconnections offers individuals the opportunity not only to reconnect but

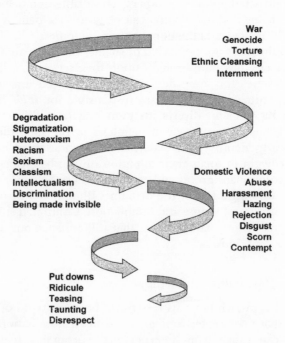

FIGURE 6.1. Acts of shame/humiliation.

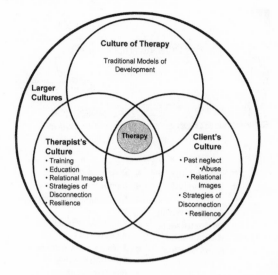

FIGURE 6.2. Relational complexity.

to move the relationship toward a new, enhanced connection. However, when shame or humiliation is the source of the disconnection, the movement in the therapy relationship may be disrupted or derailed (see Figure 6.3). The significance of this disconnection should not be underestimated. After all, if one cannot feel worthy of connection (i.e., one feels shamed)—or is made to feel unworthy of connection (i.e., one feels humiliated)—within a therapeutic relationship, with whom can one feel worthy of connection? The fear generated from these types of ruptures may prompt a wide range of difficult reactions in our clients and ourselves, arousing painful relational images or triggering perplexing strategies of disconnection. Being attuned to and accurately identifying shame or humiliation as the source of the disconnection and the source of the concomitant behavioral responses are essential to effectively repairing the rupture in the relationship.

One way of understanding responses to being shamed or humiliated is to utilize a model originally developed by psychiatrist Karen Horney (1945) as a typology of personality types. Adapting Horney's model, we can classify responses to shame or humiliation under three broad categories (see Figure 6.4). Some individuals may engage in a "moving away" strategy, separating themselves from relationships (e.g., withdrawing, silencing themselves, or making themselves invisible).

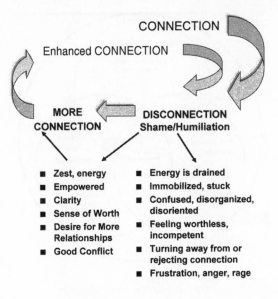

FIGURE 6.3. Movement in therapy.

Many children shamed through neglect and abuse may adopt this strategy of survival. Other individuals may exhibit a "moving toward" strategy by keeping important parts of their experience out of relationship in an attempt to earn or keep connection; that is, they may attempt to appease or please the other to secure the relationship or just to survive in the relationship. This strategy may explain the logic underlying the behavior of some individuals coping with difficult, problematic, or even abusive relationships. Finally, still others may exhibit a "moving against" strategy, directing anger, resentment, and rage against those whom they believe to be the source of their shame or humiliation. Media accounts of the recent series of multiple murders in school or workplace settings—such as the Littleton, Colorado, tragedy—suggest that the killers were retaliating against shame or humiliation in the form of ridicule or public disgrace.

In therapy, variations and combinations of these three strategies may become evident in our clients' behavior as well as our own behavior, diminishing the relationship's capacity for mutual empathy and authentic connection. Recognizing these strategies early can lead us to address the genuine source of the disconnection. Furthermore, applying the relational practices we have already identified can help us transform experiences of shame or humiliation into opportunities for growth and greater connection.

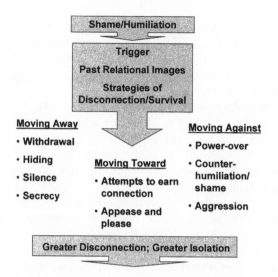

FIGURE 6.4. Strategies of disconnection/survival.

SHAME AND GROWTH IN THE THERAPY RELATIONSHIP: THE CASE OF CAROL

Wendy Rosen

My first reactions in hearing the prologue to Carol's life story were fear and reluctance, and I hadn't even heard any real details yet. She certainly wasn't the first client with a history of abuse with whom I'd worked; yet something felt different this time. I simply had the feeling that this would be a long, unnerving ride with Carol, and I felt scared. Do I want to take this on, I asked myself? Interestingly, in the first session, she asked me if I thought I could handle hearing about her history. I "assured" her that I was no stranger to hearing about abuse, and while I imagined by her question that some pretty bad things had happened to her, I thought I could bear hearing about them, despite its being painful in the listening.

Carol had tried a number of other therapists in her recent effort to resume therapy but hadn't found any therapist with whom she clicked. She described these other therapists as either too "by-the-book" clinical and aloof, too naive, not strong enough, or having had bad taste in office decor. By the end of our first hour, Carol was tearful and seemed quite fragile. It was clear to me that she was desperate for someone who felt willing and strong enough to handle her. I suggested we both think about our meeting and whether or not it felt like a good fit and suggested that she call me within a week. I knew when Carol left that she had touched me and that I was already engaged in some kind of wrenching emotional tug of war that I did not yet understand. I also believed that she really needed help right away and that, despite my trepidation, I wanted to try this relationship with her. She called shortly thereafter and set up her next appointment.

Carol was 33 years old, white, Protestant, and raised in North Dakota in a working-class family with eight children. While she identified herself as a lesbian, she acknowledged an uneasy relationship to her sexual identity. She had a twin brother, Carl, and they were the middle siblings. Her father was a laborer, and her mother was unemployed outside of the home. All of Carol's siblings have remained in North Dakota, not far from their parents. While growing up, Carol's home life was utterly chaotic and frightening. Over time and with a great deal of shame, she described her family to me, referring to them as "poor white trash." The house was typically dirty and completely cluttered. There were no clear rules in the house, such that the kids remained unsupervised with no guidance available. Fist fights and running wild were the norm. Survival relied upon knowing how to defend yourself at all costs, figuring out how to play the system, and getting whatever you needed by any subversive means possible.

Carol described her father as passive and often absent. He gave her mother carte blanche to run the house and handle the kids, and he rarely intervened. Neither Carol nor her siblings had much of a relationship with him. Her mother, conversely, was omnipresent. Carol had a lot to say about her mother, who was the recurrent menacing presence in just about all of her flashbacks and nightmares. Beginning with Carol's premature birth and continuing into adolescence, Carol's mother maintained a highly paranoid, delusional, and abusive relationship with her daughter. While she could be quite harsh with the other children, all of the siblings agreed that Carol had it the worst. The fact that she was a twin and a girl became the basis for her mother's delusional belief that Carol "came from the devil" and that there was something very wrong with her, especially with her body. Mother continuously taunted her that she was really a boy but that her body was somehow deformed into looking like a girl. She would handle her daughter's body roughly in a range of abusive ways, beginning in infancy.

Whenever I would ask Carol to tell me about some of the things that her mother would do to her, she would respond that she couldn't talk about them, and often she would have a frightening flashback of her mother threatening her in some way. Therefore, instead of having to speak of the many abusive acts she suffered, Carol eventually decided to make a list of all the words that came to mind regarding her abuse, such as "kick," "bite," "beat," "burn," "penetrate," and many others. In my mind, this list of fragmentations represented her private experience of these traumatic assaults in the form of encapsulated, codified moments of terror. To present them in sentence form would have defied the reality of her dissociated management of the events and their encoding in the form of repetitive flashbacks of images and bodily sensations. Even more unbearable, it would have forced her to become the living subject of this horror story in all of its terror and shame.

Early in therapy, Carol's anxiety was so great that it took her most of the hour to feel she could settle down and sit still. She was extremely hyper, made only sporadic eye contact, and typically would joke or be evasive and sarcastic. When the hour was over, she justifiably would feel that we hadn't really talked about anything or made any kind of connection. We both would end up feeling frustrated and incompetent in our efforts at engaging the other's attention. Carol admitted that her anxiety was so great at seeing me each time that it took her a long time to settle down and feel more comfortable. Because of this and at Carol's suggestion, we eventually decided to meet for an extended 2-hour session each week. While I was apprehensive about this at first, as I wasn't sure I could endure for 2 hours, I had this feeling that Carol was pretty adept at assessing her needs around comfort and safety. I also figured I could stand to learn something about endurance from someone whose life was a study in just that. We both needed time together, and we were both a bit afraid of actually having it. I was always exhausted at the end of these sessions, but I no longer felt that either of us parted unaffected.

Carol's "suggestions" regarding the design and direction of the therapy relationship became central to our work together. Our relationship became a forum for cycles of mutual resistance and surrender, the former leaving each of us feeling safe, smug, and out of connection, and the latter finding us feeling scared, vulnerable, and ashamed. This, of course, paralleled Carol's adaptive and miscarried lifelong efforts at survival during which she walked a fine line between life-sustaining decisions and impulsive actions. Oftentimes, this line became blurred, as an elaboration of her history reveals.

Carol learned how to survive her childhood through lying, stealing, and dissociating, on the one hand, and through humor, athletic skills, and an engaging, curious mind, on the other. She also survived through stolen moments of illicit contact, including incest with a brother, an incident of her fondling a small child for whom she had baby-sat, and an intimate liaison with one of her female high school teachers. Carol felt irreconcilable shame about the former two in that she saw herself as a willing participant, despite her better judgment. She felt no shame or remorse about the third, however, as her felt experience was inarguably one of loving comfort and growth, particularly around her burgeoning sexuality as a lesbian and the chance for a safe, sensuous physical engagement with another. When Carol ran away at age 17, this teacher had taken Carol in to live in her home with her husband and children. She sheltered, cared about, and believed in her and enabled Carol to graduate from high school and go on to college. Their sexual relationship was sporadic and short-lived as her teacher realized that prolonging it was not a good idea for either one of them and thus she ended it. It was a rather abrupt ending, which hurt Carol, but the two of them have maintained a lifelong caring connection ever since. Carol's teacher has not been able to talk about that chapter of their relationship, however, which has left Carol with a lingering curiosity about just what it was that her teacher felt with her at the time, how exactly she had experienced her emotionally and physically. She needed to know who she was through the eyes and benign touch of an intimate other. Was she tainted? Did she indeed come from the devil? Was she really a girl or a defective boy? Was she capable of being handled and held and loved?

These have been the central questions of Carol's therapy and of our relationship throughout our work together. Given her history of abuse, her own impulsivity, the sometimes muddiness of her boundaries, and her very real ignorance of what constitutes safe connection, I knew I was being invited into some really dicey territory. There was simply no good psychotherapy handbook for these issues. There were plenty of blanket rules and professional warnings, but there wasn't much in the way of a finer honing of responses to the very unique meanings and idiosyncrasies of each particular client and the client–therapist relationship. Given my own young adult history of precocious intimacy as a means of satisfying certain physical and emotional questions, I knew that some fragile territory of my own would be entered. These would be private places in me of uncertainty and shame. Added to this was the consistent driving force to all of Carol's momentum through life, that of challenge. Her life has been a series of mind-numbing challenges, and she has met and often attempted to preempt them through indiscriminately challenging just about everything in her path. I knew, then, that our relationship would very likely become one of throwing down the gauntlet over and over again, as survival and success had become defined by such victories. Whether or not I was up to the mutual challenge our relationship would be was no longer a question, as I had already accepted it. Whether or not I would be able to discern the differences between the growth-promoting challenges and the self-defeating, relationally damaging ones was the bigger concern, especially as I had to be both participant and observer. On the other hand, by being both participant and especially observer, I would have countless opportunities myself to either hide or to shame, each time "protectively" taking myself out of connection. As I was to discover, I was far from always being able to make these delicate choices with conscious ease and care.

Off and on during our relationship, Carol would complain that she had a hard time remembering me between sessions. She'd say, "I can't feel you. I can't see your face." She acknowledged how hard this was for her, as picturing me was a source of comfort to her whenever she had a bad flashback. I thought about this inability to remember, on the one hand, as her way of paradoxically protecting me and preserving our relationship from what she felt was her own toxicity, and also protecting herself from what might prove dangerous in me. On the other hand, I also knew that enduring internal connections are built on experiences of empathic love and truly being in an authentic relationship, and these were all but absent from much of Carol's early life.

Eventually, Carol began to complain further that I was sitting too far away from her and that this was part of the problem. She couldn't feel my presence. I agreed to pull my chair up more closely during our sessions, but I secretly began to feel some anxiety and the faint rumblings of resentment. I felt nervous about our physical closeness for reasons I could not clarify, except perhaps to chalk it up to my own issues about intimacy and physicality. I was also feeling challenged, however, as if Carol were testing me and taking some small delight in seeing me squirm. Carol initially described the greater proximity as helpful, but this was a short-lived remedy. She soon began to say that she needed to be better able to truly feel my presence and asked if I would sit on the couch with her. She wanted to be able to hold my hand at times when she was deeply upset and shaken or when she felt unbearably alone. While her request made me even more anxious than before, it did not irritate me as much, since I felt that I could say no and provide "sound clinical reasons" for my refusal. There ensued a protracted phase in our relationship where we focused on this very issue in an exceedingly painful, angry, and confusing series of emotional interactions and eventual negotiations at the heart of which rested some of our most shame-ridden places.

The first part of this phase consisted of my attempts to explore with Carol the reasons for and meanings behind her request. I framed them against the backdrop of her history of sexual abuse and the dismantling of traditional boundaries in her student–teacher relationship. I emphasized the importance of communicating through words and feelings, highlighting repeatedly the definition and limits of our relationship in this regard. I made clear the central importance of her emotional safety through the maintenance of clarity in our relationship, so as not to repeat past transgressions and injuries. With each explanation, clarification, and interpretation, I was met with increasing tears of frustration and anger and accusations that "you're not understanding me." I began to feel my blood pressure rising with each and every one of her imploring protests. I started to feel harassed and abused by her. Eventually, I could neither stand it nor understand it, and so I fired back my own accusations of what I perceived as her almost sadistic attempts at undermining what I also perceived to be my best therapeutic efforts. I told her that I felt as though she was relentlessly pushing me to go beyond my own comfort and what I truly believed was right. I told her it felt suspect, given her history of abuse by her mother, and also given her past relationship with her teacher. She protested that sexual feelings for me were not an issue for her, that I was treating her as if she were asking for something more than she in fact was, that I was making her feel as if she was a truly harmful person, and that maybe some of the problems we were having were mine rather than hers.

This suggestion touched a nerve in me, leaving me feeling confused and ashamed, as if she'd unearthed some ugly secret or character flaw in me. She also felt terrible and, I believe, diminished at how little I seemed to trust her. She would sometimes call me during the week, feeling utterly bereft and alone, but our conversations offered no antidote to the rupture between us. During this whole series of exchanges, I held inside the nagging feeling that there was something very wrong with this picture. I was feeling angry, hurt, defensive, stuck, relentlessly challenged, and yet emotionally detached from my many well-versed clinical rebuttals. Most of all, however, I was painfully aware of how wrenching this seemed for Carol and that I somehow was clearly contributing to it. These observations and the widening chasm between us propelled us to the next phase of interactions.

I felt thoroughly saddened by the shared challenge at this point and began to think that maybe Carol had a point, that I, in fact, was not really understanding her entirely. At the same time, in my weariness, I felt that she was not understanding me either, that at the very least there was occurring some very mutual failure of empathy. Each of us was feeling accused, humiliated, and terribly unseen in some way, but I remained thoroughly confused about where we were so tragically missing one another. What I did know, however, was what I was feeling about Carol's request that I sit with her and that she be able to hold my hand sometimes. Instead of trying to assume Carol's experience and unconscious motivations, therefore, I began to explore and speak some of my own. From this vantage point, I could at least return to some more authentic and truly present place in the hopes that Carol could meet me there and that something more clear and connecting might emerge for us. I felt immediate relief. At last, I had given myself permission to own and acknowledge my discomfort without having to understand it entirely. I could tell Carol that not only did I feel some concern about her request for such closeness due to her trauma history but that it made me anxious to think about sitting on the couch with her and for any form of touch to be a part of our relationship. I didn't know all the reasons for my anxiety, nor did I feel that she needed to be privy to all my internal processes in this regard, but I felt I could tell her some of what I did know.

I talked to her about my professional training regarding the place of touch in therapy, about my fears of how this could get interpreted, and about fears of reprisal or professional censure. In other words, I was frightened, but also I couldn't bear doing anything that in any way might harm her. Carol responded that she truly trusted me and added that she, likewise, would never choose to do anything to hurt me. In fact, what hurt her most was that I didn't trust her. I also told Carol that I thought I had some of my own issues around intimacy and physical closeness that were affecting my response to her, and while I didn't really understand them all, the important point was that they were mine and not hers and that I would keep working on figuring them out. In fact, I had begun privately to question my own sources of shame and apparent discomfort about physicality, which felt painfully deflating, yet equally humbling and personally touching. This whole process of exploration felt, in many ways, like a loving act and a shared gift. I gradually came to the conclusion that I could find no convincing reason to deny Carol's request that I sit with her and be open to touch, such as holding her hand or putting an arm around her shoulder during tearful moments of great pain. Even further, it might very well prove to be a mutually growthful move to make in our relationship. I was very clear with myself and with her about the limits of this contact, that this touch would not be motivated by or aimed at anything of a sexual nature, and if any such feelings arose, we would talk about them. I believed that Carol knew at heart what she needed and that I could challenge my own limits just a little more than I had dared before. It felt like a chance to move out of a lonely place of shame into one of mutual respect, important growth for both of us. So, I nervously moved over to the couch, with Carol nervously checking in with me about whether I was ready and okay with this. I've since never left her side nor failed to hold her in comfort when the moment called for it.

In sum, this case describes the relational process of moving through feelings of shame toward important points of connection by successfully negotiating a mutually respectful meeting place for a therapeutic relationship, a place that leads to health and growth. Over time, my relationship with Carol has become an increasingly strong one, though certainly not without its bumpy moments. These moments, however, no longer feel terribly threatening to either one of us. Our challenges to one another continue, but they have turned playful, more benign and strengthening. It feels stunningly respectful and loving, filled also with sadness, longing, grief, and quietly dissolving shame.

ANGER, SHAME, AND HUMILIATION: LEGACIES OF A "POWER OVER" PARADIGM

Maureen Walker

I am moved by Wendy's account of her relationship with Carol, as it bears witness to one of the most potent premises of RCT: that authentic relationship offers us the gift of conflict—the opportunity for the emergence of something new (Miller, 1987). In preparation for our presentation at the Summer Training Institute, we (Judy, Wendy, Linda, and I) talked at length about what happens in those moments of genuine encounter when both the therapist and the client are moved by and moved into those private spaces where shame, anxiety, and fear reside (L. M. Hartling, R. Rosen, M. Walker, & J. V. Jordan, personal communications, January–June 1999). It is likely that in those moments both the therapist and the patient experience an intense and unforgiving awareness of fragility and helplessness. In a culture that overvalues certainty and control, this awareness can trigger painful disconnections and violations.

In the course of one of our discussions about shame and humiliation in the therapy relationship, I somewhat reluctantly recounted an incident that occurred when I was in graduate school. At that time, I worked as a counselor in an inpatient alcohol and drug treatment program. In addition to being the only student clinician, I was also the only person of color and the only nonrecovering person who had been hired as a primary therapist. I fought hard to gain credibility with the patients and the rest of the clinical staff, most of whom were white, male, grizzled survivors of the "street" or veterans of well-known treatment programs. In many ways, my colleagues enjoyed a built-in status that I could not lay claim to. I had only my book learning, or (as one of my colleagues said to me) I was trying to learn about addiction "the hard way." Over time, I gained a reputation as savvy, confrontational, and insightful—an image in which I took particular pleasure as it gave me access into relationships with my patients and colleagues.

As primary therapist, my job was to lead process and education groups. On one particular Monday morning, I came in ready to "take charge." There was a new patient whom I will call Rick, who had been admitted over the weekend. According to the nurse's report, he had been disruptive on the unit, rude to the staff, and contemptuous of his peers, whom he nevertheless regaled with stories of the many treatment programs he had "outsmarted." Rick was a lawyer by training. He walked with a decided limp and was missing his right arm, having lost it, as the story went, in a drunk driving accident. The group was proceeding with usual Monday morning check-ins. Rick's check-in was quite predictably some expression of his disdain for the treatment program. I'm not at all sure how I responded to him, but I am sure it was pretty important to me to feel as if I could have some impact. So I said something. To which he responded that the last thing he was interested in was my "K-mart psychology." I have no idea what happened after that. I probably responded, or more likely issued some confrontational retort. He walked out. The group probably rescued itself and me from his withering judgment by talking about his denial—I honestly don't know. What I do know was that I was stunned and felt momentarily reduced to nothingness.

If it is true that we are at any age all of our previous ages, I was in that moment the 3-year-old kid who waited behind the fence for the older school children to walk past so that I could hear snatches of their conversation. I was still the 3-year-old who was ecstatic to figure out that y-o-u spelled "you." In my 3-year-old world, having that knowledge meant that I was worthy of connection, or at least, worthy of notice by the older, wiser 7-year-olds. Something had happened in what Klein (1991) calls the "emotionally relevant field" between Rick and me: a relational space that encompasses both the interpersonal and the cultural-collective. The critical paradox was that what is held in isolation as intensely private shame is both an impediment to and an expression of our yearning for connection. Because of the terror that often accompanies the yearning, we retreat into self-absorbed disconnection (Stiver, personal communication, October 5, 1998). It is a space where the collective dimension of the private shame is not easily recognized and named.

As Hartling and Luchetta (1999) have pointed out, humiliation involves being put in a lowly, debased, powerless position by someone who, at the moment, has greater power than oneself. In that moment, Rick and his peers—the witnesses to our exchange—held the power, and I was the 3-year-old behind the fence wanting very much to have significance and value in their eyes. In that private space of shame and fear, I lost significance and value in my own eyes when I failed to come up with the right answer, the perfect, *breakthrough* intervention that would cause some shift in Rick (and perhaps bolster my own credentials as a nonrecovering addiction counselor). The point is that my sense of connection was quite tenuous, a commodity that had to be earned daily by unerring insights and certain knowledge. My need to be right and my need to know were my defense against the fear of invisibility and the shame of nobody-ness. I have a sense that in that private space, which in my mind had been exposed to public view, my fears of invisibility, powerlessness, and nobody-ness were not unlike Carol's in her implicitly accusatory plea to Wendy: "You don't understand me."

Silver, Conte, Micelli, and Poggi (1986) have suggested that humiliation consists, in part, of a particular sort of powerlessness, in that the person lacks a quality or resource that enables her/him to achieve some goal or standard. In the culture of traditional therapy, some part of that standard has to do with certainty and control. The alarm signals from my own private defenses were compounded by the unrelenting admonitions from supervisors:

- Never get into power struggles with clients.
- Never let the client take control (along with the dire warnings that some of them would surely try).
- Maintain the therapeutic frame lest you leak away your power.

Missing from most of those conversations were guidelines, or even support for remaining authentic and present in the face of uncertainty and pain. The implicit metaphor is that of therapy as conquest—an encounter that "good" therapists always win. Indeed, the language of conquest permeates much of the discourse about therapeutic practice; for example, it is not uncommon to hear therapists speak about *breaking through* a client's resistance. Because of the exaggerated emphasis on control, a therapist is left with few options for staying in connection when she/he experiences anxiety or confusion in a session. Within the context of a "power over" or "conquest" model of therapy, there is little room for self-empathy, a quality that enables presence and authenticity. Under these conditions, the default option in conflict is disconnection, whether through rigid certainty or self-effacing avoidance. Each is a strategy of disconnection that pulls the therapist out of active engagement with the client, thus depriving both of the opportunity to use anxiety and conflict as paths to expanded awareness.

Rick and I were situated in a traditional "power over" model of psychiatric treatment; within this frame I felt sorely exposed as lacking the power (e.g., insight, confrontation skills, control) I should possess. The public-ness of our encounter posed an additional threat: that in losing "control" of the session in front of other patients, I would be exposed as unworthy of connection not only within the group but also in the larger culture of psychologists that I was training to join.

Humiliation is endemic to "power over" cultures. Klein (1991) describes such cultures as humiliation-prone. Interestingly, power-over cultures are likely to view this humiliation as prosocial. That is, after a series of ritual humiliations a person is somehow transformed and achieves fitness for membership and belonging. The unfortunate byproduct of prosocial humiliation is that it instills a lasting sense of vulnerability (e.g., fear of censure and exclusion), as well as a penchant for imposing such humiliation onto others. Again, Klein describes the phenomenology of humiliation as something akin to one's losing face or sense of identity. Whether in the case of a fledging graduate student or an accomplished therapist, that sense of identity has much to do with the relational images we form of what a good therapist should be. Our investment in holding onto those images is meant to ensure our survival in the professional community.

Humiliation can be traumatic (witness my dissociation during my "public shaming" by Rick). It brings with it the threat of being "turned away from" (Klein, 1991), of being publicly exposed as unworthy of connection. Add to this individual trauma the impact of social marginality. Whether by reason of race, sexual orientation, gender, or some temporarily disabling condition such as grad-student-hood, the threat that one's collective identity might be besmirched heightens the potential for trauma.

I started this talk by mentioning a relational conception of conflict as an opportunity for transformation or the emergence of something new. I think Wendy has provided a reassuring example of the growth-fostering possibilities through her relationship with Carol. Over several months, we often talked about paths to reconnection, or—as Linda has put it—transforming humiliation into humility (L. M. Hartling, R. Rosen, M. Walker, & J. V. Jordan, personal communications, January–June 1999). When I told this story, Judy asked a playful but poignant question: "So what would be so bad about being a K-mart psychologist?" We all laughed. What would be so bad about providing a serviceable product at a reasonable price to large numbers of people? Her question brought into clear view the relational images that are part and parcel of nonrelational training in psychology. Implicit in those images are elitist fantasies of being perhaps "Armani" psychologists, or better yet one of those exclusive salon purveyors whose customers come only by appointment. Judy's question facilitated renewed awareness of the healing power of humor, especially as it helps us to explore the hidden relational images that constrict our capacity for mutuality in relationship.

At the time of the telling, my memory of my encounter with Rick seemed to come completely unbidden. Such is the power of relationship to awaken, renew, and transform. Rick and I brought into the room our common humanity, the needs and vulnerabilities that become the substance of growth in relationship. We brought with us our yearning for meaning and connection, as well as our very powerful strategies for staying out of authentic connection. From our own private spaces we brought relational images that defined safety as maintaining dominance and control over the other, thus postponing for at least one more day the threat of nobody-ness. He bolted from the room. I dissociated. The lesson of my dissociation is that in my attempt to save face, I lost touch. It is probably a safe bet that now, 16 years later, Rick is not sitting in some parallel universe in a room with his colleagues talking about his encounter with me. But maybe he is. Such is the gift of conflict and the possibilities for transforming reconnection.

RESTORING EMPATHIC POSSIBILITY

Judith V. Jordan

In an earlier paper on shame, I suggested that shame is an essential relational affect and I defined it as a sense of unworthiness to be in connection, an absence of hope that an empathic response will be forthcoming from another person (Jordan, 1989). There is an ominous and despairing feeling that one is beyond empathic possibility. Furthermore, shame is a sense of unworthiness about one's very being, not just about one's actions. Traditionally, guilt has been described as involving discrete acts of transgression or violating standards of behavior; the experience of shame is global and immobilizing. It is a ubiquitous human experience, and it often leads to withdrawal and isolation accompanied by an immobilizing sense of self-blame and an inability to move back into the very connections that could provide repair.

Shaming, unlike the spontaneous arising of shame from some sense of inadequacy or failure of our being, is done to people by other people, usually to control or disempower them in some way. It plays a role in almost all socialization to greater or lesser degrees. Socialization toward independence and socialization toward gender role compliance are among the areas where the most stringent shaming typically occurs. It is used by parents, and it is used by peers. Shaming serves to disconnect people from themselves, from their real feelings, and from others. It also serves to silence and isolate people. Shame is directed at marginalized groups and serves to put and keep them in a place of disempowerment and silence; they are made to feel that their reality is deficient or lacking. Dominant groups characteristically use shame against subordinate groups to keep them from expressing their reality in a way that would threaten the dominant view of reality.

Healing the shame that spontaneously arises in us—or that is done to us by others to control or disempower us—involves reestablishing a belief in empathic possibility. That is, the person struggling with shame must come to believe that another person can respond empathically to her/his experience. The shamed person must come to know that she/he is respected and matters to the other person, that her/his efforts to bring her/himself more fully into relationship will not be met with severe judgments and rejection, and that there will be the possibility of mutuality. Relational therapy, with its nonjudgmental stance and its emphasis on mutual empathy, provides an opportunity for the deep healing of shame.

Helen Lynd (1958) wrote a wonderful book on shame in which she noted "enlarging the possibilities of mutual love depends on risking exposure." Both Wendy and Maureen have spoken about opening themselves to being responsive to their clients and to their own deep feelings and uncertainty. They describe a kind of emotional vulnerability and exposure that does not necessarily involve personal disclosure of facts about their lives. In Wendy's case, she acknowledges how afraid and uncertain she felt and how these feelings threatened to take her into the safety of a nonresponse, into disconnection. But her handling of the potential disconnection leads us to think about how shame can serve as a signal to move toward deeper connection rather than moving us into disconnection. It is often unacknowledged shame that leads to disconnection. Maureen touches on the issue of shame, of not wanting to be seen as foolish by her client or others (including herself), and she embraces the often painful growth that happens in conflict. The relational model, with its emphasis on mutual empathy, supports the therapist in staying in her/his vulnerability, which also takes us closer to an edge of uncertainty and possible shame. There are no easy, pat answers in this territory.

Linda beautifully outlined for us the strategies of disconnection, of shaming and humiliation. She referred to Karen Horney's work on "moving toward," "moving against," and "moving away from." Our model offers another way: that is, "moving *with*." We suggest that in therapy it is important for the therapist to be moved by the client's experience, to be moved with the person. In order to do this, we must be open and vulnerable. We must struggle with our own images of perfection or with images of what constitutes an ideal therapist—all knowing, always in charge, always empathic.

Mutual empathy involves allowing our clients to see, know, and feel that they have moved us, that they have had an impact on us, that we are vulnerable, open, in process with them. The therapist's authenticity and vulnerability, necessary to mutual empathy, provide invaluable information to the client and they contribute to building reliable, trustworthy relationships, which lie at the heart of real safety and growth in therapy.

Wendy addresses the disconnections and threatened disconnections as she struggles to stay present with her client, particularly when she's struggling to discover what will be in the best interest of this client. It is a challenge to stay in empathic connection when, as a therapist, you feel pushed to an edge with which you're not comfortable. And part of staying in connection is staying in touch with and being aware of what's arising in you, what's coming from the client, what's in the relationship, as well as what's in the context, what's coming from the culture of therapy. The culture of therapy often permeates the therapist's thinking, sometimes supporting our work and sometimes creating doubt or shame. Are we doing what our supervisors taught us, right or wrong? Our work occurs behind closed doors, with few clearly defined procedures and techniques. There is much room for self-doubt, a secret belief in difficult moments that someone else would surely be better serving this client than we are. Or in Maureen's experience as a graduate student, there is the very real concern about being evaluated by peers and supervisors. We have many questions: Is this helpful to the client? Is this deemed useful and ethical by the psychotherapy culture I belong to? Does what is deemed useful and ethical by the surrounding psychotherapy culture match what I, as a therapist, have found effective and healing? If not, how do I deal with that dilemma?

I believe that empathic possibility is the antidote to shame. Clients must develop empathy with others and with themselves. The dominant, white, middle-class culture overvalues control and certainty; not to be in control is to be vulnerable to shame. We are shamed when we are told we are not separate and autonomous enough, not contained enough, not neutral enough, that our boundaries aren't good enough. Typically, as therapists (and as people) we become armored, we get defensive, and we get rigid (i.e., disconnected) whenever we're ashamed and anxious. The challenge is to work with and transform the disconnection of potential shame, vulnerability, and exposure, being caught in the headlights, as Linda notes. How can we stay open and responsive in the face of shame? As therapists we need to know when we are disconnecting in shame.

Shame involves judgment and blame. The person suffering with shame feels self-blame or turns the blame against others. The challenge is to take appropriate responsibility for the uncertainty that occurs around vulnerability without moving into blame of other or self. The question becomes: How can we look together at what's happening in this relationship? How can we bear the uncertainty and vulnerability together?

As therapists we need to examine our own shame and vulnerability. I think we need to ask ourselves: What are the places of our own fear of exposure and sense of unworthiness? What do we value? What happens when clients seek to meet us psychologically where we feel most vulnerable? Wendy addressed the areas of professional boundaries and values around touch, but she also examined her own personal vulnerability around intimacy and closeness. As therapists, we have a responsibility to be acquainted with our own vulnerabilities. We have an opportunity to possibly recognize our own vulnerabilities more clearly and transform some of them. We can look at how to transform shame, which is potentially a source of terrible disconnection and isolation for all of us. And in so doing we can contribute to the reworking of the shame of our clients.

Humiliation is often public, clear, and sharp. It is done to us. We are seen in, or put in, a humiliated position. Shame can also be done to us and can be public. Although shame is often subtle and private, arising within an individual, one person or group often does it to another. It is silencing and disempowering. The dominant culture, for instance, develops standards of behavior and shames those who do not match those standards. Similarly in therapy, the dominant therapy culture develops standards of practice and if therapists don't subscribe to those standards, if therapists practice from a different model, they may be shamed. Therapists who question some of the more stringent rules of being objective, neutral, and nongratifying sometimes feel shamed into silence. Therapists sometimes are shamed into not communicating what they're actually doing in therapy because they fear censure and shaming from colleagues. Clearly, ethics and standards of practice that are instituted to protect the safety of clients are necessary. We must adhere to ethical and legal standards in our professional work. But there are also therapeutic opinions of what constitutes "good treatment," often unproven biases that are presented as "good practice," that are then used to shame practitioners into a kind of constricted and disconnected practice of therapy. To the extent that therapists feel they must adhere to a dogma or rigid set of practice principles which they may not feel are truly healing for their clients, they are silenced and possibly rendered less effective. Tracy Robinson and Janie Ward (1991) have written beautifully about bringing African American adolescent girls into voice and into resistance for liberation. It is a guide to survival and transformation for African American adolescent girls growing up in a racist culture. A large part of their strategy is to point out that there is not just one reality but many different views of reality, that the dominant reality is not always right, and that it is important to think critically about any dominant reality. These authors also suggest that alternative models of healthy development and points of view need to be created and enunciated. This is true in the field of therapy as well.

Therapists, too, need to construct new paradigms of development and treatment. We must struggle with the mainstream tenets rather than simply accept them and/or be shamed by them. We can be interested in these principles of treatment, question them, learn from them, try to understand their possible usefulness, and be empirical about them (do they work?); but we need to keep representing an alternative view of healing where it seems appropriate. Let's think critically about therapy, about what heals, about our own practices. We don't just have to accept the values of the dominant culture, whether it's the dominant culture at large or the dominant therapy culture. We need to seek change in the context that shames or disempowers us.

One path to transforming shame is increasing empathic responsiveness and rebuilding a sense of empathic possibility. Courage, too, can function as an antidote to shame. Courage is about bringing oneself more fully into connection. It involves finding out that you're not alone. It answers the lonely question, "Am I the only one?" with a resounding "No, you are not alone." Can we share our vulnerability and be strong and stay integrated in the face of shaming strategies? In her work, *Feminist Theory: From Margin to Center,* bell hooks (1984) looks at the strengths that are developed at the margins of societal power structures. To the extent that we participate in the power and privilege of the center, each of us needs to look to the paths of courage and wisdom that the people at the margin have developed, often in response to extreme oppression. People of color, lesbians and gays, people in classes other than the middle class, and people outside the dominant power dynamic often develop a wisdom, an awareness, and the ability to resist the dominant paradigm. The dominant culture is preoccupied with control, with certainty, rationality, and predictability. There is a perpetuation of the meritocracy myth, that people get what they deserve, that it's a "just world." Unfortunately, sometimes therapists engage in shaming; therapists can shame one another, and supervisors have the power to shame students. Strengths (defined in a narrow and autonomous way) and separation get idealized. Much energy goes into keeping the voices of people who are shamed and humiliated from uniting, from coming together to express and create an alternative reality.

Joining together, hearing each other into voice, coming out of the isolation that keeps us in doubt and shame can lead to transforming the dominant values of both therapy and the larger culture. It takes courage to work with new models, to challenge the old. The growing edge is not always totally safe or clear. There is vulnerability at this growing edge. Together we need to work on developing protected vulnerability and prudent trust. Therapists should not practice without a network of colleagues with whom they can share new insights about practice, uncertainties, and difficult therapeutic decisions. In such a supported and witnessing context, therapists like Wendy and Maureen will find the necessary and safe-enough freedom to explore and be responsive to learning about what actually heals the disconnections, shame, and pain that bring our clients into therapy.

REFERENCES

Barnhart, R. K. (Ed.). (1988). *The Barnhart dictionary of etymology*. New York: Wilson.

Gilbert, P. (1997). The evolution of social attractiveness and its role in shame, humiliation, guilt, and therapy. *British Journal of Medical Psychology, 70,* 113–147.

Hartling, L. M. (1995). *Humiliation: Assessing the specter of derision, degradation, and debasement.* Unpublished doctoral dissertation, Union Institute, Cincinnati, OH.

Hartling, L. M., & Luchetta, T. (1999). Humiliation: Assessing the impact of derision, degradation, and debasement. *Journal of Primary Prevention, 19*(4), 259–277.

Horney, K. (1945). *Our inner conflicts.* New York: Norton.

hooks, b. (1984). *Feminist theory: from margin to center.* Boston: South End Press.

Jordan, J. V. (1986). The meaning of mutuality. *Work in Progress, No. 23.* Wellesley, MA: Stone Center Working Paper Series.

Jordan, J. V. (1989). Relational development: Therapeutic implications of empathy and shame. *Work in Progress, No. 39.* Wellesley, MA: Stone Center Working Paper Series.

Klein, D. C. (1991). The humiliation dynamic: An overview. *Journal of Primary Prevention, 12*(2), 93–122.

Lewis, H. B. (Ed.). (1987). *The role of shame in symptom formation*. Hillsdale, NJ: Erlbaum.

Lynd, H. (1958). *On shame and the search for identity*. New York: Wiley.

Miller, J. B. (1987). *Toward a new psychology of women* (2nd ed.). Boston: Beacon Press.

Miller, J. B. (1988). Connections, disconnections, and violations. *Work in Progress, No. 33*. Wellesley, MA: Stone Center Working Paper Series.

Miller, J. B., & Stiver, I. P. (1994). Movement in therapy: Honoring the "strategies of disconnection." *Work in Progress, No. 65*. Wellesley, MA: Stone Center Working Paper Series.

Miller, J. B., & Stiver, I. P. (1995). Relational images and their meanings in psychotherapy. *Work in Progress, No. 74*. Wellesley, MA: Stone Center Working Paper Series.

Miller, J. B., & Stiver, I. P. (1997). *The healing connection: How women form relationships in therapy and in life*. Boston: Beacon Press.

Miller, J. B., Jordan, J. V., Stiver, I. P., Surrey, J. L., & Eldridge, N. S. (1999). Therapists' authenticity. *Work in Progress, No. 82*. Wellesley, MA: Stone Center Working Paper Series.

Robinson, T., & Ward, J. (1991). A belief in self far greater than anyone's disbelief: Cultivating resistance among African American female adolescents. In C. Gilligan, A. Rogers, & D. Tolman (Eds.), *Women, girls, and psychotherapy: Reframing resistance* (pp. 87–103). Binghamton, NY: Harrington Park Press.

Silver, M., Conte, R., Miceli, M., & Poggi, I. (1986). Humiliation: Feeling, social control, and the construction of identity. *Journal for the Theory of Social Behavior, 16*(3), 270–283.

Sullivan, H. (1953). *The interpersonal theory of psychiatry*. New York: Norton.

Tangney, J. P., & Fisher, K. W. (1995). *Self-conscious emotions: The psychology of shame, guilt, embarrassment, and pride*. New York: Guilford Press.

Wurmser, L. (1981). *The mask of shame*. Baltimore: Johns Hopkins University Press.

This chapter is based on a session presented during the 1999 Summer Advanced Training Institute at Wellesley College. © 2000 by Linda M. Hartling, Wendy Rosen, Maureen Walker, and Judith V. Jordan.

7

Racial Images and Relational Possibilities

MAUREEN WALKER *and* JEAN BAKER MILLER

In this conversation, we are trying to understand further the ways in which cultural and relational influences affect each other. Specifically, we want to address how sociopolitical factors shape psychological development. We explore some of the ways that rigid patterns of inequality and nonmutuality have a destructive impact on all participants in a relationship, restricting possibilities for movement and creativity.

We are talking especially about cultures that first define certain groups of people as less valuable and then oppress and restrict these people. In these cultures, persons who are deemed less valuable suffer both visibly and invisibly. Although persons who have the power to restrict and oppress the "less valuable" groups tend to suffer less visibly, participating in an oppressive sociopolitical system wreaks damage on relational functioning.

Our conversation rests on the belief that connections with other people are the source of growth for all people and that disconnections are the source of major problems. In order for connection to occur, each person has to be able to receive—and respond to—the experiences of other people.

Out of her/his history of these interchanges, each person constructs a complex set of relational images that constitute her/his picture of what happens in the world. Based on these relational images, each person then creates beliefs about her/himself and her/his characteristics. The background for these concepts can be found in many of the working papers and books produced by the Stone Center—for example, see Jordan, Kaplan, Miller, Stiver, and Surrey (1991), Jordan (1997), and Miller and Stiver (1997).

CONVERSATION

JEAN BAKER MILLER: In talking about the need in this country, you recently said, "It's more than 'diversity'." Can you tell me more about what you meant?

MAUREEN WALKER: Diversity implies that all we're talking about is difference and that there is equality among the different groups of people. But in this culture people are assigned to categories that aren't just different, they are subordinate or dominant. There are inherent power differences in these categories and political inequalities that have an impact on how we are with each other. If we truly believe that we grow in relationship with each other, then this situation of cultural and political inequality will have an impact on human development and human functioning.

To use the language of diversity is to imply that we are talking about simple difference when we are in fact talking about politicized and "problematized" difference: difference that translates into "more than" and "less than" or "better than" or "not as good as." That's the fundamental level of naming and acknowledgment. The second level is to recognize that under conditions of political inequality, gross and subtle power distortions have a critical impact on relational development and functioning.

In much of the popular conversation about so-called diversity, we focus on those people who have been socialized as "less than" and we try to address and understand what we call internalized oppression (meaning how oppressed people begin to believe the false images of themselves that the oppressor group creates). However, there's not much talk about what happens to the members of the dominant group. The situation of "structured-in" inequality also distorts the dominant person's sense of who she/he is in the world, whether in the smaller immediate world of friends and family or in the larger society. A person who is socialized to believe that she/he is "better than" can have a sense of identity that is built on relational images that are malformed and misguided. When we talk about simple diversity, I don't think we get a sense of that. Because this structured inequality is not named most of the time, people in the dominant group end up with problems they don't understand.

MILLER: So are you saying that those people who are socially defined as the more privileged are led to have distorted images of who they are and what should be coming to them?

WALKER: Yes, and these distortions set up unrealistic expectations. There are many times when these expectations are not fulfilled because they were unrealistic in the first place. However, if a person has been socialized or "trained" to accept all of the little convenient categories that are set up around difference, she/he sort of misses all of the distortions.

MILLER: Will you say more about that?

WALKER: Well, when Joan D. Chittister (1998) talks about patriarchy, she says something that rings true to me: "Patriarchy humiliates women all the time, but it kills men" (p. 27). Now I would say that patriarchy also kills women, in obvious and not so obvious ways.

I think her point, however, is that the entitlements of socially constructed maleness lead men to an early death: either through the thoughtless violence of legalized or street warfare, or by goading them to participate in a culture of "get more," "have more" in order to "be more." Men haven't been socialized to look at how they've been set up by patriarchy. They don't learn to question the game or the rules of the racist, classist, consumer-driven society that governs their lives—get more, have more, and be more. They are always out there having to measure themselves and compete against other (usually) men and compete, whether in a violent situation like war or whether just about who is accumulating the most stuff in a very materialistic culture.

They don't see that we have an economic situation that sets them up. Only a certain number of people are going to win by the rules of a class-based, consumerist society. The social hierarchies provide them with convenient categories of "less than" people to identify as "others"—"minorities" (whether by virtue of race, ethnicity, gender, or sexual orientation). These "other" people then are often scapegoated as the ones who are preventing them from moving forward and attaining whatever heights and privileges are "due to them" by virtue of their whiteness and their maleness.

MILLER: When you say that, are you thinking that white men, for example, are led to believe false notions about themselves such as that they are better than other groups of men, are never vulnerable, and the like. Then the relational images that many white men create lead them to expect that they should get much more than most of them will receive because these images are unrealistic in the first place?

WALKER: Men are constantly having to measure themselves against other men as a way of searching for their value: "Am I doing better than you?" They are not encouraged to see the economic structure that sets them up to do this. They don't look at that but see only themselves competing with the men nearby.

There's a quotation from Lyndon B. Johnson that's something like "If you can convince the poorest white man that he is better than the richest black man, he will never notice that his pocket is being picked."

That's an earthy, LBJ sort of saying, but I think it speaks to the power structure that keeps us looking through relational images at convenient categories of people without noticing what sets these images in place.

UNDERLYING FORCES

MILLER: So it's not diversity but an understanding of a whole system.

WALKER: Yes. Patricia Hill Collins (1990) talks of "the matrix of domination," acknowledging the many categories of stratification. In the matrix, people are "better than" or "less than" along a number of dimensions and different levels of power inherent in each category.

There is a tendency in this culture to portray some of the results or manifestations of stratified difference, but not the underlying forces. An example of this tendency would be the conventional interpretations of violence. For example, the media show crime-ridden neighborhoods or barrios that are imploding, but they don't show those banks that redline and participate in the creation of desolation and nihilism. Another example would be the common depiction of poor and working-class, predominantly white neighborhoods as "racist." These neighborhoods bear the stigma of political deviance without an analysis of the oppressive and violating effects of the matrix of domination on poor whites.

MILLER: I've thought that dominant groups in this society tend to project the parts of life that they devalue onto others—for example, people of color or poor or working-class people. They portray others as more sexual or more physical and brawny or more violent. In doing this, dominant groups deny large parts of their own experience. They don't find the ways to integrate these parts of life into growthful cultural images.

Another feature is that such a situation keeps dominant group members from knowing the effects of their own actions. We've said that people learn about themselves (and others) only as they engage in interaction with others. If dominant groups interact with others in only very limited and restricted ways, they don't learn.

Do you think that's so, or is that too much "psychologizing"?

WALKER: I think what you're saying is true on a lot of different levels. If we were to talk about racial violence, for example, the images that typically come to mind involve some conflagration of dispossessed people throwing rocks and burning things, usually their own surroundings. We are less likely to surface images of those powerful white men redlining in banks, charging unfair and disproportionately high interest rates on loans, or refusing to give loans, decisions based only on racial categories or sometimes race and gender. These are forms of racial violence, but they are not the images we usually construct.

Because of the power they have, these men have what we might call "other ways of doing violence." People who don't have the means to perpetrate invisible violence are more easily seen, more easily scapegoated. The dynamic of invisibility works within as well as across racial groups.

Again, for example, talk of racial violence by whites usually centers on those with the least economic clout. We rarely identify more economically privileged neighborhoods or suburbs as centers of racial violence. Are we then saying that people in the less privileged areas are inherently less enlightened than people who are in more privileged neighborhoods? So the projections you talk about sort of get booted downhill, so to speak; so that whoever are those in the least powerful position are going to have all of that stuff projected onto them.

MILLER: And it allows the top people to not really see or admit to what they participate in—another way of living without knowing.

WALKER: Right. There's a theorist, Joel Kovel (1984), who talks about the aversive and the dominant forms of racism. I think you can probably do that with any form of "ism." The aversive racist is the one who can perpetrate violence invisibly. The dominant racist is out there throwing Molotov cocktails or marching in protest against desegregation or some other form of power sharing. Kovel maintains that the person with the power—the aversive racist—will always prepare the blow that is delivered by the dominant racist. Another scholar who talks about these patterns is Dr. Kenneth Hardy (1996). He says that people who have power are able to perpetrate racism without leaving their fingerprints on it. Those people can then talk about the less powerful people—either within their own race or not—as unenlightened or racist. They never have to face those parts of their own being. Thus, they never take the opportunity to grow and come into a fuller humanity by owning these parts of themselves.

MILLER: Also, if you teach disconnection as part of your culture, which you do as soon as you have these categories, it warps your own people. Inevitably, you can't be teaching people to find the fullness of love or justice. This is complex because, for example, some white people can be aversive or dominant racists and can seem to be very good to their own children. But it seems to me that can be true only up to a point because they are teaching hate.

WALKER: And when you get to that certain point, you can see how true that statement is. Maybe that point is reached when you try to push beyond a certain image that a person holds dear; then it takes very little to get to a place of violence. You can see this dynamic working in the family or in the little community that the person seems good to and tightly bonded with. You can't really build sustainable bonds around hatred and disconnection. A piece that makes the disconnection intractable is that it is not named. When it's not named, people learn to do disconnection and hatred without talking about it. So it's not available for examination.

"DOING DISCONNECTION"

WALKER: There is a powerful example that speaks to the complexity of teaching people how to *do* disconnection based on categories of difference. I've had the opportunity to do work with many white people who grew up going to Catholic schools in the 1940s and 1950s. Many of them reported that on Fridays they would all bring in "pennies for the black babies." In some cases with enough pennies you could "buy" a black baby. That was sort of like getting a gold star. People from different schools in different cities and countries talked about this practice. One gentleman went so far as to describe a statuette in his school that was rigged up so that when the pennies were dropped in, a black child figurine would nod a silent "Thank you."

Now the power of that image is this: There were children who were supposedly being taught really good things about love, charity, caring for the stranger, enlarging a sense of social and faith-filled responsibility. Those were very positive, very powerful messages, but at the same time those children were being taught to problematize a whole group of people and see them as "less than," inadequate, inferior, incapable.

MILLER: That's a striking example. Teaching or doing a supposedly good thing is so contaminated . . .

WALKER: So intertwined. It's no wonder that people end up feeling split and confused. Janet Helms (1992) did some research on that. One of the outcomes she talked about is that because of being systematically socialized to have more power, or think they are "better than," lots of white people are filled with ambivalence. She says that white people learn a lot about being white but don't learn much about how to talk about it. I imagine this is true about any group socialized to think they are "better than" other groups.

MILLER: In these times, when a dominant group is oppressing people, there's a whole denial of what we're doing. I mean it's rarely said in the media or other places that that's what they're doing.

WALKER: In fact, there are whole sets of myths set up to perpetuate the denial: meritocracy, for one example; individual endeavor is another.

For example, affirmative action is associated with powerless people. It's not called affirmative action when a powerful man hires another man who reminds him of himself—or someone with whom he feels socially or politically compatible.

MILLER: In current times, nobody says, "We're a racist society" or "We oppress poor people."

WALKER: No. In fact, it's usually the opposite. What is said are things like "Everybody can make it who really tries."

MILLER: That's the individual endeavor and meritocracy part of it. I've been reading a book that's very enlightening on this topic, *How Jews Became White Folks* by Karen Brodkin (1998). She and others have described how "affirmative action" programs existed historically although they were not called that. For example, after World War II the GI Bill made it possible for many men (and the women vets) to go to college and to own a house through low-interest mortgage programs. But African Americans and some other ethnic and racial groups of people often were systematically excluded from these programs.

You were saying earlier that members of a group that is defined as "better than" need to uphold certain images of themselves. This then affects their images of what can happen in their relationships.

WALKER: Yes. There's a movie, *The Long Walk Home,* in which a white woman gives a ride to her maid during the Montgomery bus boycott. Her husband finds out and says, "Here I am trying to hold up my head as a white man and you're carting around a nigger maid. She's our maid; we don't know her. And we can't know her. She is as different from us as a cat is from a dog." Much of his oppressive behavior (toward his white wife and black maid) was directed toward maintaining an image of himself. Even the stereotypes, the negative images of others, are juxtaposed against images he is trying to maintain of himself.

MILLER: I wanted to return to another point. An effect of all the myths we've been talking about is that they keep the more privileged people from knowing the effects of their own behavior. They're participants in the system, and they don't know it.

WALKER: And don't want to know it. It might be life changing. So there are a lot of systems in place to keep people from knowing.

MILLER: It's again about keeping people from reality.

WALKER: And it's institutionalized in inauthentic relationship. The privileged person never wants to hear from the less privileged person because it shatters whatever myths he has constructed about who he is in the world. To have to hear something different and really get it, I think could catapult a person into a kind of chaos and eventually a real grief process.

RELATIONAL IMAGES AND SOCIETAL EXPECTATIONS

MILLER: We've talked a bit about how the whole overall system operates and a bit about what therefore happens to dominant or privileged groups. We want to discuss further what happens to people who are defined as "less than."

I think you have discussed some of the things that affect children growing up in a group described as "less than" in the United States. You said that inevitably children grow up with a lot of fear. And you related this to how this situation affects their entering into connections—or disconnections. I know you said that children would experience, for one, a huge blow to their sense of fitness for connection.

WALKER: I think I was talking about the fact that from an early age children can get a sense of being defined as a problem. These can be in ways you might not think about, just in ways that say to them, "You are different, and your difference is a problem." Some of that message is delivered just through living in a world where the prevailing images (of what's normal) are different from who the child is. Many people have used the example of "flesh-colored" Band-Aids. The big question is: Whose flesh?

Of course, it's much more than that, but we can't ignore the significance of sensate experience. Take, for instance, hair texture. My son has grown up in predominately white neighborhoods. He could not just walk into any of those many shops lining the streets of our town—as his friends could—to get a haircut. As a youngster, getting a haircut meant giving up an entire Saturday morning and driving 17 or 18 miles into the city to find a skilled barber.

After a while, and many Saturday mornings spent in the car, he became quite fearless (much to the chagrin of his friends) about walking into a suburban shop and asking, "Can anyone here cut my hair?" The reason that's problematic is, first of all, it takes quite a bit of courage for a kid to walk into a place and ask the question: "Can you cut my hair?" Then if the answer is "No," it's not really seen as lack of skill on the barber's part. It's your hair that's problematic, so different, so out of the ordinary that all of us who are skilled in this trade don't need to know how to do it.

That's such a primitive level of being problematized, but when that starts when the child is very young, he is susceptible to taking in the notion of himself as problematic. That's not to say there aren't countervailing forces in the child's supportive relationships; that goes without saying. But that doesn't take away from the fact that there are these kinds of devaluing, sensate experiences.

Then there are other experiences. In one of her talks, Beverly Tatum (see Ayvazian & Tatum, 1997) mentioned the plight of young black males such as her sons, who might be described as rambunctious, spirited, or energetic. Her experience, however, was that teachers were prone to describe the young black boys as angry or aggressive—consistent with the prevailing images of "the angry/violent black male." This description was in stark contrast to the child's white counterparts, who though they were exhibiting similar behaviors, were more likely described as spunky.

How confusing and violating to the child's experience! This misattribution can be done even by well-meaning people: for example, the nice, smiling teacher who's teaching you to read and who seems to care about you. What happens to relational confidence when these images jump up so readily to make her misinterpret a possibly benign action and view behavior as "aggressive" rather than spirited?

MILLER: It's such a big thing. You raised a son. It's constant, right?

WALKER: A constant. A struggle for survival. The child (and the parent) walks around not knowing when the next blow is going to come. I don't know any black parents who don't prepare their sons for the day that they will be stopped and harassed. There is a joke about it; we call it "driving while black." Everyone prepares for that moment. We have to ask what it's like to grow up with awareness that you're under suspicion for being "not as good as," as moral, as unable to contain one's impulses—all those dirty things that are projected on to "lesser" beings.

MILLER: The next thing you talked about was the hypervigilance, the wariness.

WALKER: Well, I think that follows from what we've just been talking about, this expectation that at some point you'll be targeted and for no other reason than the racial categories and the acculturated images associated with them. One lives with the knowledge than the images exist and that they carry profound meaning and expectation.

MILLER: You said that there's even a joke about it, "driving while black." Would you say that that's one of the ways that families and the community give children some strength to deal with this?

WALKER: Yes. Some of the ways are (1) naming it and (2) I think you're right, humor is huge. I think in some ways it breaks the isolation of it, the belief that it's me and I'm a problem. To be able to joke about it collectivizes it. I guess, in a sense, the person doesn't end up carrying this sense of deficiency and defectiveness as her/his own private burden.

MILLER: It's not that it makes it go away or that it's less hurtful.

WALKER: It's just a way to try and understand the "not understandable." A way to frame it. I think about one mother who says that she always told her son to put his hands up over his head when he walks into a store. Jokingly, the point is well made. But it expresses a real sense that things will be really tough for you if you come up against these images in this world. There is always the expectation that you're going to do something that is illegal, that is immoral. It will not go well for you. It won't be seen as a childish prank; it will be seen as the "criminal impulses in you" or something like that.

Unfortunately, the prevailing relational images are such that the experience is almost clichéd. My son was searched one morning when he went into a supermarket to buy a protractor to use in his geometry class. There were so many interesting parts of that experience. One was the way he told me about it. He didn't tell me on the day it happened, nor did he mention it as a "headline" comment. He told it almost as a sidebar remark. I think this way of recounting the experience spoke to the shame and ambivalence he was feeling, as well as the self-doubt. I think he felt he had done something wrong even though he clearly knew he hadn't. It spoke to that notion of disconnection from self. In one of the early papers, you wrote that under conditions of systematic inequality, the person violated will often feel at fault for the disconnection.

A couple of interesting things happened after we learned about his experience. We were able to connect with him and support him so that he got reconnected to *himself* and could talk with clarity about what had happened to him. That was such a striking example of how connection with others leads to better connection with oneself, with one's own experience.

He knew that we were going to follow up and talk about it, make it a larger discussion. He knew that it wasn't just an interpersonal event but one that had community consequences. We went to the head of the corporation and requested a meeting. One part of the response was quite disturbing. Perhaps because the corporate management was fearful of litigation, they proceeded to scapegoat the young assistant manager who had subjected my son to the search. As a family, we were not the least concerned with anything litigious; we were focused on education, recovery, and prevention.

My concern was this: "What is going on in your organization that led your young manager to think he was doing the right thing by searching my son, a young black male standing in the aisles gazing at school supplies?" The organization pulled out the young manager and they were ready to publicly castigate him as an aberrant person (again the least powerful singled out for "deviant" acts). They wanted to show us what they had written in his personnel file. We refused to look at that.

Our objective was to facilitate a conversation between the manager and our son in the interest of relational clarity and confidence. We also wanted to talk about what should happen in the organization so that other young people would not be subjected to similar mistreatment. The management didn't get that, but conveniently targeted a relatively less powerful young manager and hung him out to dry. To do otherwise would have forced corporate management to acknowledge that powerful cultural systems were in place that led the young manager to expect that he would be rewarded for his vigilance in protecting the store against the likes of this young, presumably larcenous black male.

MILLER: Did talking about that get anywhere with them?

WALKER: I don't think that went anywhere. The young manager got the incident on his record and eventually got transferred out of the store. It was an unsatisfactory outcome because vengeance was not the goal.

MILLER: Did your son feel supported?

WALKER: My son felt very, very supported because we had that conversation. The director of personnel came, the manager came, and I'm sure they were very rehearsed. The assistant manager who conducted the search was forced to give an abject apology, to say (1) that he didn't intend any harm and (2) that what he did was not a racist act. Of course, that's a classic tactic of domination: "Now that we've done what we've done, let's mystify what we've done." My son accepted the apology and said, "I do want to understand what 'it' was then." You know, please explain the "it" to me and tell me what "it" was if not racism. What was there in my behavior (being) that led to my being searched? Although there was no response to that question, it was good that in spite of the "apology," my son could stay connected enough to know that there was some level of mystification going on. Under other circumstances, the mystification could work to make him unclear about what he was feeling and thinking. That's getting back to the receptivity issues and the images issues.

MILLER: So a big thing for him was to know he could count on you.

WALKER: He could count on family and also he could count on the process of dialogue. He could also know not to have big expectations of dialogue but just to go through the process. I think the process of going through it was really important, of having a place to push for clarity. Clarity may come to different people in different conversations. It's back to that notion of how growth occurs. We don't always see it at the same rate in all parties. It may be in a few events later or further removed that whatever learning there is can take hold or get clearer. Probably, something transformative happened for everybody, just different things.

MILLER: So putting this in terms of the impact on connection, you also said that these threats have a big impact on receptivity.

WALKER: Right. And I don't think we can underestimate the amount of shame that these threats and negative expectations engender. We know that shame has a big impact on receptivity. One way of dealing with shame is to try not to feel what one really feels in those circumstances. Sometimes there may be collusion with the mystification. Sometimes in the midst of such disconnection, all that can be expressed is the anger or the contempt or the joke, and not the shame or the extreme weariness. In such instances, one is not open to one's own experience, sometimes because it's too much to bear in the moment. The fatigue, the disappointment, the wariness, and the sense of hopelessness in some instances hang like a shadow over interpersonal encounters.

The novelist Bebe Campbell-Moore describes it well. In response to the horror of the Holocaust, many Jewish people say, "Never again." In response to the repetitive trauma of racism, she suggests that a more appropriate saying among African Americans would be "When will it end?"

I remember once feeling quite indignant that the receptionist at a gym I frequented was an older white man who would invariably speak to me if there were no other white people around. If there were white people around he would ignore me and act as though I wasn't coming through the door. The contrast was striking. We were both part of a system stratified along dimensions of class, occupational status, and race—probably along with many others. Although my professional status was culturally constructed as "better than," my racial status was clearly "less than." And in all instances, it was the "less than" that defined the interactions. Now this wasn't new learning for me. I had experienced such feelings before. It took me a while to recognize and name something more than anger about this situation. I realized, when I was able to really stay with the feeling and really keep connected to what was going on, that I had no ill feelings toward him at all. What I really felt was extreme weariness. I felt pain and sadness at how much our relationship embodied the pain of the world.

MILLER: When you stayed with your feelings, you reached a new view?

WALKER: Whatever relief comes because recognition breaks isolation. The pain is bigger than the dyad, even though we are live embodiments of it in the moment. And by staying alive to and connected with our feelings—thoughts in those moments, we have an opportunity to change them.

CONTROLLING IMAGES AND RELATIONAL IMAGES

MILLER: You were saying also, "When will it end?" This just goes on and on in large and small ways, and it's exhausting.

WALKER: It's hard if there is an expectation of harm; then it's going to be very difficult to be open—either to your own experience or to being transformed by other people. I think that's a huge piece. I think it's scary to talk about. We sometimes get rutted in disconnections because the possibility of connection does bring with it vulnerability—the challenge to let go of the relational images that seem to provide a protective function. It is sometimes quite difficult to talk about transformation and mutuality on all sides of the structured-in inequalities. I guess in some instances, it is not always politically expedient to talk about how anyone in the relationship has to be open to change.

Typically what we get in much so-called diversity training is that the people who inhabit the more powerful categories need to behave better. That's certainly true. However, relational–cultural healing is also about how everybody needs to be open to *movement*. The gross and subtle inequalities of a stratified culture inhibit our willingness to receive and to allow and show others that they have an impact on us. We get stuck with these images of the other person or of ourselves that make it hard to move or to be open to any kind of movement. I think it's just all related.

MILLER: You're saying that RCT holds that mutuality is the basic force that leads to something happening between people that we call transforming. If you have relational images that make you not as receptive as you could be, immediately that's going to interfere with that mutuality—and therefore with movement, change, growth, or transformation.

WALKER: Right, it affects what you hear, how you hear, how you receive—sometimes hearing through the layers of historical images rather than being active and aware in the moment.

MILLER: You've mentioned a fourth factor, that these experiences then shape the images of relational possibility.

WALKER: I find myself thinking more about Patricia Hill Collins term "controlling images" and the images we get from the dominant culture, both individually and collectively. According to Collins, controlling images have the effect of making oppression appear to be a normal, natural part of everyday life. They take on special meaning because the power to define the images resides with the dominant group. These images are then key in maintaining interlocking systems of race, class, and gender oppression even when the political and economic conditions that originally generated the images disappear (Collins, 1990).

I am particularly concerned for young people who get so many images coming from the dominant culture, very few of which are about how to be in mutually empowering relationship—I should say, how to be in relationship in more liberating, transformative ways. The images promulgated through the media are about how to establish dominance and subordination. And I think they cripple people a lot.

Recently, I was having a conversation with some young people about the images that come through music. There's a very popular song by a young woman, "I Was Born to Make You Happy," or something like that. We were saying, "Wow. What an image that is for an 11-year-old to hear about who she can be in the world and who she can be in relationship." I think it is important for families and courageous communities of people to say something different. It's crucial for the family and caring communities to be cognizant that when she's grooving to a song like that, she's getting images of relational possibility, not just cognitively but also on an emotive and sensate level. I think we deal with those images and we have to have ways to make them conscious. In the course of our listening to the music, I don't think such images are even conscious.

In terms of race relationships, a lot of the images that come through affect us in ways that are not conscious, in ways that we sort of swallow without thinking about what we're swallowing. An advertising campaign by a major automotive company exemplifies this issue. The ad was trying to show the car company as one that valued diversity and employed different kinds of people. There was also a theme about total quality assurance and about how decisions can be made on the spot. The purpose of the ad was to show that any employee is empowered to stop the assembly line to correct a defect, so that we consumers can have confidence in the quality of their product. The scene unfolds with an African American man on the assembly line; he's looking at the product with a really studied focus. He sees something wrong and stops the line because he spies a defective molding of some sort. He holds up production until the problem is corrected.

On one level the image is of this African American male who's making the decision that helps us to have confidence in the quality of the product. However, the commercial doesn't end until a white male comes over, places his hand on the black worker's shoulder, and pats him with a silent message: "Good job." So the message was loud and clear that we still needed the white male voice-over before something can be defined as good and trustworthy.

I think that's an example of an image that comes in quite unconsciously and that, unless we talk about it, can provide a distorted response to the questions: "Whom can we trust; who is capable, and who gets to say what knowledge or what expertise is, and how does it get sanctioned in this society?" It was done in such a seductive and slick way that it would be hard to know what it was conveying.

MILLER: And this is the new way to make a car youthful and "with it."

WALKER: These are examples of controlling images that tell us what to expect of ourselves and of other people. Put another way, the images seek to define the roles that people can take in relationships. With sufficient proliferation, the very limited roles seem natural and necessary rather than socially ascribed.

MILLER: You were starting to say this is about the images and how few we have that are about good connection.

WALKER: And how many images we have that are about dominating something or someone, or being dominated by someone. The images may also be about being seen as a product or a prize. These are images that support inauthenticity, images that support strategies of disconnection. Sometimes the images are about "having" relationship as a possession or a prize. What we see in media is that relationship is not a way of being. It's something to have, with connotations of "power over." The images do not help us develop good connection practices.

This feels quite important because I think it addresses how we want to be with people. What is the quality of relationship we seek? Far too often, when the emphasis is on having "power over," we behave in relationships in ways that seek to maintain stasis, that keep our cherished images in place even if they are destructive ones.

MILLER: It seems to me that you're developing a very helpful linkage using the concept of "images." Patricia Hill Collins (1990) has spoken of "controlling images," which the dominant groups in a culture impose. We've spoken of relational images that people construct from their experiences in relationships. I think you're spelling out some of the ways that the culture's controlling images become internalized in the individual's relational images, that is, how the external becomes the internal or how the cultural becomes the psychological.

Controlling images based on dominance and subordination affect the relational images of both the dominants and the subordinates but in different ways for each group. Most importantly, they create a mode of operation, a *modus vivendi* that hinders openness to the influence of others, to receiving the experience of others—the openness that is essential for connection. And connection is the source of growth for each group and each person in the group.

WALKER: Yes, the culture itself becomes an agent of disconnection and distortion, proliferating images that undermine mutuality and authenticity. So much of what we deal with are power distortions that interfere with relational development. Growth and healing take us back to the notion of mutuality—not sameness, but openness to influence on both sides. Growth-in-connection means recognizing that everybody lives under a culture that prescribes relational violations: a culture that says, "this is how to survive under these conditions" and so forth. Nobody walks out unscathed, and everybody has to be open to transformation.

Further, if I spend so much of my time and energy scanning the world for possible trouble, I can lose touch with my own desire. An Afro-Caribbean business student once said to me, "I spend so much time playing defense here that I forget where I'm going." When focused on survival and defense in a "power over" relationship, whether organizational or personal, strategies for disconnection become standard operating procedure. To merely survive, a person may set up so many conditions for connection that make authenticity all but impossible. The relational damage is obvious; it is impossible to focus on objectifying the other without doing the same to oneself.

MILLER: Can you explain that a little more?

WALKER: I'm thinking about how dehumanizing the whole process of stratification and power distortion can be so that as a way of surviving one might say, "Men are like this," or "White people are like this," or "Republicans do this, and Democrats are like this—whatever." To the extent that I have captured them in an image, there's a complementary image of myself that doesn't allow for shades of gray, doesn't allow for ambivalence, doesn't allow for movement. Those stances are all about blockages to mutuality and to movement and growth. The movement really happens in the gray. Disconnection also happens in the gray, in the subtleties.

An interesting by-product of social progress is that the universe of relationships is harder to scan. That was illustrated in the automobile commercial we talked about earlier. There have been times when the inequities were gross and blatant. Most often that's not now the case—at least in the professional and social arenas where a lot of us are operating. (When I say that, I realize how class bound what I just said is. I'm sure there are places where the inequities are as gross as they have ever been in the past, but for the people who've been helped by all the civil rights progress, all the middle-class and upper-middle-class people, the relational arena is larger and larger. (There certainly are other places you can be where the relational world is quite small.) But there's the danger that the relational arena is getting larger and larger and our connection practices haven't kept up with the arena. Our relational practices can get smaller and more restricted.

MILLER: So would you say it's harder or more confusing and mystified today?

WALKER: Maybe I'd say it's more complex. It's different for each generation. The black sons of this generation are probably less likely to suffer the fate of Emmett Till, getting beaten and lynched and thrown into a river. However, I do think this generation has to figure out more ambiguities without having a lot of cultural support. This generation has to figure out how to do connection practices in a culture that does not support authenticity and mutuality. If you have a relational arena that is large and filled with ambiguities but you have relational images that are tight and don't allow room for movement, then you have the possibilities for lots of disconnection. That's where I see the room for healing.

And I think it is a part of this current patriarchal setup of disconnection, this need to have categories based on this notion that somebody's got to be "better than" and somebody's got to be "less than" in order for the world to go on—or the world, as it is constructed, to go on. It really is about connection and about what derails connection. Intuitively, when I talk about this topic, I say it's about healing the world. And I believe it; I believe it. But I think we have to clarify and define further just how it is.

REFERENCES

Ayvazian, A., & Tatum, B. D. (1997). Women, race and racism: A dialogue in black and white. *Work in Progress, No. 68.* Wellesley, MA: Stone Center Working Paper Series.

Brodkin, K. (1998). *How Jews became white folks.* New Brunswick, NJ: Rutgers University Press.

Chittister, J. D. (1998). *Heart of flesh: A feminist spirituality for women and men.* Grand Rapids, MI: Erdmans.

Collins, P. H. (1990). *Black feminist thought: Knowledge, consciousness, and the politics of empowerment.* Boston: Unwin Hyman.

Hardy, K. (1996). Unpublished results of a symposium. Maine Institute for Family Therapy, Portland, ME.

Helms, J. E. (1992). *A race is a nice thing to have: A guide to being a white person or understanding the white persons in your life.* Topeka, KS: Content Communications.

Jordan, J. V. (Ed.). (Ed.). (1997). *Women's growth in diversity: Writings from the Stone Center.* New York: Guilford Press.

Jordan, J., Kaplan, A. G., Miller, J. B., Stiver, I. P., & Surrey, J. L. (1991). *Women's growth in connection: More writings from the Stone Center.* New York: Guilford Press.

Kovel, J. (1984). *White racism: A psychohistory.* New York: Columbia University Press.

Miller, J. B., & Stiver, I. P. (1997). *The healing connection: How women form relationships in therapy and life.*. Boston: Beacon Press.

8

Women, Race, and Racism
A Dialogue in Black and White

ANDREA AYVAZIAN *and* BEVERLY DANIEL TATUM

*B*EVERLY DANIEL TATUM: We're very pleased to be here this evening. This presentation is the outgrowth of a paper I presented at the Stone Center in 1993 entitled, "Racial Identity Development and Relational Theory: The Case of Black Women in White Communities." That paper (Tatum, 1993) was based on my research with black women in predominantly white communities. One of the themes that emerged repeatedly in my data was how difficult it can be for black women in white communities to find the kind of mutually empathic relationships that lead to the emotional growth described by the Stone Center theorists (Jordan, Kaplan, Miller, Stiver, & Surrey, 1991). During the discussion that followed my presentation that evening, a white woman in the audience asked, "How can a white woman genuinely befriend a black woman? How can that kind of relationship be nourished across racial lines?" That is the question that we intend to address here.

Jean Baker Miller (1988) has written eloquently about the constructive power of relational connections and the potentially destructive force of relational disconnections and violations. This theme of connections, disconnections, and violations is certainly central to our thinking about how we can connect across racial lines. What happens when our experience is validated by another in a mutually empathic relationship? We feel a strong sense of connection. But when we have experiences that are not validated, for example, when I as a black woman encounter racism and I am unable to talk about that experience with white colleagues, I may feel a sense of disconnection from them. Or should I choose to share those experiences and in fact find them invalidated by my colleagues, I may question my own perceptions. Without validation from others, I may choose to deny my own perceptions in order to avoid the isolation that comes from disconnection. Repeatedly separating myself from my own experience in order to stay in relationship with others ultimately results in a psychological state of violation. Negotiating the choices involved in maintaining connections across racial lines is a central focus of our dialogue (presented in this chapter).

ANDREA AYVAZIAN: I want to add my welcome and my greetings to Beverly's, and I want to say that for both of us, although we travel nationwide and do work on issues of racial justice offering consultation and seminars together, we have decided to take a personal risk tonight by offering a look into the issue of connections across racial barriers by using our own relationship as the basis of our talk. Beverly and I are venturing into new territory by offering an analysis of our own relationship as a case study of women connecting across racial lines. We want to speak very personally tonight because, as Bev said, this question was asked when she was here a year ago. I can also add that in traveling and doing speaking with Beverly, white women often stop me in hallways and restrooms and at the coffee machine and say, "You two seem so close. How did you create that bond?" So we want to look at our relationship in the light of Jean Baker Miller's work. We are going to focus on the following three areas, which we call the critical junctures in our relationship: how the relationship was established, the theme of mutuality in our relationship, and difficult periods we have faced. A thread that is also woven into our talk is what we call "common differences," areas where there is sameness between us, where we have similar feelings, viewpoints, even experiences, and yet these similarities are expressed in different ways in our lives. We will close by talking about our friendship as a work in progress. So with that background and appreciating you all for sharing in what is a new venture for us—to speak about these issues very personally—we want to begin by discussing the critical junctures in our relationship within the framework of this theme of connections, disconnections, and violations.

CRITICAL JUNCTURES

AYVAZIAN: When I think about some of the critical junctures in our friendship—for example, how we met and how the relationship began—I am reminded of an article by Joe Wood (1994) that I read in the *New York Times Magazine*. In the article, Wood, who is black, was talking about his friendship with Dan, who is Jewish. Wood said of the relationship: "Our kinship is not easy."

In many ways, my kinship with Beverly is *very* easy. Deep affection and admiration flows between us and the friendship is strong, nourishing, and treasured. However, it is also fair to say that nowadays any adult relationship that crosses racial lines is "not easy." If the friends are conscious of the social, political, and economic realities in this country today, their "kinship," as Wood states, will inevitably have times that are "not easy." And we have faced those times.

To put this in perspective, let me back up and provide some of the details about how our relationship was formed. Our relationship was established on a professional basis. Beverly and I do not live in the same neighborhood, although we live in the same town, and we do not work in the same place. Our children do not attend the same schools. We were brought together by an agency that does antiracism education, paired up as a biracial team to do some antiracism training at a college in the Boston area. We were brought together initially on a professional basis and immediately had the experience of preparing to work together as a team. Also, because the job in Boston involved a series of workshops, we had the experience of traveling to and from our area in western Massachusetts to Boston, a 2-hour car ride each way. Beverly and I call that first professional collaboration, during which our relationship was formed, our "trial by fire." The group of college students with whom we were working proved to be a very challenging group. It was a difficult training because of so many what we call "Yes, buts." The students were resistant to hearing our material and working with the concepts and the framework for understanding race and racism that we were offering. Yet, this adversarial experience actually pulled us together as a twosome. Going into what turned out to be a hostile environment forced us to really scrutinize the material that we were presenting to the group.

Consequently, Beverly and I had the experience of talking very deeply about painful issues around race and racism very early in our professional/personal relationship. We had potentially difficult conversations analyzing racial inequity because we had to scrutinize the material we were presenting to this challenging group. These conversations in the first days of our relationship, we have discovered, are of the sort that biracial friendships sometimes avoid for months or years. Looking back on it now, we believe that this process was a bonding experience.

We also found that our rides to and from Boston were opportunities to talk not only about our work but about our personal lives. We discovered some common ground as women, as mothers, and as professionals in our community. Early on, Beverly was very helpful to me as I was going through a difficult period with my then 1-year-old son. We forged close personal ties through what was initially a professional connection.

TATUM: As Andrea has said, our relationship did form in the context of work. This is an important observation because one of the things that we know about our society is the fact that it is still quite socially segregated. As Andrea has told you, we don't live in the same neighborhood, our children don't go to the same school, and we don't worship in the same places; our lives are separate in many ways. Even though we frequently work together and certainly spend leisure time together now that our friendship has developed, our paths would not likely have crossed in other ways. Given the reality of social segregation, work does provide one of the few places where women of color and white women may come together across racial lines. So, it is not an accident that it was our work together that laid the groundwork for a friendship to develop.

As Andrea mentioned, one of the things that has been very important is that at the beginning of our relationship there was an examination of our values as they related to the work that we did. We were forced to talk at a deeper level—not the superficial chitchat that you might engage with someone over the coffee machine—regarding what we thought about a very significant issue, in this case race relations in the United States. The mutuality that evolved in that relationship was very much in keeping with what Jean Baker Miller calls the "five good things." When a relationship is in fact mutually reinforcing, it gives you a feeling of increased zest, a sense of empowerment, greater self-knowledge, increased self-worth, and—most important in the context of a friendship—a desire for more connection (Miller, 1988). Certainly as the mutuality in the relationship became apparent, we did seek each other's company outside of work situations, and we have been fortunate to have been able to share life experiences, as Andrea has said, around issues of parenting and personal relationships of a wide variety. That has been very important.

But as in all relationships, conflict arises. There certainly has been some conflict in our relationship, which we want to talk about, too, because it is also an important part of how one negotiates relationships that are going to be genuinely mutual. The most significant conflict, a real test of mutuality in our relationship, occurred when Andrea and I were conducting a workshop in St. Louis about 3 years ago. At that time, we were facilitating a workshop with a group of clergy on racism and, as we often do, we made reference to other "isms," including heterosexism. This topic, in the midst of a roomful of clergy representing a variety of religious traditions, triggered a rather heated discussion about homosexuality in which a range of religious viewpoints were expressed. As we struggled to deal with this issue in the context of our workshop, Andrea and I became aware of the fact that we had differing strategies for interacting with our participants on this issue. While we were able to deal with that difference productively in the context of the workshop, as we were processing the event on the flight home we had a conversation that led to a real test of the mutuality in our relationship.

As background information for this incident, I should say that I had just become very involved in a worship community in Springfield. I had just joined a church, which was a very important and significant step in my personal life, and as we talked about the controversy that had arisen in our workshop, we talked about the positions that our own religious communities had regarding homosexuality and heterosexism in the church. I am a member of a Presbyterian church. At this writing, that denomination is in the midst of a struggle around whether or not to ordain gay men and lesbian women. Andrea is a Quaker and belongs to a Meeting that is openly gay affirming and sanctions and supports same-sex commitment ceremonies. So our two worship communities have very different positions.

Andrea said to me that she didn't understand how I could be a part of a religious community that was exclusionary in the way that the Presbyterian church currently is, and in fact suggested that I should find another church. When she first said it, I was taken aback by the comment but had some trouble figuring out exactly what it was about it that bothered me. In fact, I shared her concern about the heterosexism in my denomination and in my local church. I have raised, and continue to raise, questions about this issue with my pastor and with fellow parishioners. On the other hand, my local congregation is a relatively progressive, predominantly black, Afrocentric congregation that is very affirming of my racial and spiritual identity in many ways. I experienced Andrea's suggestion that I should leave this congregation as an affront. I did not express this initially but withdrew into reading a book, and we completed the plane ride in relative silence. I continued to think about the conversation and later realized what was most offensive to me about it.

It occurred to me that there was really a lot of white privilege in her statement. As a black woman living in a predominantly white community, there are not many opportunities for me or my children to be part of a community where our African American heritage is explicitly affirmed. Consequently our Sunday worship experience in a congregation that defines itself as "unashamedly black and unapologetically Christian" is extremely valuable to me. I did feel that her statement that I should withdraw from this community was a statement of her white privilege. In fact, she was taking for granted the many churches or worship communities that she can choose from because almost all of them are predominantly white and will affirm her racial identity. She can easily choose to be a Quaker without worrying that she and her family will again be one of few white families present. Her statement to me was a failure to recognize that privilege.

I felt that I had to say something to her about this. At the same time, I hesitated because this relationship was important to me and I did not want to alienate our friendship. Yet, it was a real juncture in terms of this issue of connections, disconnections and violations, because I could feel myself disconnecting. Was my spirituality an aspect of my life that I would not be able to share with this person? In order for us to be able to maintain the growth and development of our relationship, certainly being able to talk about my spiritual journey and my worship community was an important point of connection that I needed to be able to maintain. I decided to share my perspective with Andrea, and I am happy to report that she responded in a very validating way. She simply listened to what I had to say and then said, "You're right."

AYVAZIAN: I want to speak to this because a potentially serious "disconnection" threatened our relationship—a relationship that had developed strong bonds, one that had become mutually important. When Beverly raised her feelings and concerns with me, two things went through my mind—two things that I knew she and I had said specifically to white people many times in the past! One was that when a person of color tells you something you have said or done is racist or reveals your inattention to white privilege, take a deep breath and begin by assuming she/he is correct until proven otherwise. The other point is that as white people strive to be strong white allies, we do not have to hold ourselves to a standard of perfection. It is impossible, given our socialization, our background, the struggle, the sensitivity, and the pain surrounding these issues, that we can be perfect white allies. I try to remember that I am not called to be perfect, I am called to be faithful and consistent on these issues. Beverly was exactly right. I remembered all the times I have said to white people: "When your racism is pointed out to you, when your privilege is made evident again, just listen, listen undefensively, and take a deep breath and respond in ways that will further your progress along this difficult journey." I tried to follow the very advice that I had given to others. I tried to follow the advice I heard from a man of color who, when I asked him what he most wanted from his white allies, he responded, "I want them to be consistently conscious." I believed that this was an opportunity for me to not attempt to be perfect or defensive but to say, "I'm on a journey and have not yet arrived." That was an important juncture: a disconnection threatened, but we managed to talk it through.

There was another time that a disconnection threatened but was overcome by both of us being aware of what was going on in the relationship. This happened around the time of the Rodney King beating and the Simi Valley verdict in which the four Los Angeles police officers were acquitted. After the Rodney King beating, both Beverly and I were shaken by the videotape, and we were stunned by the news of the acquittals. But again, Beverly and I responded in a manner that we had actually talked about with other groups. It was a surprise, but in some ways not a surprise, to find ourselves experiencing it. In our shock and grief following the Simi Valley verdict, we essentially separated for a period of time and turned to different communities for comfort and support. Bev talked about her reactions to the events primarily with other African Americans. I suspected that she would want to immerse in the black community, and then I witnessed it. In my own state of pain, shock, and anger, I found myself talking to two white men who I specifically called and met with, two men who identify as white allies. Meeting with them was the appropriate place for me to take my grief and do some healing and action planning in order to move forward.

In fact, one of the meetings that I had following the verdict was with a minister in our community, the Reverend Peter Ives. During those meetings in which we grieved and expressed our despair and outrage, we also said to each other that we needed to do something that was proactive, visible, and long term to bring issues of dismantling racism into the centerpiece of our community. From those meetings, something very positive was created—the Committee for Northampton.

Taking a moment to explain what was born from this time of upheaval and pain might be instructive. The Committee for Northampton began with just two people, quickly grew to two dozen, and soon encompassed hundreds of people in our community who joined together to bring issues of dismantling racism into every conceivable aspect of community life. The committee designated 1993 as the year when "dismantling racism" would be the overarching theme for our small city of 35,000. A committee that included parents, teachers, city counselors, business owners, members of the clergy, students, and others spent the second half of 1992 organizing activities that would happen in 1993—including hanging a banner across Main Street with our goal, "Dismantling Racism, Building Community." In fact, we were very successful. During 1993, the Committee for Northampton organized or cosponsored 54 events in 52 weeks. These included speakers in the service clubs, pulpit exchanges, dismantling racism workshops, film and video series, cultural events, dinners and picnics, photography exhibits, and special events in the schools. The year culminated with eight performances of Langston Hughes's play, *Black Nativity*. The Committee for Northampton grew out of our response to the atrocities in California.

Following the Simi Valley verdict it was appropriate for Beverly and me to separate for a while and immerse ourselves in our own groups to work on these issues. We recognized that the separation did not need to be a disconnection. We maintained the connection between us, but we recognized then, as we do now, that there are times when it is more appropriate to seek the comfort, support, and planning time with, in my case, strong white allies; in her case, members of the African American community. I bring this up now because I have heard so many white people talk about periods when they feel separated from their friends of color who go without them to a meeting, an event, or an empowerment group. This is an important point because white people can feel a loss, and even a sense of personal rejection, when this happens. I don't think these periods of separation should be interpreted in that fashion. Beverly and I see these as normal, necessary, and even predictable after racial trauma. The bridges that have been built may be perfectly strong, but there still may be a need to separate for a time.

TATUM: I want to add just a few comments to what Andrea has said. In fact, the weekend when the events following the Simi Valley verdict were unfolding, I was at a small women's conference, a gathering of about 20 women, to which I had been invited. The only person I knew in the group was the woman who had invited me, and I was the only woman of color there, As we were arriving, everyone was very much aware of the riots that were unfolding in Los Angeles following the acquittal, and what struck me was the reluctance among the group to talk in any serious way about what was going on in Los Angeles. A few people expressed a need to talk about what was happening and what it meant for the country and for their own particular communities, but generally speaking the majority of the participants seemed to disregard these events as someone else's problem, not of concern to us as a group. I felt very alienated by that response, I have to say. Perhaps because I was with white women I didn't know, it did not feel like a safe place for me to completely engage. I was quite concerned about what was happening in communities of color in Los Angeles and in other parts of the country in response to this verdict. Yet I felt that my concern, a part of who I was, a part of my own perspective as an African American woman, could not be safely brought to this meeting. I certainly experienced that as very disconnecting, and in fact I went home early from the conference and declined the invitation to attend the following year.

AYVAZIAN: Beverly and I also want to talk about other ways that we feel connections and to respond to a question that is often asked of us about our relationship. White people often say to me, "It sounds like you two work together on issues of racism and talk about them very openly in your friendship, but are you, Andrea, always in the position of learner?" Beverly and I want to take a moment to remind all of us that each individual has multiple social identities. We feel this point is important because there are ways that Beverly and I are, in some areas of systematic oppression, both in the dominant category. We both receive the privilege or advantage, and we support each other in being strong allies. I am not always in the position of being dominant, and Beverly is not always in the position of being targeted. In the area of race inequity and racism—in that form of systematic oppression—I am clearly dominant. I receive the privilege, the unearned advantage and benefit of being white, and Beverly is targeted.

But there are other areas where Beverly and I are both targeted and areas where we are both dominant. We're both targeted as women, and we're both dominant as Christians, as heterosexuals, as able bodied, as middle class. We felt it was useful to remember that as women we both feel targeted in groups of men where we are negotiating around money, for example. We are both disadvantaged systematically in a society that overvalues male attributes and characteristics. Again, the writing of Jean Baker Miller (1987) is useful here as she discusses the experience of gender domination and subordination in her book, *Toward a New Psychology of Women*. The fact that we are both practicing Christians and women of faith and identify very strongly and publicly in that way means we are both dominant. We are not Jewish or Muslim. We are both able-bodied, both heterosexual, both middle-class women, and we offer each other support in remembering that we have a responsibility to interrupt anti-Semitism, to interrupt homophobia and heterosexism, to interrupt classism, and so on. We thought it was necessary to bring our attention to the fact that because each of us has multiple identities and plays multiple roles in a multilayered fabric in society, we offer each other support and connection around being allies in areas where we are dominant and in the area where we are both targeted as women.

TATUM: Obviously in any relationship the kind of support you receive from the person with whom you are in relationship is significant. As Andrea has discussed, we do support each other in our own journey toward understanding the implications of our social identities, both in those areas where we are dominant and where we are targeted. But I want to also speak about another place where I have felt a great deal of support in our relationship. This has been around a personal experience of loss. As I have indicated, my worship community is a very significant part of my life, and 2 years ago we experienced the loss of our pastor. For those of you not involved in a worship community, that may seem like a minor thing. Suffice it to say, that it is a lot like losing your therapist. It was a very difficult and painful loss for me to lose the opportunity to regularly meet and talk with someone who had been very influential in my own spiritual development. What I really appreciated was the fact that I was able to share my own grief about this loss with Andrea, who—because she also is a person of faith—was very understanding and appreciative of the significance of this loss for me. Sharing this loss has been a very important and significant part of our relationship. It has been a real source of connection, and I certainly have felt some empowerment in dealing with this transition in my life and the life of my church community through our relationship.

COMMON DIFFERENCES

AYVAZIAN: Given the foregoing discussion of the formation of the relationship, the developing of strong mutual support, respect, and affection between us, and the difficult periods that we have gone through, Beverly and I wanted to move into talking about what we call our "common differences." These are areas where there is sameness between us, yet where our sameness is expressed or manifested differently in our lives because of our racial difference.

Beverly and I are both mothers of sons. One of the areas that has been a strong connection and a source of mutuality is that we have shared considerable dialogue about our children's growth and development over the past 5 years that we have been friends. Beverly has been extremely supportive of me as I have faced challenging periods with my feisty and assertive little boy, who has at times taxed my ability to know what is best for him and how to move forward. My friend Beverly, who happens to be a clinical psychologist, has been very helpful.

We are two mothers with school-age children who have many similarities but who have made some different choices, we believe, because
of our racial difference. In particular, we have made different choices
about the schooling for our sons and the environments we feel they
need in order to thrive. My son is in a public school in our town and
fits in well in his kindergarten class and in his school. During a parent–
teacher conference this past spring, his teacher said to me, "Andrea,
your son is just like a thousand other rambunctious, big-for-his-age 6-
year-old boys that I have had in my teaching career." And I thought to
myself, "I'm sure he is. I'm sure he doesn't stand out in very many ways.
He's like a thousand other children that this woman has had in her
long career of teaching kindergarten." In our predominantly white
community, the same could not be said about Beverly's sons. Her two
African American boys are in a private school setting. I will let her
speak to why that decision was made for her children.

TATUM: It's true that I have chosen to put my children in private
schools. Like many of the black families I interviewed and wrote about
in my book, *Assimilation Blues: Black Families in a White Community*
(Tatum, 1987), I have worried about how my children will be responded to by what has been to date an entirely white teaching staff
(with the exception of an occasional student teacher of color). Though
it may only be an illusion, I believe I have been able to exercise more
control over my children's classroom experiences as a result of enroll-
ing them in private schools. There have been times when I have felt
that racial issues were present in both peer and teacher interactions,
and both my husband and I have been actively involved in negotiating
those issues with the school and our children.

The task of raising young African American children, especially
boys, in contemporary society is not an easy one. My children are also
big for their ages, but unlike for white boys for whom physical maturity
is often a social advantage, being black and big for your age places you
at some psychological risk: 7-year-old black boys may be thought of as
cute; 14-year-old black boys are often perceived as dangerous. The
larger you are, the sooner you must learn to deal with other people's
negative stereotypes, and you may not yet be cognitively and emotionally mature enough to do so effectively. The smallness of their private
school environment, where I can easily make myself known as a parent
and where my children may be seen as individuals rather than representatives of a racial group, may offer some small margin of protection
for them. They will need all the margin they can get. Though I am a
product of public schools myself and I support quality public education, I have not regretted our decision to send our children to private
schools.

AYVAZIAN: There are two other areas we want to talk about in terms of "common differences." As Beverly and I have mentioned throughout our talk, we both identify as women of faith, specifically as Christians, but we express our faith in very different ways. Beverly is a member of an Afrocentric Presbyterian church in Springfield, Massachusetts. I am a member of a Quaker Meeting in Leverett, Massachusetts. The experiences that we are having during the same hour on Sunday mornings are markedly different. When Beverly and I visit each other's houses of worship, we stand out as visitors. I have been to Beverly's church a number of times, and I have been the only white person in the room on a couple of occasions. Beverly has been the only person of color at Quaker worship when she has come to visit my Meeting. At Beverly's church, I have been moved and inspired by the singing, altar calls, testifying, sermons, and other vocal expressions of faith. My Meeting is essentially 80 white people sitting in a room being silent. It is a very different experience. Although comfortable worshiping with each other, we have been struck by the ways that each of us stands out as being a visitor and how we have chosen such different paths to express our faith.

Although I identify as a white antiracist, my "church" experience is very monocultural, and it strikes me as a very "white" thing to do, to sit there in silence. Occasionally people are moved by the Spirit to stand and speak, but it still feels like I am having a very white experience on Sunday mornings. Beverly's worship experience strikes me as being grounded in her African American heritage. Also, when I visit Beverly's church, I am reminded of what it is like to be in the statistical minority. When visitors are recognized during the service at her church and asked to introduce themselves to the congregation, I say my name and that I am there with the Tatum family. Following the service, more than a hundred African Americans come over to greet me by name, "Hi, Andrea. Welcome back." It has been a reminder for me of what it is like to be very visible in a group or community.

TATUM: Another area where our common differences have emerged, and one that actually has been an important aspect of our relationship, is that we have sought different kinds of experiences and some of those have been a point of separation. At one point I decided that I really wanted to have an opportunity to talk about faith in daily living in my own town during the week, rather than always having to drive 30 minutes on the highway to Springfield. So I could have this opportunity more conveniently, I thought I would invite a small group of women to come to my house and talk about these issues. My idea to start such a group was very much influenced by two books I read, *The Monday Connection* by William E. Diehl (1991) and *The Dream of God* by Verna J.

Dozier (1991). I was inspired to call my group the "Dream of God" group.

As I talked about my idea with Andrea, she was very excited about it and wanted to participate. This was a point of discussion because in some ways I had envisioned this as a group of African American women, yet at the same time I did not want to exclude Andrea. We talked about the fact that maybe it could be an "African American women and Andrea" group. In fact, I was willing to do that and discussed it with the other women I had in mind, because I knew she was a woman of faith who would appreciate this opportunity as much as I would. But as circumstances would have it, or perhaps by God's grace, Andrea's schedule conflicted with mine and it was very difficult to find a time when we were both free. So she has not participated in the group. Retrospectively, we both look back on it and agree that perhaps this is how it was meant to be. My group consists of three black women, and it has been a very satisfying experience just as it is.

AYVAZIAN: On this point, with the Dream of God group, and the retreats organized by and for black Christian women that Beverly has also participated in, I have struggled with a certain level of envy, which we have talked about. Beverly has gone away on religious retreats specifically for black women, and she has told me about them in some detail. The reports have been very moving. I have found myself wishing that I could be a part of them and join with her in these experiences, but I know that I can't. Again we have tried to look these times of separation as periods that do not need to be a source of division or disconnection between us. I can hear about the retreats that she's attending without me, support her, and our relationship need not be threatened.

CHOOSING THE MARGIN

The last point that we want to talk about as another example of common differences is what Beverly and I have come to call from "margin to center" or from "center to margin." Both of us have been influenced by the works of bell hooks, particularly *Feminist Theory: From Margin to Center* (1984), and Audre Lorde's work, *Sister Outsider* (1984). Beverly and I have been influenced by these women's writings and the concept of moving from margin to center or, in my case, from center to margin. Let me clarify this further. Beverly and I have remarkably similar political views. We share very similar progressive politics, but again in this area of common differences we have expressed our personal politics in different ways. I am a person who appears to start at or near the center of acceptability and power in our society. As a white, middle-class, heterosexual, able-bodied person, I receive considerable privilege in society. (I'm in so many dominant groups.) I start at the center where social, political, and economic power rests. Consequently, bell hooks's book, *Feminist Theory: From Margin to Center*, speaks to me, but in the reverse. I recognize that I start at the center and I feel called to move to the margin.

As I move to the margin, I try to take other progressive people, specifically in my case well-intentioned white people, with me into more progressive politics, living a more progressive agenda, choosing the margin. To accomplish this, I have made decisions like choosing, since 1981, to be a war tax resister, which means I don't pay a portion of my federal income tax every April; I make a public protest, objecting to the priorities reflected in the military portion of our federal budget and our ongoing preparation for and involvement in war. Also in my journey from center to margin, my life partner (who is male) and I have chosen not to sanctify our union and our love of each other in a formal wedding. Instead we had a ceremony of commitment that could be replicated exactly for same-sex couples. We made this decision so that we can advocate as allies to gay, lesbian, and bisexuals as a couple that has chosen in one small way not to accept heterosexual privilege. Because I start with so much privilege—so clearly at the center—these are two ways that I can move to the margin, stir up good trouble, and invite other people like me to question their politics and live their commitments to the principles they hold dear. However, I have not lobbied for Beverly to make those same choices. There are ways that because of my privilege I've had the luxury to step out of the center, to do what is unexpected and in some ways unacceptable. But I have not during the last 5 years suggested that Beverly make the same choices. For example, with war tax resistance, Beverly supports me. She hears about it all the time; she hears about my latest traumas with the Internal Revenue Service, but we don't have conversations about how I feel she should make the same choice. I recognize that my daily life is more advantaged and more comfortable than hers because of my color. Consequently, I do not advocate that she should choose war tax resistance. She expresses her political convictions in other ways. The same is true around formal marriage and same-sex unions. It has not been an issue for me and it has not been a source of disconnection for us that Beverly has made different choices for her behavior as a strong ally to gay men and lesbians. Her allied behavior is evident in other ways. These are examples of how I believe it is my task to move from center to margin and to take other people with me, as I often say, to stir up good trouble.

TATUM: As Andrea said, this idea, from margin to center, has been important and I'd like to refer to a reading that I found very helpful from Letty M. Russell's book, *Church in the Round: Feminist Interpretation of the Church* (1993). She refers to the work of Audre Lorde and bell hooks, and uses this idea to make the following point. She says, "We make choices about moving from margin toward center or from center toward margin according to where we find ourselves in relation to the center of power and resources and the cultural and linguistic dominance in any particular social structure. Our connection to the margin is always related to where we are standing in regard to social privilege, and from that particular position we have at least three choices, not to choose, to choose the center, or to choose the margins" (p. 192).

As Russell points out, our first choice is not to choose. If we make this choice, if we choose not to choose, we are essentially saying that those of us who are marginalized by gender, race, sexual orientation, class, or disability have the possibility of doing nothing. But, as she says, in so doing we internalize the oppression. I think that if we consider not choosing, if we think about internalizing our oppression and allowing ourselves to be defined as marginal, then we have in effect been psychologically violated. Referring again to Jean Baker Miller's (1988) discussion of disconnections and violations, it seems clear to me that to not choose is in essence a choice of violation, because it forces us to disconnect from our own experience, to try to ignore and not name the particular alienation that we are exposed to in our society.

Our second choice, Russell points out, is to choose the center. She says, "those on the margin choosing the center do so by emulating the oppressors and doing everything to pass or to be like those who are dominant and be accepted by them" (p. 192). Whenever we make this choice we are choosing disconnection in the sense that we are saying, "Yes I want to be in relationship with you. If I have to deny certain aspects of my experience to do so, then I will. I will disconnect from that part of my experience in order to maintain my connection with you." Certainly some black women may choose to do this so the relationships that they develop with their white colleagues will be, by definition, somewhat incomplete because there will be this kind of distancing, or disconnection from one's own experience, or at least those experiences will be kept separate from the relationship.

Our third choice is for the margin. Here Russell says, "Those on the margin claim the margin by working in solidarity with others from the margin as they move toward the center. They seek a transformed society of justice where they will be empowered to share the center and no one will need to be marginalized" (p. 193). As I reflect on this choice, it seems to me this is the choice of connection. This is the choice of saying, "1 will be connected to those who are able to acknowledge and affirm my experience in the world, who are able to stand on the margin with me." As I look at my own situation relative to these choices, I am proud to say that I choose to be an African American woman. You may say, "That is not a choice! You were born an African American woman." By saying I choose, I am saying I claim that identity and my own definition of it, rejecting those that others may impose upon me against my will. Society can be transformed by those on the margin only if we "choose" the margin. Otherwise we collude in our own oppression and the oppression of others.

I choose to stand on the margin as someone who is defined by society as marginal in terms of my race and in terms of my gender. I also recognize that there are places where I am in the center and need to choose the margin because, as Andrea has already pointed out, there are places where I am dominant. But the primary point here is that those of us on the margin—or in the center—claim the margin by working in solidarity with others from the margin as they move toward the center. It is in this context that I can warmly embrace Andrea as my friend, as someone who has chosen to stand on the margin with me. I am proud to claim her as my friend.

AYVAZIAN: Beverly and I want to close by sharing some of our thoughts about what we call our friendship as a work in progress. We have said that we recognize the challenge of continually joining together and being apart, joining together and being apart. We have forged a relationship that is not based on the false goal of color blindness. We recognize the differences in our life experiences and the difference that race makes in a relationship, and we have built a sturdy bridge across that divide.

In closing I want to share with you two lines of a Pat Parker poem called "For the White Person Who Wants to Know How to Be My Friend." The first two lines are as follows: "The first thing you do is forget that I'm black. Second, you must never forget that I'm black." Do I forget that Beverly is black? Sure I do. She is a dear friend with whom I spend time. Love, admiration, and affection flow between us. Do I ever forget that she's black? Sure I do, she is my friend whom I care about; there are times that I totally forget that she's black. But do I really forget that Beverly is black? Yes and no. Sure I do, and no I don't. That is who she is in the world, and yes it is forgotten, and no it is not actually ever forgotten. But in the end, I have discovered that the issue is not how I respond to Beverly's blackness. It is how I have come to understand my own whiteness. In the end, I believe the issue for me is how I have come to understand social, political, and economic power and my unearned advantage and privilege as a white woman in a racist society. I believe the strongest thing that I bring to our friendship, our relationship, and our connection is an understanding of the significance of my own whiteness. I come at long last to our relationship with an understanding of my whiteness, something that for several decades I was helped to not see or to not recognize its significance. It is my understanding of my own whiteness, not my response to her blackness, that allows me to interact with Beverly in a way that continues to foster mutuality, connection, and trust.

I have a mental image that Beverly has heard before. I see both of us marching on the long journey toward racial justice. We are there on the road, walking shoulder to shoulder toward the promised land we cannot yet see. But we have strength and courage and faith in the journey. Others are marching with us, and many have gone before. We have not arrived but we are well on our way, and we celebrate each victory that moves us forward. Beverly calls us "partners in justice": shoulder to shoulder we move toward our goal.

Thank you!

REFERENCES

Diehl, W. E. (1991). *The Monday connection: On being an authentic Christian in a weekday world*. New York: HarperCollins.

Dozier, V. J. (1991). *The dream of God: A call to return*. Cambridge, MA: Cowley.

hooks, b. (1984). *Feminist theory: From margin to center*. Boston: South End Press.

Jordan, J. V., Kaplan, A. G., Miller, J. B., Stiver, I. P., & Surrey, J. L. (1991). *Women's growth in connection: Writings from the Stone Center*. New York: Guilford Press.

Lorde, A. (1984). *Sister outsider*. Freedom, CA: Crossing Press.

Miller, J. B. (1987). *Toward a new psychology of women* (2nd ed.). Boston: Beacon Press.

Miller, J. B. (1988). Connections, disconnections and violations. *Work in Progress, No. 33*. Wellesley, MA: Stone Center Working Paper Series.

Russell, L. M. (1993). *Church in the round: Feminist interpretation of the church*. Louisville, KY: Westminster Press/John Knox Press.

Tatum, B. D. (1987). *Assimilation blues: Black families in a white community*. Northampton, MA: Hazel-Maxwell.

Tatum, B. D. (1993). Racial identity development and relational theory: The case of black women in white communities. *Work in Progress, No. 63*. Wellesley, MA: Stone Center Working Paper Series.

Wood, J. (1994, April 10). What I learned about Jews. *New York Times Magazine*, pp. 42–45.

This chapter was originally presented at a Stone Center Colloquium on May 4, 1994. © 1994 by Andrea Ayvazian and Beverly Daniel Tatum.

Part II

Applying the Power of Connection

9

Couple Therapy
A Relational Approach

STEPHEN J. BERGMAN *and* JANET L. SURREY

*F*or almost a decade we have been working mostly with heterosexual men and women, applying the relational model in gender workshops, couple therapy, and couples groups. We have found that the
model—which emphasizes holding awareness of self, other, *and* the relationship—is a powerful framework for guiding couples therapy. The
therapist's primary work is to help each member of the couple hold
this relational awareness. Sitting with a couple, one can begin to "see"
the relationship as it exists between and around the two people and to
work on the qualities, dynamics, and history of the relationship, and
the vision of the relationship in the future. The therapist also "sees"
this specific relationship being shaped by a web of others—in the extended family, the culture, the historical context, and in the larger
world.

As an example, in our couples groups, we begin by asking people
to introduce not themselves nor their spouse to the group but their relationship. Here are examples from three couples in the same group:

A couple together for a year and a half: "It's very young, like a fawn, a lot of innocence, great potential. But it's fragile, tenuous, easily hurt, and could easily go in the wrong direction."

A couple married 7 years, with two young children: "It's reliable and there, like the sky or maybe the moon. But it's clouded over, hard to see. Too many conflicting obligations—kids, work. There's no time for us. We're in parallel play."

A couple married almost 50 years: "Very old and solid, like a deep river or a porcupine. A long history of doing things a certain way, so now it's hard to move."

Images of nature are often used, as if in the human imagination the relationship is some being, alive in the natural world.

The work we discuss in this chapter is based on our experience with more than 5,000 men and women, including children and adolescents, in our workshops; 50 couples in couples groups; and approximately 30 couples in therapy. Steve has done most of the work with individual couples, which he will be describing. While there has been some diversity of race, ethnicity, class, sexual preference, and age in our workshops, our couples in therapy are mostly white, heterosexual, middle class, and privileged. We are continuing to broaden our work to address the intersections of gender with race, class, ethnicity, and sexual preference, which *must* be addressed if differences are to be used for building connections rather than creating disconnections that lead to isolation, abuse, and violence. We try to hold and integrate this larger context in our clinical work.

We intend to explore in this chapter how the nature and content of the gender impasses that we discuss change in other relational configurations, such as same-sex couples or heterosexual couples of different class, race, or ethnicity. This sample is relatively high functioning and generally seeking gender equality. This is a select sample, but we feel it offers new perspectives for couples and family work. While we may talk about "men" and "women," no particular man or woman fit our gender descriptions exactly.

The zest and vitality of a couple's relationship comes from *movement*— not from connection alone, but from *growth* in connection. We have found that using the relational model and bringing a sustained seriousness to the challenge of mutual relationship creates an urgency, if not an imperative, for a couple to move one way or another—either to connect and shift toward mutuality, or to disconnect, which may mean separating. In an honest encounter with the psychological facts of the relationship, couples often are able to separate without being crippled by shame or guilt. As one woman put it, "I don't hate him. I hate the relationship with him." In Steve's experience, often the movement one way or the other happens quite rapidly—within four to eight sessions. Sometimes couples do not move but stay entwined in nonmutual, growth-stunting, and barren relationships. For example, a couple described their relationship as follows:

WOMAN: We're like two branches of a tree, growing together. I realize that the other branch is there, but I don't really see the trunk at all.

MAN: An electric power tool, which you plug into a battery pack to recharge. Then you go off and come back when it's ready to use.

Our work is guided by the Stone Center model of relational mutuality: that respectful engagement and movement around difference can ultimately lead to growth. As Surrey writes (1987, p. 3):

In mutual relationships each person can represent his or her feelings, thoughts, and perceptions in the relationship, and each person can feel that they can *move* or have impact on the other and on the flow of the relationship. The capacity to be moved, to respond, and to move the other represents the fundamental core of mutually empowering relationships.

In describing relational movement, Jordan (1986, p. 5) writes:

One is both affecting the other and being affected by the other; one extends oneself out to the other and is receptive to the impact of the other. There is an openness to influence, emotional availability, and a constantly changing pattern of responding to and affecting the other. The movement toward the other's differentness is actually central to growth in relationship.

The Stone Center theory has been evolving to a greater focus on the dynamics and development of the *relationship*, rather than on intrapsychic or individual change alone: "The relationship, then, comes to have a unique existence beyond the individuals, to be attended to, cared about, and nurtured. The development and movement of relationship becomes the central challenge" (Surrey, 1985, p. 7). Miller and Stiver (1992) write that growth-fostering relationships are characterized by movement—out of isolation and disconnection and into *new* connection.

There are strikingly different "relational paradoxes" in "normal" male and female development: young boys becoming agents of disconnection to preserve themselves (Bergman, 1991); adolescent girls disconnecting from their authenticity to try to maintain relationship (Gilligan, 1990; Miller, 1988).

Growth through and toward connection in couples involves working together on all the challenges to mutuality inherent and inevitable in male–female relationships. We have found it to be central for us to hold the belief in this inevitability as well as in the vision of relational mutuality. After working with thousands of men and women, we are sobered by the depth and universality of these challenges yet continually inspired to see what is possible and how far we can move together when a sustained context and commitment are present.

A FIRST THERAPY SESSION: FROM IMPASSE TO RELATIONAL MOVEMENT

Tom and Ann—a mythical couple made up of our experiences with many couples, a couple with whom some of you may already be familiar from Jean Baker Miller's aptly titled paper, "What Do We Mean by Relationships" (1986)—come into the office so angry at each other and so discouraged about their marriage that they cannot even look at each other, so they face me, the therapist (Steve). Tom is a tall, athletic-looking middle-aged WASP with greying blond hair and horn-rimmed glasses. He owns a small computer software company. Ann is a youthful-looking, dark-haired Jewish woman with intense dark eyes. She is headmistress of a private school. Both wear business suits. They have two teenage sons. Immediately, they start talking about the faults of the other person, referring to each other in the third person pronoun:

TOM: Nothing I do is enough for her.

ANN: I'm tired of taking care of this relationship.

TOM: She's so demanding! And oversensitive. I try and try, and nothing seems to work.

ANN: He's so closed; he never talks. If we start to have a discussion that involves feelings, he changes the subject or gets angry and walks out. I feel shut out and alone. I told him that unless he came to therapy, the marriage is over.

TOM: Nothing I do is enough. I even went into individual therapy for her—to try to work on myself.

They fall silent. The relationship is stuck. I get a sense that this is the end point of an impasse, the result of many painful attempts to connect. I feel for them.

A traditional couple therapy approach is to try to have each person stay in the "I," first person, rather than to be in the "you," second person. This couple, however, wasn't even in the second person, but the third: "he" and "she." My initial attempts to get them to stay in the "I"—making statements such as "I feel" or "I think"—fail miserably.

TOM: I feel that she always makes me feel like a failure.

ANN: I feel that he's treating me like his mother!

I could follow up on "mother," which might lead to a significant family history. Using the relational model, however, the first priority is the quality of their connection, which is always in the present moment. And so I actively try to shift the paradigm away from self and/or other to the relationship. There are three reasons for this: to see what the relationship, in fact, is, its potential, and its history as seen by each of them; to shift away from the idea of "psychopathology" residing in one or the other; and to see if this paradigm shift might help move things in the present moment.

With a sense of concern, I say that they are stuck, in an impasse, not moving, and that this stuckness is not because of a "sickness" in him or her, not the fault of either, but rather a difficulty in how they are meeting. I introduce the idea that in addition to "self" and "other," maybe we can also look at "the relationship," almost as a "thing" with qualities, a past, and quite possibly a future. I ask what they can say about the relationship.

TOM: What relationship? There's no relationship here.

ANN: (*starts to cry*) It feels dead. Boring and dead. So different from where we began.

This may not seem like much, but in fact it is a relational statement, the first time that either has used the "we" and referred to "it," the relationship. I say, "I know it seems pretty hopeless right now, but maybe you can describe what the relationship was like when you met."

ANN: He was different—so open and trustable—

BERGMAN: (*interrupting*) Sorry, I didn't mean to ask about him. I meant the relationship.

This surprises them. For the first time they look at each other. They begin to talk, more and more animatedly, about how the relationship in the past was, in Ann's words, "safe and loving, a lot of trust, and we used to be really free, do the wildest things—go to concerts, go dancing." Tom talks about how he was attracted to Ann's depth of feeling and how, wanting to impress her on their first date, he got tickets to Symphony Hall—only to find that it was "Barbershop Quartet Night." Now there is a palpable shift in the room, making eye contact. They laugh. They are talking about the past history of the relationship, but they are not in the past—they are in the present moment, making contact, in connection. There is a real sense of things coming unstuck, things moving.

What is moving is the relationship. I begin to sense their potential.

After a while, now that they are connected, I try to build on this relational awareness, asking them to do a "qualities of relationship" exercise. Each tries to get an image of the *color* of the relationship, the *texture*, the *sound*, the *climate*, the *animal*:

color:	*Ann*	red, cool blue
	Tom:	black, purple
texture:	*Ann*	lumpy, mud
	Tom	it started out smooth, now it's sandpapery
sound:	*Ann*	ocean
	Tom	distant rain
animal:	*Ann*	cat
	Tom	tiger

I point out how there are real similarities in their images, as well as clear differences, and say that the shift back—smooth to sandpapery—will happen again. I tell them that the problem isn't the shift or the conflict; it's how to be in creative movement rather than in deadness, stuck.

ANN: I guess we really don't know each other.

BERGMAN: I have a sense that you really do know each other pretty well. What you don't know right now is how to move in the relationship.

The session ends with my affirming that there is in fact a relationship here, a "we" with a history. Ann says that she knows it but that Tom often seems to forget. Coming back from a business trip recently, he hung up his coat on the rack at the door and walked past her to his answering machine without even saying hello. I suggest that they can try to be creative, even playful, about working together on the relationship. For instance, they might try putting up a sign over the coat rack inside the door: "Danger: There is a relationship here." They laugh. Now we are, to a certain extent, all on the same side, all three of us working together for the sake of the relationship. I feel empathy with the pain in each of them and with the way they are connecting and disconnecting.

I say, "You're both very vulnerable right now, and the relationship is vulnerable too. It's important that each of you take care right now not to do more harm, not to hurt each other or the relationship any further."

They sense my concern, agree, and ask how they can do that. I suggest two tools they can use: the check-out and the check-in. The check-out can be used when the couple is in a fight and one person wants to stop. He or she says so but then has to say when they will bring the subject back up again. Either person can call for a check-in, which consists of each person in turn telling what he or she is feeling in themselves and in the relationship. The other listens, without asking for elaboration, and just says, "I hear you." The check-in is a simple but powerful way to make a connection in the moment. I ask if they would like to try a check-in right now, suggesting they look at each other as they do it:

TOM: (*looking at Ann directly*) I'm afraid to say anything because we might start up again. I feel shell-shocked.

ANN: I feel you're really trying, Tom, but. . . .

BERGMAN: Can you just stay with your own experience for now?

ANN: (*pause*) I feel kind of lost and scared to trust you again. But I hear you, Tom.

TOM: And I hear you.

There's a palpable shift at this, an *authentic* statement from each of them to the other.

Finally, I suggest that before the next session they try to write a "relational purpose statement." Together, on one sheet of paper, write down the purpose of the relationship and the purpose of their "we." This is a way of seeing whether or not a couple shares the same basic worldview and values—on which much can be built. We've found that how far a couple gets on this shared project is a fairly reliable predictor of how the therapy will go.

As they are leaving, Tom says, "Thanks. You brought back the idea that there is a relationship here and that it does have some good to it."

ANN: Yes, it helps to keep the focus on the relationship, not just on him.

BERGMAN: Yes, and right now each of you have to take care of it.

TOM: (*joking, with a poignant truthfulness*) So it'll take care of *me*!

They leave with a sense that together we three have broken through an impasse, a first step has been taken, a feeling that they are moving again in however tenuous a connection—which builds greater faith that this is possible. They have a sense of greater *relational resilience* (Jordan, 1992), of *relational presence*, and that someone is really with them and with their relationship, which helps *them* to have a sense of the reality of the relationship, too, and its potential. A seed has been planted that they *can* act together to move to greater connection. This we call "relational empowerment" (Surrey, 1986), that is, locating the power or capacity to act *in the relationship*.

AN EXTENSION OF RELATIONAL THEORY TO COUPLES

Impasse

Miller (1986) has written that relationships are always in movement— either toward better connection or increasing disconnection.

In all relationships, minor disconnections are inevitable, a sign of life and change. In growth-fostering relationships they become a stimulus for relational growth. There is a challenge to move out of the past and into new connection. We have called this growth through and toward connection, or relational development.

Over time when disconnections cannot move in this way, there is an experience of impasse. Stiver (1993, p. 3) writes:

> In an impasse, both people feel increasingly less connected, more alone and isolated, and less able to act effectively in the relationship. This can be experienced by either or both people as frustration, anger, confusion, boredom, disappointment, loneliness, hopelessness, or personal failure.

When an impasse persists, there are negative psychological consequences for both people (the negatives of Jean Baker Miller's [1986] "five good things"), and they contribute to the occurrence of depression, substance abuse, and violence.

An impasse begins to have a repetitive, spiraling quality. You step into it and become less and less able to keep from going down the same path. There is a feeling of being trapped or taken over by this habitual, stereotypical movement, less sense of freedom or range of motion, less space and energy for any creative insight or action, a feeling of being locked into a power struggle. Finally the same impasse begins to show up in many areas of the couple's life together, for example, in sex.

Invitation to deep connection can provoke impasses. As Miller and Stiver and write, "When yearnings for connection are stimulated, so are all the protective strategies each person has developed to stay out of connection based on past relational experience and cultural learnings" (1991, p. 2). In heterosexual couples these are often interlocking or complementary strategies based on past relational images—of what happens and of what can or cannot happen in relationships. That is, a woman might unconsciously assume, "If I ask him to move with my feelings, he will ridicule me or leave," while a man might assume, "If I ask her more about her feelings, things will get out of control and I won't know how to deal with it." When one person meets fear and protection in the other, each becomes more locked into the past, more into protection, and less capable of opening or expanding.

Such assumptions keep both people from moving more fully into the relationship and contribute to the sense of constriction or diminishment of relational possibilities. In therapy, impasses have been called "the royal road to change" (Atwood, Stolorow, & Trop, 1989), as there is a great *challenge* for both people to create a *new* way of being and moving together. In working with men and women, we have found it helpful to explore how each person's past experiences in relationship—and especially around the *nature* of the relational paradox for each gender—contribute to the development of impasses, but we also work to find the ways the differences can contribute to growth. We work by building on qualities that support creativity in relationship: curiosity, flexibility, persistence, playfulness, paradoxical thinking, risk taking, openness to the new, patience, and capacities for sustained attention and imagination.

Core Relational Principles Guiding Couple Therapy

Holding Relational Awareness

While it is necessary to work on connection to self and other, it is also essential to work on staying attuned to the relationship. Facilitating awareness of interest in and caring for the relationship are powerful ways to help couples move out of self-centered or other-centered positions and perceptions. Introducing new positive imaginal ways of describing and naming the "we" makes more available in the moment the whole history, energies, and resources of the relationship.

The language of connection and disconnection is exceptionally useful in helping couples describe their experiences and helping to move out of the blaming or pathologizing mode—either directed at self or other. Learning to see impasses as attempts at connection which then lead to greater disconnection can be very useful.

Working toward Mutually Empathic Connection

As the therapist works toward empathic connection with either person, and each person with the other, she/he is facilitating movement out of impasse. As either person moves into greater authenticity, both are moved to a new level of clarity and energy. The movement into connection moves everyone; often one feels a palpable shift in the room. Holding an empathic understanding of each person's experience and vulnerabilities provides a template for the process of mutual empathy. The therapist holds the possibility of connection and enlargement in places that feel impossible, places of disconnection—when the woman or man loses the empathic connection to the other or loses touch with her or his own authenticity. By deepening the understanding of each person's experience, we move from "difference," which is still a self-centered perception, to an authentic connection to the *person*; this moves the relationship. When the therapist supports the process of mutual empathy and mutual authenticity, she/he is helping to support the creative tension of holding different perspectives simultaneously, which is basic to the creative process of growth in connection.

Mutual Responsibility and Mutual Impact

The therapist always works to facilitate mutual responsibility for the relationship. This is especially important for women, who often feel alone, angry, and burdened with this. When the therapist continually focuses attention back on the responsibility for relationship, women begin to feel supported and freer to try out new ways of moving. The language of "we" is very helpful here. As one man said, "We're hanging out in the disconnection here, trying to find a way back into connection." And another put it, "We got *into* this together, and we have to get *out* of it together."

The concept of mutual impact is helpful in guiding movement out of power or control struggles. When each person feels that they are having an *impact* on the relationship, we are moving from a "power over" to a "shared power" or "power with" paradigm. Gendered experiences of power must be explored in couples. Men need to acknowledge the enormity of their power in the world and their often invisible power in relationships. At the same time, men often feel women have enormous power and competence in relationships and, feeling quite vulnerable, keep themselves out of real relational process. This is a huge topic. For now, let us just say that introducing this new paradigm as a way through power struggles can be helpful.

We emphasize that each person is responsible for their own behavior but also responsible to each other and to the relationship. Mutual responsibility is the key to working through impasse. As a couple or group struggles to understand and move together through an impasse, the relationship grows toward what Jordan (1992) calls "relational resiliency" (the energetic resources to move) and what Surrey (1986) has termed "relational empowerment" (the shared sense of effectiveness or ability to act to move the relationship toward connection). These qualities reside not just in the individuals but actually *in the relationship*.

The Gendered "We"

Over time, working together, we have discovered that the way we work with this model can be quite different. This may reflect gender differences, especially in the notion of the "we."

For me (Janet) as a woman, the "we" is built on a sense of relational movement—of how we are and move together, of two voices in dialogue—something greater than the moment, greater than the sum of the parts, informing and being informed by each person. It's the *between*, the movement that connects. As the notion of "self-in-relation" is contextual, fluid, and moving, so is this conception of relationship.

For many men, the notion of the "we" seems more to be a "thing," with properties and qualities, perhaps even with "boundaries" of what is "inside" and what is "outside." Of course it is not a "thing" any more than "self" is a thing, but I (Steve) have found that men may find it very useful to have this "thing-ish" orientation. One man talked about "taking the relationship on our vacation." For better or worse, it can also be an enlargement of a man's "self" boundary to include the "we." One man may see himself as the family's "Chief Executive," his wife as "Secretary of Health and Human Services." The downside of this is that the "family" can become as isolated, protected, and static as the "self." As one man put it, "I want the 'we' to mean only us—the hell with your friends!" For women, this "we" is not easily trustable, as it can simply be a projection of the man's values, perceptions, and decisions, such as in "We vote Republican." But I have found that many men are helped by this concept of the "we" and actually become more open to mutuality when they can center in something larger than themselves. It can be a step *toward* true mutuality.

For a month Janet has been asking me (Steve), "What do you mean by the 'we'?" We have spent an enormous amount of time trying to grasp our own differences in what we mean by the "we." In writing this paper, as whenever we work together, we wanted to make sure we remained differentiated and also flowed between our shared voice, our gendered voices, and our personal voices—all of which have emerged more clearly through this dialogue.

THE COURSE OF A COUPLE'S THERAPY USING THE RELATIONAL PERSPECTIVE

Ann and Tom came back to the second session saying that things were better but still difficult. Both felt that getting in touch with the history of the relationship had been useful. But as they had started to work on a relational purpose statement, they had gotten into an impasse:

TOM: We started out well enough, and decided that one purpose was "to provide a loving environment for the growth and protection of our children and ourselves." That was easy. But then she wanted more and got into her "we're not close enough" issue—

ANN: Wait a sec—I didn't say "not enough." I just want it better.

TOM: You're insatiable—as you said—"The sky's the limit."

ANN: What's wrong with that?

TOM: There's no limit to the sky! Nothing's ever good enough.

ANN: You just want to stay stuck in the mud—as if mud's good enough!

I stop the process. This may seem like bad news, but in fact I was delighted. In the first session, they were totally stuck in an impasse, not even looking at each other. Now they are in an impasse, but engaged, on a growing edge, trying to move. There's more to work with. They are actively struggling with each other. And they actually had started to work on their relational purpose statement. I have a sense of liking them.

Now that they are connecting, there is room for me to start to use all the various ways to work empathically with each of them and with their relationship. I acknowledge to them that this can be really hard work and that both of them are trying their best. I say that it's not unusual for impasses to come up around trying to do the purpose statement. I ask them to tell me more of what happened.

It turned out that their relational styles in doing this were much different: she wanted to toss things around in dialogue and then write something down at the end; he wanted them each to make a list and then put them together. He'd felt lost in her "looseness," and she'd felt shut out by his structure. He'd stormed out and then come back, ready to work on the purpose again. She said she couldn't work on the purpose until they processed their fight. He said he didn't want to waste any more time on the fight but wanted to get down to the task. This got nowhere. Each was trying to connect in his and her own way, each feeling that the other was in the way.

Movement around Gender Difference: Engagement around Difference to Mutual Empowerment

I talk about this being another example of a relational impasse, one which we have labeled the "product/process impasse." It is not unusual for men and women to split this way.

I say to Tom, "In these kinds of situations, we men often seem to get all hung up on getting it done, getting to the bottom line, 'fixing it,' and don't pay attention to the process—which is her style. You know what I mean?"

TOM: Do I ever! I want to fix it, get it done. And, as she says to me, "Don't just do something, stand there!" (*They laugh*.) First, her process around writing this drives me nuts, and then, we have to process that process! I had to fix both! But what you're saying then is that the only way to fix it is to stop trying to fix it? (*more laughter*).

I say to Ann, "From my experience, women often want to think in dialogue to get clearer. And men have a difficult time believing that such a process can actually get anywhere. Right?"

ANN: In fact, it works better!

I am thus able to reframe their impasse in terms of how what each of them is doing is influenced by the different ways each *gender* has learned to move in relationship. The problem isn't difference itself; it's not being able to see difference clearly and without judgment, to work with and move with difference in relationship. Engagement around difference moves a couple from self-centered perceptions to a fuller awareness of the whole person and the potential richness of the relationship.

Picking up on my saying that men are taught to fix things, Tom talks about his work (he's an executive in charge of hundreds of people) and about his family (he's the only son of a distant, reserved father and a depressed mother). I spend time exploring his family history, knowing that Ann senses what I'm doing: making an empathic connec-

tion with Tom by taking a "we men" stance toward his vulnerabilities. I
ask Ann about her listening to Tom.

ANN: I feel touched, but I feel angry too, about—

TOM: Oh Jesus! I'm spilling my guts here.

BERGMAN: Can *you* listen, Tom? (*to Ann*) It sounds like there's also a lot
of pain behind that anger.

ANN: Yes. I guess I'm angry that he won't talk like that to *me*, when I
need it so much.

I'm trying here to move toward each person's experience, to hold
the pain each feels and the pain in the relationship, helping them to do
the same. We go on to look at his pain at feeling controlled by her and
her anger at not wanting to be seen as a monster trying to control him:
his dread, her anger. We get into Ann's family history here as well.

The gender of the therapist may be important in this process. I, as
a man, taking the "we men" stance, can often make empathic connection with the man, sensing that often the woman is understanding what
I am doing in paying attention to the man's experience in this way. She
knows that I'm doing it not just for him, I'm doing it for the relationship and for her. Often she appreciates the man opening up, and so it
also helps me connect with her. When I turn to her, she is more connected to me. A woman therapist, working with a woman in this way
with the man watching, may be seen by the man as "ganging up" on
him. That is, he may not be able to see it as in the service of the relationship and him, to his benefit.

Other important examples of engagement around gender differences are in educating a couple to the different emotional timescales of
men and women; the different abilities to focus on many things at a
time (women) and one thing at a time (men); the different awareness of
the relational context, of anger, the different relational curiosities; the
different attentions to maintaining the continuity of connection; and,
of course, the differences in power both within and outside the couple.

As we have described in our earlier paper (Bergman & Surrey,
1992), these differences in the relational field may be much more visible to women and more invisible to men. Making them visible to both
genders can bring rapid movement. For instance, Tom was slower to describe his emotional state, something both of them had to take into account. If Ann felt that Tom was trying to let her in rather than avoiding
the subject or seeing her as a monster, she could relax and even enjoy
this shared process of finding a resonant frequency of emotional dialogue. Difference can be a blessing to a relationship. Learning to work

on difference of gender helped Ann and Tom to learn to use difference in general. For instance, each has a different attitude toward illness: Tom is a hypochondriac, and Ann is a stoic. Each's attitude could be of great use in dealing with ideas of illness in the other. Ironically, once you feel understood and accepted for who you are, you feel ready to change.

Movement through and toward Connection

By the end of the second session I am moved by how much they have moved, and I tell them that. To give words to what they've done, I mention the notion of connection and disconnection:

BERGMAN: Our priority together has to be, first and foremost, connecting. If we're not in connection, there's room for all kinds of trouble to creep in: the past, accusations about family (you're like your father; you're like your mother), gender stereotypes (you're like all men; you're like all women), and ethnic issues (you're like all WASPs or Jews). In connection, we can talk respectfully about any of these differences, such as religious, ethnic, and class differences, without stereotyping. Today, by hanging out through this disconnection, you've managed to make an even better connection. Doesn't it feel that way right now?

ANN: Yes. In the middle of a fight, I lose sight of Tom as a whole person and of the whole history of the relationship. He seems so diminished—like my father.

TOM: And *you* get bigger—like my *mother*. (*They laugh.*)

To strengthen Tom's not feeling so alone with his difficulties, I ask if he'd like to read something on "male dread." He says, "Yes," and I give him my paper (Bergman, 1991).

I mention the idea of the *continuity of connection* (an awareness that the relationship continues to exist even when they are apart or feeling disconnected) and that there may be gender differences in this sense of continuity. For instance, I point out how rare it is for a man to spontaneously say, "I was thinking about what we were talking about yesterday."

Check-ins can be helpful in maintaining continuity, although, as one woman said, "We have to be careful not to let our check-ins degenerate into conversations." Finally, I ask if they'd like to take another shot right now at writing a purpose statement. They come up with the idea of writing in dialogue, a line from him, then her:

ANN: To provide a safe environment for each other.

TOM: And—wait for it!—for the relationship!

This is more than compromise; this is creativity.

In the next session Tom said that he read my paper six times. "It was like you were talking about me. It was a big relief!" Ann, too, thought it helped her to understand his dread and the dread/anger impasse.

For several weeks things went better and better. They cooperated around the house; with their teenage sons, they were saying, "We're trying to find out how the 'we' will draw the line with them, together." They started to use the language of connection with each other: "Our connection right now is good." Being in better connection, they could go back over the hard things in the relationship. Humor, which had first drawn them together, made a comeback. Tom talked about "the big D—Dread," saying, "God I'm in dreadlock!" or "Lookout! Here comes another dreadattack!"

TOM: All this talk about the importance of relationship is getting to me. Annie, if you could have on your tombstone: "She was superb at relationships," would that be enough?

ANN: Absolutely! Although I'd also like a second line. And maybe a third too. Something like, "And she pitched in the World Series."

TOM: Can you understand that I can't even *imagine* that that would be enough? For me it would seem a humiliation—a failure—and that makes me feel ashamed to say it.

Reframing Autonomy

The fifth session started as a disaster. They came in angry and discouraged, unable even to look at each other, back in the third person accusatory: "he said"/"she said." Nothing I tried helped. The issue was money for a vacation, a fight about he being tight, she being extravagant.

I have learned that in a deadlock such as this, attention must be paid first not to the specific issue but to the state of the connection. I ask, "What does the 'we' need now?"

ANN: (*replies angrily*) I can understand what you're doing, asking about the "we," and that may be okay for him, but I'm frightened by the "we." My whole life has been in the "we." When I hear you ask me about the "we" now, a red flag goes up. I'm going to lose the "I." In fact, I don't feel you really understand it from a woman's point of view, what that's like. Maybe we should go to a female couples therapist.

BERGMAN: I can see how, as a man, I might have some trouble seeing it from your side. But can you try to tell me about it?

ANN: I'm frightened that my concerns will get lost in my work on the "we," that if I'm empathic to him, I'll accommodate to him, and I'll lose. You're asking me to settle for too little.

I respond to her concerns, saying, finally, "It's important for you to keep speaking up about what you need here, and that *all* of us pay attention, so you gain, not lose. We're all on the side of not settling for less."

ANN: I'm not so sure Tom is.

TOM: If you're so good at this, why can't you stop me from feeling dread?

ANN: I'm not an expert in this stuff either, and I'm tired of taking care of you and it.

TOM: Look—I've just got to work on my *own* crap, get my own crap together first, that's all. Maybe then I can get into this, not before.

This is such a dramatic change. A light bulb goes on. I ask about his own psychotherapy, with a well-known psychologist who—I know from an initial conversation with him at the beginning of my couples work with his client—works in a more traditional, self/other paradigm. It turns out that his therapist has been on vacation for 5 weeks (ever since we'd started meeting) but had come back last week. Tom had had an intense session that focused on his childhood and ever since had withdrawn from the relationship.

Individual therapy of one or both members of a couple who are also in couple therapy can be extremely useful if it works toward enhancing relationship. Most of the time it does. However, Tom's stance in the couple therapy is not unique. A more self-centered individual psychotherapy may accentuate, codify, and entrench self-centeredness. Despite a man becoming familiar with every nook and cranny of himself, he may be left with a profound unfamiliarity with the pathways of mutual relationship.

Couple therapy, with its frank clear presence of a relationship, may make it easier to work on men's relational skills—bringing male strengths into relationship—and ultimately teaching men mutual empathy and movement through and toward connection. In couple therapy, men may more easily move, first from the "self" to the "we." The "we" may be safer to explore than the "other." Once in the "we," a man may then be able to move to ask about differences, about the "other," and then by facing these differences move toward mutuality, with empathy. Women's path toward mutuality in couples work may be different.

And so now with Tom I say, "I can really feel for you, knowing something of the pain of your past. I guess you feel that if you go into this relationship fully, you'll be less yourself?"

TOM: Less, hell—lose myself completely. She's so controlling!

BERGMAN: I know you feel that way. But haven't you had the experience, when you've been in a real connection with Ann, you've been *more* yourself? More alive, more full of zest, you can go out and do things better?"

TOM: (*thinks it over, sighs, and says sadly*) Yes, that's true.

BERGMAN: So what keeps you from being in good connection with her?

TOM: I'm afraid. It's like if I go into something with her, I'll get lost. She sees it as "the sky's the limit," and I see it as "the tip of the iceberg." I've gotten so I keep everything secret from her, do everything alone. You only achieve things alone. Like climbing Mount Everest.

Ann is moved and says, "Honey, no one ever climbs Mount Everest alone." Tom smiles.

BERGMAN: Maybe the healing for you can be right here in this relationship. Maybe you should focus on where you are in this relationship here and now, and let the individual therapy work go for a little while.

ANN: I want to help, Tom.

TOM: I thought you said you were tired of helping.

ANN: If you're open to me, if we do it together, I won't be tired. You don't have to do it alone.

For the first time in years, Tom starts to cry. He reaches for Ann's hand, and says, "I don't know if I can do it."

At the next session, Tom is buoyant and announces, "I fired my therapist—as a gift to her!"

My heart sank. It wasn't exactly what I'd had in mind. And my subsequent chat with his therapist was not exactly what you would call a meeting of the minds. But we did agree on a sabbatical.

After that, the couple therapy went well. My first priority—and theirs—is holding the relationship. This is not behavioral or systems theory. The priority here is not the theory but the therapist's relational presence. Mutuality is two voices in dialogue. As one woman said at the end of a workshop, "You gave me the other half of the string, and now we can make a tie." As we've said, mutual empathy is a central part of this process. But in some sense the process is more than mutual empathy or perhaps a further reflection of mutual empathy. I not only try to hold each individual empathically, but my holding their relationship empathically helps them to hold their relationship in a similar way. It has to do with being related to the relationship. As a couple said to another couple in one of our groups, "Your holding your relationship helps us to hold ours."

How does holding the relationship help people to connect mutually? I think it may have something to do with offering something startling and new, something creative, beyond the usual, conditioned, past ways of seeing. Men often feel stuck in a relationship, focused on self versus other, trapped between the dread of connection and the fear of disconnection or loss. Afraid that "something might happen," they may defend the status quo. Women may more easily initiate relational movement. Women, seeing a man move from a self-centered perspective and start to come alive more mutually, may be able to join this movement empathically and feel more fully themselves in the relationship.

With the man of the couple, I am usually working to help him move off of a self-centered way of seeing, opening up the idea that men can attend to the "we" and to the *different* experience of others, that he can move the relationship and the other, and *be moved* by the other and the relationship. I am trying to move men from a notion of equality and justice—or equal opportunity and justice—to mutuality (Gilligan, 1982). I am less concerned with "male role" or "male identity" than with "male relational skills."

With the woman, I usually work on her doing less of the relational work for the couple, on her understanding differences in dread, emotional timing, and talk, and focusing on herself. I help her to represent *her* experience in conflict, say what she feels and what she wants, and to hold her ground when she feels strongly about something—for instance, with Ann, about her work as a headmistress, her family history, and her not being a defender of the status quo but on the side of change and growth.

Three Enlarging Movements in Therapy

All the while I am using three enlarging movements in therapy, which help to open the focus, in the present moment, into new, creative ways of seeing:

1. *Relational movement*: moving back and forth from self and other to the relationship.
2. *Gender movement*: moving back and forth from "I, Tom," to "we men," and from "I, Ann," to "we women." This is not to say all men, or all women, are the same. But for men in particular, it is a chance to enlarge from self and link to a larger group. Given the current epidemic of violence and abuse by men, this is a complex linkage.
3. *Movement through and toward connection*: moving back and forth from connection to disconnection to reconnection, impasse, and breakthrough.

Things went well with Tom and Ann. I liked them. The therapy was fun. They were able to hold the relationship between sessions, that is, keeping in mind that there is a "we" here, bigger than both of them, with a vital history and future. I began to see them less frequently—about once a month. For a while they would call me up in a "crisis." First, I dreaded these calls, but I came to see their "crises" as signs of life out on the growing edge of the relationship and I began to enjoy helping them reframe impasses, getting them moving. Let me mention briefly a few of these reframings.

Reframing Depression

They called up in a crisis. When they came in, Ann said she was feeling very down. Tom, frustrated and worried, asked, "Do you think she needs a little Prozac?" I said I thought not. "How about a little Zoloft?" he asked. "How about a little reframing?" I said. I helped them to look at Ann's "depression" as a sign of movement in the relationship. It turned out that Ann, more connected to Tom, was paying more attention to her own feelings.

TOM: But when she gets this depressed, how do I know when I should just let her cry and when I should try to do something about it?

BERGMAN: You could *ask*. (*Tom is stunned by this idea.*) Why not ask her where she is, how you can help?

Tom does so. Ann doesn't respond. I ask what keeps her from answering.

ANN: I'm stopping myself, like I feel dread too. I want to tell him, but I don't trust his response. I've been left so many times.

BERGMAN: All of us have to hold what's new in the relationship, now. Maybe, right now the way out of this depression is through the relationship.

This helped. Men often have a hard time *asking* about another's experience. This, a gender difference in *relational curiosity,* is a key element in *power inequalities* in a couple. Power is not only about cultural systems but also relationally determined by whose experience is attended to.

Reframing Dependence and Independence

Tom often felt entrapped in the relationship. He had a recurrent dream: he was a boy, and his mother was tying him to a tree to keep him from running out into the street. They called me up in crisis. Awakening that morning they had felt close and made love, and then Tom, obsessed with a deal at work, had rushed to get out of the house and hadn't even said good-bye. He was driving their son to work when the car phone rang. It was Ann, feeling very hurt that he had just left without even saying good-bye.

TOM: Here we go! Whatever I do, it's not enough. You always want more.

ANN: I don't think it's too much to ask you, especially after being so connected, in sex, to say good-bye.

TOM: I can't be myself in this relationship. You're so damn dependent on me, and you want to make me just as dependent on you—trying to "feminize" me. All day long you've been bugging me, calling me, interrupting meetings, and it's kept me from really focusing on my work.

BERGMAN: Let's try to reframe this. Tom, what would've happened if you had stayed in connection and said good-bye this morning?

TOM: She wouldn't be bugging me.

BERGMAN: So you'd have *more* freedom, not less?

TOM: (*thinking it over*) You got me. But that's so damn hard for me to stay with. It's such a big job!

BERGMAN: Maybe not. It wouldn't have been such a big deal just to say good-bye, and that would have altered the whole day. We men have this mental image that to deal with a woman's feeling is an immense thing, but it's not.

TOM: (*smiling*) You mean the real iceberg is in my head? (*We all laugh.*)

BERGMAN: This isn't about the "feminization" of us men; it's about the "relationalization" of us all. If that's taken to mean "feminization," we—and the world—are in big trouble!

The false dichotomy of dependence–independence causes much grief in couples. Relationship is not a zero-sum game. If Ann feels Tom is attending to the relationship, she can attend to other things. She feels less anxiety if she's not watching all the time, thinking all the time. In her words, "If I focus outside this relationship—on my work, on my self—it and he will disappear." She feels more able to initiate things and have her own life. It's not her "learning to be more independent." It's both of them learning to hold the connection, the "us," and having the faith that the connection will sustain and hold each of them in their own lives and creativity. Her calling Tom up on the car phone was something new. She never would have done that in the past.

As she put it, "I'm not settling for less anymore, and *we're* not either."

Reframing Obsession

Tom became obsessed with a stressful work situation. All he could talk about was work, and he didn't want to be this way. Ann was fed up. They came in, and this time Ann suggested that *Tom* might need a little Prozac. "I hear it's good for obsessive–compulsive people too," she said. As we worked, I tried to reframe obsession in terms of relationship, that is, that the way out is neither in medication nor in getting more into the analysis of the obsession, but rather by moving more fully into relationship. Any obsession is a turning away from living in connection. I suggested that by putting the relationship as a priority, Tom could let go of his obsession with work. Ann agreed, saying that if she felt connected to Tom, she would be glad to listen to his work: "If *you're* interesting, your work is interesting to me." We talked about ways to make the transition from work to home—how to connect after a long hard day.

A month later, in their last session with me, Tom and Ann said that reframing the obsession had helped.

TOM: I'm pretty much over my dread now. I can attend to *her* experience and ask about it. I feel more able to nurture the relationship now.

ANN: It's amazing. I feel listened to now. Not that there aren't troubles. Last week we got into a hassle. He was at work and kept me waiting for hours. I started to get angry, but then I wasn't all that mad because I figured that *we* got into this and now *we* are going to get out of it. The incredible thing is that I feel that his empathy all of a sudden has me thinking, "Hmm. What has *my* part been in not having enough power in this relationship in the past? Maybe *I* haven't been initiating enough here. Not that I'm a victim, but rather what part have I played in this?"

TOM: When we're in conflict, I feel I can *do* it now, that my whole ego isn't on the line. In the past, I felt that I had to have the right answer, that what I did was a reflection on what I was worth. Now I know that's got nothing to do with it, in terms of Ann. I can let go of my self-centered thinking about this by asking about her. (*to Ann*) I used to think you were so damn oversensitive. Now I see that your sensitivity can be useful in this relationship. (*joking*) Especially given mine.

ANN: Neither of us has to do it alone. We do it together.

TOM: We do it together.

They've come to a place not only of mutual empathy and mutual authenticity but of mutual empowerment. I called them up a year later, and while money is still an issue, they're doing well.

COUPLES GROUPS

In working with heterosexual couples in a group setting, I (Janet) continue to prefer working with a cotherapist of the other gender for the very reason that it is difficult to get couples to join a group in the first place. The extraordinary isolation of most couples around what really happens in their relationships is a great problem, as both people are deprived of the gifts of observing and working with other couples experiencing similar struggles and impasses. Feeling less alone with their struggle and having the opportunity for enlarged relational perspectives are profoundly helpful in moving out of impasses.

Seeing similar issues in others and being there *for* others create a context for growth, not only for individuals but for relationships. A context which supports and values relationships is also enormously helpful. One man said, "In our lives today we're surrounded by couples getting divorced, and it makes me feel so much stronger being with others who are staying with it."

As a woman, Janet feels supported and less burdened by working with a male cotherapist and other men in the group. Men are often able to make important empathic connections with each other, and we are increasingly convinced how much men need each other to feel understood, to increase trust, and to feel permitted, if not encouraged, to take a more relational stance. This support often helps equalize the genders around a major imbalance frequently seen in male–female relationships. Often men are envious, at times angry, about a woman's strong relationships with others—especially her friends—and thus feel more emotionally dependent on her than they perceive she is on them. This creates feelings of greater vulnerability and more dread. As one woman described in a couples group:

> "One of the most profound moments for me in this group was seeing Michael [*her husband*] flanked by all the other men in the group. Not so alone—supported and enlarged—more himself. I've always been afraid of men in groups, but here, feeling we were working together, I felt strangely comforted and deeply loving of him."

Sexual Impasses

One of the most isolating areas for most couples is their sexual relationships. Gender differences are highlighted in sexuality, and all the gender impasses we have described previously (Bergman & Surrey, 1992), dread/anger, product/process, and "power over"/"power with," may be seen here. In our workshops with men and women of all ages, curiosity about the others' sexuality abound. All of us have many unanswered questions and not a lot of opportunity to discuss these together.

In all our workshops, women's questions center around the urgency and meanings of sex for men, how men can separate sex from emotional relationship, how men can want sex when the relationship is in a bad place, and how men connect violence and sexuality.

Men's questions center on the mysteries of women's sexuality: What turns you on? Do women fake orgasm? Why don't you initiate sex? What's it like to be touched by a man? Why do women need to talk before sex? Why do women need to talk after sex? During sex?

Moving into Connection

Sexual impasses can be reframed from the perspective of movement in relationship. The sexual impasse around *moving into connection* is typical. Men see physical connection as a means to relational connection. Women want sex to be an expression of relational connection. Often, over time this difference leads to impasse—less of either kind of connection (sexual or relational), anger, resentment, disappointment or blaming, or giving up on the sexual and focusing on other areas of the relationship. Reframing these impasses as difficulties around movement into connection may open a couple to new perspectives and sometimes to new ways of moving.

In the opportunity for deep connection that sexuality offers, the longing or yearning for connection is stimulated and so are all the protective strategies evolved through past experience of pain and failure in relationships—in this and others.

One man described this: "What has to happen for a woman in that 15 minutes of emotional foreplay? I feel like all our personal and collective histories of sexual abuse and power violations have to be worked through, and all the ways we have failed each other, the ways our parents failed each other—and maybe even our grandparents too. It's overwhelming! I don't know how to do it."

A woman described this: "I feel I have to get into the present moment, to be here. I need to feel safe but also *real*. All the feelings I've been avoiding start to rush in: anger at you, things that weren't said, all my pain and disappointment in you and in myself. Tears come. I don't always feel up to it. I guess I have my own version of dread."

Another man said, "It's such a shift from the rest of my life where I'm in charge, hyperactive, hyperbusy. Here I'm supposed to slow down and listen to her, attune my movement to hers. I can't do it. I go too fast, and she gets hurt. So I tend to avoid the whole thing."

In the movement of getting connected, the resistances we all have to slowing down, being real, in touch, and connecting come to the fore.

Men and women often split responsibility for different aspects of the relationship. Women tend to feel angry and alone in tending to the emotional part of the relationship, where men feel the responsibility for initiating the sexual part. Again, working toward mutual responsibility is helpful.

The different sexual rhythms of men and women make moving together a great challenge. Men's more linear movement and product/performance orientation may seriously collide with women's more process/dialogical way of moving. Women often say that they want to feel that neither person is leading, but rather that both are in a simultaneous movement. Women often avoid any form of initiation which feels like "power over," that is, asking the other to follow or be with her in her movement. Men may have more difficulty following or moving with the other.

The Process of Disengagement

The process of disengagement creates a final challenge: once connected, how to disengage without disconnecting. Men are likely to end more abruptly, moving to the next thing, which may be sleep, even showing intolerance for sustaining the connection as long as a woman may want. Women need more movement around separation—like saying good-bye at a party—a more gradual, back-and-forth process, feeling a wish to move together through the disengagement.

SOME PRINCIPLES OF COUPLE THERAPY FROM A RELATIONAL PERSPECTIVE

Let us summarize principles we've illustrated in working with Tom and Ann:

1. *Holding the relationship*: with awareness, faith, and "in process."
2. *The priority of maintaining connection*: connection comes first.
3. *Three enlarging movements in therapy*: reframing in terms of relational movement, gender movement, and movement through and toward connection.
4. *The concepts of impasse and breakthrough.*
5. *Strategies and tools to create mutuality*: check-in, check-out, purpose statement, creativity.
6. *Working in the present moment*: we have found that the greatest barrier to movement toward mutuality is the ego, or ego-centeredness. In a larger sense, the ego is the past, all the conditionings of the human past and the individual past. The way out is in the present.
7. *Engaging around difference*: creating mutual empathy.
8. *Reframing depression, obsession, autonomy, and dependence in terms of the movement or stasis of the relationship.*
9. *Working with continuity and transition*: the ongoing struggle for mutual authenticity.
10. *Working with spirituality*: one way that the idea of "the relationship" helps people is that it suggests something greater than self and other. Many people we've worked with have made the link between the relational model and their own spiritual connection or practice, the capacity to be part of something greater than the self. For example, often we have found that men who are in a 12-step program, who have had an experience of spirituality involving movement out of self-centeredness, may appreciate this approach and move with it quickly. It is often helpful to address the individual and shared spiritual dimension with a couple.

The creative movement in connection, toward mutual relationship, greater than self and other, brings us to an awareness of a connection with a dynamic and interrelated whole of which we are part. This is at the heart of helping people—and couples—to heal.

Let us close by reading Ann and Tom's relational purpose statement: "Providing a safe and 'growthful' environment for each other, our children, our friends, and for our relationships. Trying to provide financially so we don't have to worry—trying to have more fun anyway. Living together in a peaceful and compassionate way, bringing that to others and to the world."

REFERENCES

Atwood, G., Stolorow, R., & Trop, J. (1989). Impasses in psychoanalytic psychotherapy: A royal road. *Contemporary Psychoanalysis, 25,* 554.

Bergman, S. J. (1991). Men's psychological development: A relational perspective. *Work in Progress, No. 48.* Wellesley, MA: Stone Center Working Paper Series.

Bergman, S. J., & Surrey, J. L. (1992). The woman–man relationship: Impasses and possibilities. *Work in Progress, No. 55.* Wellesley, MA: Stone Center Working Paper Series.

Gilligan, C. (1982). *In a different voice: Psychological theory and women's development.* Cambridge, MA: Harvard University Press.

Gilligan, C. (1990). Joining the resistance: Psychology, politics, girls and women. *Michigan Quarterly Review, 29,* 501–536.

Jordan, J. V. (1986). The meaning of mutuality. *Work in Progress, No. 23.* Wellesley, MA: Stone Center Working Paper Series.

Jordan, J. V. (1992). Relational resilience. *Work in Progress, No. 57.* Wellesley, MA: Stone Center Working Paper Series.

Miller, J. B. (1986). What do we mean by relationships? *Work in Progress, No. 22.* Wellesley, MA: Stone Center Working Paper Series.

Miller, J. B. (1988). Connections, disconnections, and violations. *Work in Progress, No. 33.* Wellesley, MA: Stone Center Working Paper Series.

Miller, J. B., & Stiver, I. P. (1991). A relational reframing of therapy. *Work in Progress No. 52.* Wellesley, MA: Stone Center Working Paper Series.

Stiver, I. P. (1992). A relational approach to therapeutic impasses. *Work in Progress, No. 58.* Wellesley, MA: Stone Center Working Paper Series.

Surrey, J. L. (1985). The self-in-relation: A theory of women's development. *Work in Progress, No. 13.* Wellesley, MA: Stone Center Working Paper Series.

Surrey, J. L. (1987). Relationship and empowerment. *Work in Progress, No. 30.* Wellesley, MA: Stone Center Working Paper Series.

This chapter was originally presented at a Stone Center Colloquium on March 2, 1994.
© 1994 by Stephen J. Bergman and Janet L. Surrey.

10

Relationships in Groups
Connection, Resonance, and Paradox

NIKKI M. FEDELE

Jean Baker Miller has described an important relational paradox: In the face of profound yearnings for connection and in order to
connect to the only relationships available, we develop strategies that
keep more and more of ourselves out of connection (Miller,1988;
Miller & Stiver, 1991; Stiver & Miller, 1994). This paradox is also at the
heart of a group experience. The ongoing process of connection, disconnection, and reconnection with the aim of enlarging relational possibilities is the very essence of group work.

In this chapter, I review first the relational model developed by
Miller, Jordan, Stiver, and Surrey as it applies to group work. Second,
I touch on traditional and feminist theories of group therapy, empha-
sizing the contributions of a relational group theory. Third, I examine three important relational concepts: paradox, connection and resonance. Finally, I give two clinical examples of relational group
process.

The journey that Miller began with the publication of *Toward a New Psychology of Women* (1976, 1987) and that continues in the work at the Stone Center has helped me understand relationships in both personal and professional settings. As a therapist, group therapist, teacher, consultant, and supervisor, I have found the relational model extremely helpful in understanding the relationships, conflicts, and dynamics that are fundamental elements in any group. This includes group therapy, supervision groups, working groups, training groups, consultation groups, and larger communities such as the feminist community. A model of relationships in groups is enhanced by a feminist perspective but is applicable to all types of groups, including groups with men.

As a community, women have learned the powerful impact of groups, ranging from consciousness-raising groups of the 1970s, therapy groups, 12-step groups, support groups, self-help groups, peer groups, supervision groups, and training groups to politically active groups like Mothers Against Drunk Driving (MADD) and the Children's Defense Fund. Over the years, I have seen the need for all women to connect with other women in order to develop an adequate support network and to deal with the severe pressures women face each day in a societal structure that devalues them. These women include mothers, secretaries, therapists, homemakers, administrators, lawyers, academics, teachers, and technicians. They are a true cross section of women representing several racial and ethnic groups as well as heterosexual and lesbian women.

One significant example of the importance of networks is the development of support groups for battered women. One way these groups help women is by assisting them through the intricate maze of the legal system, which is extremely male-biased since patriarchy is at the heart of the judicial system. How many times have we been demoralized? How many stories have we heard about judges who were racist, sexist, classist, or homophobic? How many of us know how awful it feels to support women through a system where the safety of the outcome is uncertain at best? How many times must we hear about women as victims of domestic violence? And yet, over and over again the power of women connecting and resonating with each other gives us hope in the midst of such danger. At this very time, women are confronting the inequities and irresponsibility of the judicial system by coming together and demanding changes.

At the same time, there is a growing movement among men to use groups as supportive relational structures. An article by Krugman and Osherson (1993) on men in group therapy illustrates this trend. In fact, it has become increasingly clear that old models of development and relationship do not address men's experience any more than women's.

RELATIONAL DEVELOPMENT AND MOVEMENT

But how do relationships in groups provide a potential for healing and empowerment? In order to examine a model of group work enhanced by a relational perspective, I will review the key points of the relational model developed by the scholars at the Stone Center (through clinical understanding of women's development) and by Carol Gilligan and her colleagues at the Harvard Project on Women's Psychology and Girls' Development. The desire to make connections and the movement toward mutuality in those connections are at the heart of relational development as described by the Stone Center group. This relational movement is the focus of the group therapy model discussed in the present chapter. Jean Baker Miller (1986) in her paper "What Do We Mean by Relationships?" describes five qualities of growth-enhancing relationships that can also be evident in therapy groups: (1) women together experience a high level of energy, or what she calls zest; (2) women in a group who were stuck become empowered and get unstuck; (3) women begin to understand themselves and other women with more clarity; (4) all the members develop greater authenticity and self-worth; and (5) because of the positive experience in a group, women experience a desire for more connection, both within the group and outside of the group.

Relationships in groups are fertile with the relational paradox Miller (1988) first described in her paper "Connections, Disconnections and Violations." This paradox states that during the course of our lifetime, in the desire to make connections and be emotionally accessible, we all experience harm or violation that leads to a need to develop strategies to keep large parts of ourselves out of connection. In the face of intense yearnings for connection and in order to remain in the only relationships available, we develop strategies that keep more and more of ourselves out of connection. Simply put, the paradox is that in order to stay in connection, we keep parts of ourselves out of connection.

Gilligan (1990) enhances our understanding by describing the central paradox of girls' development at adolescence: girls are cut off from their own experience by taking themselves out of authentic relationship for the sake of what looks like relationships (Gilligan, Lyons, & Hammer, 1990). Stiver (1990a, 1990b) elaborates upon the strategies for disconnection in families with secrets like sexual abuse or alcoholism. The strategies, though preferable to isolation, carry a big price tag—disconnection from one's self, lack of clarity about one's feelings, and a sense of inauthenticity. Jordan and colleagues describe the shame that accompanies the disconnection as the loss of empathic possibility, the loss, therefore, of the full potential to develop oneself (Jordan, 1989; Jordan, Surrey, & Kaplan, 1983; Surrey, Kaplan, & Jordan, 1990).

Stiver and Miller, in their two papers "A Relational Reframing of Therapy" (Miller & Stiver, 1991) and "Movement in Therapy: Honoring the Strategies of Disconnection" (Miller & Stiver, 1994), summarize the implications of the relational paradox for the therapeutic encounter. They emphasize that the therapist must be open to, and empathic with, both sides of the paradox: the client's desire for connection and the client's need for strategies that keep large parts of herself out of connection. The therapist need not value the strategies themselves but must respect, and be empathic with, the woman's need for the strategies. At the same time, the therapist must be aware of her own paradox and strategies for disconnection. This openness, awareness, and empathy allows for the central process of therapy: the movement of relationships from connection, through disconnection, to new connection (Miller & Stiver, 1994).

Miller and Stiver (1994) elaborate the impact of this relational process on the therapeutic relationship: a client begins to bring more and more of herself into her own awareness and into the therapeutic space. She feels more authentic and, at the same time, she feels a new way of being in the relational world. If a person feels connected, without feeling helpless, she can rely less and less on her strategies for disconnection. Jordan has further elaborated upon the process of therapy by examining the need for shared vulnerability (1992), mutuality (1993), and empathy (1989). Group work, with its focus on relationships, provides a special forum in which to address this relational restructuring. In an empathic, supportive group, women remember and talk about things they have never shared before. Women in relational groups develop clarity about their experiences and their resulting strategies for disconnection. They experience hope about mutually satisfying relationships and expand their relational opportunities.

Bergman and Surrey (1992, 1994), in their work with couples, emphasize teaching them to be in connection by "holding on to the 'we.' " Their experience is that couples in true connection can talk about extremely difficult issues. This is an important aspect of relationship that is also apparent in group work. Members who remain connected in the group discuss difficult issues and experience a sense of perspective about their strategies within their connection.

HOW DO OTHER MODELS FRAME THE GROUP THERAPY PROCESS?

Traditional theories of psychoanalytic groups, while mentioning relationships and intimacy, emphasize a sense of self as the ultimate goal because of their reliance on traditional understandings of development. In contrast to seeing relational movement as the focus of psychological growth, the literature is peppered with notions of "hostile dependent needs," "dependent pre-affiliative stages," or (in a recent description of progress through an adolescent therapy group) "an innate need for autonomy which is countered by a greater dependency on the group, coupled with an ambivalence about autonomy, that creates hostile dependent relationships" (Alonso & Swiller, 1993, p. 230). Ultimately, autonomy is revered; relationships, though given lip service, take a backseat. Relationships and intimacy happen on the road to the true pot of gold—the self. Even efforts in group work to shift from content to group process ignore the primacy of relational movement as the task of development. Because of this misprioritizing, group therapy interventions often ignore the honest desire for connection, the true relational process that is the heart of group work.

Many group therapists (e.g., Pines & Hutchinson, 1993) view the leader's tasks as relational: they talk about maintaining boundaries (or, using a relational reframe, setting a consistent relational space), establishing the therapeutic norm of validation and mutuality, increasing member's participation and expression, and enhancing communication. But the fundamental distinction between traditional models and the relational approach to group work is the focus on developing a self as the primary goal or drive—the ultimate reward, if you will— rather than on development through relational movement and connection.

In the same multiauthor book on groups, Doherty and Enders (1993) critique the relational model without a thorough understanding or current review of relational writings. They describe it briefly as "the dichotomous structuring of affiliation and autonomy, " a very early version of relational work dating back to Gilligan's book *In a Different Voice* (1982). Since the most recent source cited from the Stone Center writings was 1986, the importance of the relational approach, though dismissed, was not adequately examined. The principal critique was an old one (Lemer, 1988): that the relational model looks only at mother–daughter interaction instead of the whole family system. Since there are a number of articles written about the relational model that examine family systems (Mirkin, 1994; Stiver,1990a, 1990b), this is clearly an outdated as well as a misinterpreted issue. The relational model, in its current level of sophistication and its current point of evolution, has not been incorporated into mainstream writings on group psychotherapy.

Yalom has written about the interpersonal school of group therapy (1970, 1983). This view of group therapy has contributed a great deal to a relational understanding of group dynamics. Group work in this approach addresses interpersonal dynamics and content by focusing on group interactions and process. A peer theory of group interaction (Grunebaum & Solomon, 1982; Solomon & Grunebaum, 1982) integrating Sullivanian concepts about the healing power of relationships, consensual exchange, and an emphasis on mutuality also contributes to an interpersonal theory of true relational movement in groups. The ideas developed by the Stone Center enhance this understanding and help us evolve a clearer view of what is healing about group work.

The curative factors that Yalom elaborates have relational equivalents in a relational model of group psychotherapy. In a relational view, we have called the curative factors *healing factors* (see Fedele & Harrington, 1990). This is indicative of a shift in focus from a client who is cured or acted upon by a therapist or by the group to one who is healed because of an interactive process with another member, the collective group, or the group facilitator. This seemingly small change in one word signifies a major addition to Yalom's perspective.

In an article entitled "Feminist Therapy in Groups," Marilyn Johnson (1987) describes a research project that integrated Yalom's curative factors with a feminist perspective. A population of feminist therapy collective clients ranked the curative factors that seemed most salient to them from a list incorporating Yalom's 10 curative factors and a number of feminist factors designed specifically for the study. Johnson found that the women clients valued four aspects of group work: three from Yalom's list and one feminist factor.

The healing factor that the feminist therapy collective clients ranked highest was group cohesiveness: the feeling of belonging to, being understood by, and accepted by a group (Yalom, 1970). In relational terms, this healing factor might translate to each members' feeling of connection within and to a group. Using this term allows for the members' *interactive experience*, rather than simply referring to a quality of the group. Members in groups do talk about group cohesion, but it is also important to describe each person's experience in the group. In a relational view, connection is the experience while validation is the process.

The second healing factor that Johnson found salient in her population was input in interpersonal learning (Yalom, 1970). This is learning how to take in information about other people that helps you to relate to them. Using a relational approach, this factor could be termed "achieving clarity about others." Group members can go beyond seeing another member's actions by beginning to resonate with, empathize with, and understand the meanings and feelings of other participants. The process experience of the members involves resonance and empathy.

Another curative factor that Johnson found is what Yalom (1970) describes as insight, that is, the ability to understand why one thinks and feels the way one does. In shifting the focus from a cognitive process, such as insight, to a more relational one, a relational view suggests that this healing factor entails an ability to integrate understanding with clarity about feelings as an ever-changing dynamic process. For example, if a member's feelings are validated and understood to emanate from the cultural or social context, it is more productive to focus her efforts to change the context or work around it, rather than attempting to change herself. This is clearly exemplified by work on battered women reported by Swift (1987, 1990). In order to have clarity, we need to work toward seeing the world as accurately as possible. And vice versa: in order to see the world clearly, we need to work at having as much clarity about ourselves as possible. This interactive process can happen in a mutually validating and clarifying relational space. The factor could be termed clarity about oneself; the process is validation and self-empathy.

Johnson (1987) also reported that the women found seeing a successful, competent woman as the leader of the group an important healing factor. This was not a sense of identification with a woman (that was also on the list), but simply experiencing competence in a woman as possible and seeing a woman as having the potential of leading a fulfilling life. Group therapists often hear despair about finding a loving partner, about being respected as a woman or as a person by coworkers, about going beyond the pain of abuse or loss. Sometimes, by our very existence and our commitment to respect and connection, we engender hope and catalyze empowerment. In the spirit of inclusion, this could also be applicable to a men's group where seeing a nurturant, warm, successful man could be a novel and empowering experience. This factor, which I would term empowerment, speaks to moving beyond the limited societal constructs available for both women and men.

Recent feminist writings on group work include two books on the subject: Butler and Wintram's *Feminist Groupwork* (1991) and Brody's *Women's Therapy Groups: Paradigms of Feminist Treatment* (1987). The therapists who contributed to these books address women's psychological development in a way that validates the feelings and experiences of their women clients. They listen to their voices, their ways of knowing, their real-life experience of the world, rather than trying to fit women's experiences into already developed and severely deficient theoretical frameworks. Feminist perspectives provide major contributions to our understanding of women in groups by recognizing society's impact on women and the social context within which all women live.

One of the contributions from feminist group work that draws on work by Miller (1976) in her book *Toward a New Psychology of Women* is the issue of power differentials between a leader and members in a group (Burden & Gottlieb, 1987; Lazerson, 1991). Burden and Gottlieb (1987) offer suggestions for reducing the power differential between the leader and members. Lazerson, in an article on feminism in group work, suggests a focus on mutual empowerment and collaboration (1991). This feminist view of power relations in group work is enhanced by the relational model's movement from a model of "power over" to "power with" and toward a sense of mutual empowerment (Surrey, 1987).

RELATIONAL CONCEPTS: PARADOX, CONNECTION, AND RESONANCE

Using a relational lens, then, we ask: What is group therapy? What are the relational dynamics of a group? How do we understand what is healing about groups? At this point, I discuss three concepts that appear over and over again in the relational literature and that are useful in framing a relational approach to group psychotherapy: paradox, connection, and resonance. These general principles of relational theory can help us understand group process in all types of groups along many continua of group work. They are applicable to structured or unstructured groups, short term or open ended, the entire inpatient, day hospital, and outpatient continuum, and in issue-focused or general groups. The activity of the therapist changes in these different groups as an empathic response to the relational movement available to the group members, but the principles remain the same.

The three relational concepts are as follows:

1. *Paradox*, defined in the *Oxford American Dictionary* as a statement that appears to contradict itself but that contains a truth (Ehrlich, Flexner, Carruth, & Hawkins, 1980)
2. The experience of *connection*, that is, a joining in relationship between people who experience each other's presence in a full way and who accommodate both the correspondence and contrasts between them

3. *Resonance*, defined as a resounding; an echoing; the capacity to respond that, in its most sophisticated form, is empathy

Paradox

Using the relational model, the ongoing dialectic between the desire for genuine, responsive, and gratifying connections and the need to maintain strategies to stay out of connection is the pivotal experience of group therapy. I find that this paradox offers the most helpful approach to understanding group process and to promoting healing interactions in a group. In an earlier paper (Fedele, 1993), I have discussed the many paradoxes in therapy: vulnerability leads to growth; pain can be experienced in safety; talking about disconnection leads to connection; and conflict between people can be best tolerated in their connection. Another paradox, that between the transferential relationships and the real relationship, is a crucial healing aspect of therapy. The challenge of establishing a mutual, empathic relationship within the context of the unequal therapist–client relationship is another primary paradox of the therapeutic context.

These dilemmas are dramatically apparent in group psychotherapy. The therapist and group members collaborate to create an emotional relational space that allows the members to recapture more and more of their experience in their own awareness and in the group. The feelings of the past can be tolerated in this new relational space. It allows us to reframe the experience of pain within the context of safety. The difficulty of creating an environment that allows vulnerability in a group format involves the complexity of creating safety for all participants. Some of the following paradoxes speak to this task.

The Basic Paradox

The basic paradox evident in group work is the simultaneous yearning for connection, on the one hand, and the need to maintain strategies for disconnection, on the other. This plays out as the tension between wanting one's feelings understood and the fear that people will not empathize with those feelings. One can protect oneself by using strategies for disconnection while participating in the group in a limited way. A group therapist needs to empathize with the intense yearnings for connection (rather than the need for separation or the drive for autonomy), as well as the need for strategies that derail connection. If the therapist does not do so, the group member will feel misunderstood and invalidated because only her strategies of disconnection would be seen in the many relational interactions that a group provides and highlights.

The Paradox of Similarity and Diversity

The next paradox, the tension between connection around universal feelings and the fears of isolation because of difference, can be translated to similarity versus diversity. Most models of group process employ similar understanding: group identity requires conflict as well as cohesion. Butler and Wintram (1991) view the experience of paradox and contradiction, as well as safety and acceptance, as central to group identity formation and change in women's groups. The particular tension of a particular group is unique to that group of people and their salient issues. This idea applies to larger groups, such as women's organizations, as well as smaller groups (e.g., therapy groups).

The fluctuations between diversity and similarity create a rhythm that permeates every facet of a group's behavior. The goal for group work is to choreograph that rhythm into movement through a mutual empathic process. The experience of similarity allows the group to hold feelings of diversity within the connection. The role of empathy is crucial to hold divergent realities within an empathic relational context. The mutuality of the empathy allows all participants to feel understood and accepted. The leader, in creating a safe relational context, fosters connectedness within that safety by working to enlarge the empathy for differences.

In women's groups, connection is enhanced when women can share a particular experience of growing up female in this culture. However, issues relating to race, class, and sexual orientation indicate that not all women's experience is shared. This is also evident in therapy groups. We don't yet have enough literature on groups of women of all races, classes, and sexual orientations, but the literature on African American women tends to favor homogeneous groups (Boyd-Franklin, 1987, 1991; Trotman & Gallagher, 1987) in order to provide a validating and empowering experience. Dowd and Forstein (1993), in commenting on issues of diversity, find that it is particularly difficult for one or two women who experience themselves as different to have a space for their experience within a larger group (e.g., one or two lesbian women in a group with five heterosexual women). Dowd and Forstein has observed this disconnection in groups where the differential was around race or sexual preference in women. However, if you move toward integration by equalizing the difference (e.g., three African American women and three Irish American women), it seems impossible to create a sense of connection or cohesion.

This paradox of diversity and commonality is a dilemma reflected in the woman's movement. In the women's community, there was a sense of solidarity until issues of diversity brought to light conflict that threatens to splinter the power of the feminist community. This conflict centers around the recognition that a false solidarity exists because all women's experience has not been represented. The important challenge here is to learn from our diversity and to maximize the potential for enormous growth and enhancement or be faced with a conflict that overwhelms our important feminist and social agenda. Safety is a focal issue here because it is in the creation of a context of safety that women who experience similarity (e.g., African American women or poor women) can remain in connection, can feel strengthened and empowered to find their voices, and can move into the integration work with women who are experienced as different.

This kind of relational movement is reflected in the work of Julia Kristeva, a feminist philosopher who describes three stages of feminism (see Lazerson, 1991). The first stage was concerned with notions of inequities in society. The second dealt with differences: different voices and different ways of knowing. The third and current stage involves an integration of the first two because both areas of inequities and differences are still of concern. It is concerned with understanding the societal constriction of an overemphasis on categories of race, gender, and class because these are false categories that conceal unique individual differences within groups of people, particularly marginalized people. These feminist considerations are important in understanding issues of diversity versus similarity, and bring us to the next paradox.

The Paradox That Sharing Disconnection
Leads to New Connection

Each women's group creates a unique environment but with similar themes. There is a unique pattern of relationships, but there are certain universal elements. An essential relational component of groups is the need for the discussion of disconnection in the group. When members phone the leader to report anger or dissatisfaction with the group, the leader can encourage them to share this experience in the group. Often, if one member feels the disconnection, it is very likely that one or more of the other members experience similar feelings and resonate with the feelings of dissatisfaction. When people begin to discuss their feelings of disconnection or isolation, they are often mirrored by other members who hesitated to introduce these feelings. A sense of connection around these experiences causes the members to feel reconnected in the group. This allows for safety and counters isolation and shame.

Members can empathize with the feelings of disconnection, even if they themselves do not experience the same feelings. The group process can validate and accept the range of feelings from negative to positive. This experience of connection with others around the disconnection gives women the power to move out of their disconnection and continue to engage in mutual relational movement. It also allows the group to work together, to experience a sense of being moved by each other, and to effect a change in their relational space so that the members feel more connected. The challenging process of creating a relational space that is responsive to the changing needs of each of the members is an evolutionary and dynamic one. It leads to the powerful experience of people understanding how they are different from others by experiencing these differences in the group; at the same time, they connect around their similarities and understand how they might be the same. Both are valuable forms of self-knowledge that flow from relationships, and they allow people to encompass the extraordinarily important experience of being different or unique but even *more* connected to others. The feelings and group culture around this process are so positive that one of my groups generated this group norm: "If you feel disconnected, talk about it and you will feel connected."

The Paradox of Conflict in Connection

A relational approach to managing conflict in a group entails creating a context of safety and empathically understanding and containing divergent realities even when they conflict. To do this, one must also keep the experience of anger within the connection. Group members attempt to explore the feelings of anger, to trace the roots of internal judgment, and to understand how the present group experience can be different than previous experiences in relationships. Holding on to conflict in connection helps us define and understand ourselves and our differences from others.

Our own reactions to the differences between individuals can help us understand personal conflicts, while feeling connected can help us deal with external conflict (Miller, 1983). One deals with conflict by making and holding connections between apparent opposites. In the larger picture, building bridges means confronting prejudices rather than ignoring them to create an illusion of solidarity. In fact, raising differences will further the development of a group. The paradox is that people can tolerate diversity by becoming more connected.

One way to view anger is to see it as a reaction to the experience of disconnection in the face of intense yearning for connection. In a group it is often the very strategies that a person has developed to participate in some limited way in relationships that interfere with that person's ability to connect more fully. By empathizing with those strategies, we can help each participant become aware of them and the impact upon the relational experience. When two members' strategies collide with one another, resolution of the impasse can ensue when the group recognizes each person's need for strategies and provides the mutual encouragement for each person to understand the force of those diverging needs and strategies. This allows for conflict in connection.

Connection

Connection is the second important concept of relational group work. While many group therapists would say that the group should create a feeling of belonging and acceptance, they do not say that the primary task of the leader and the group members is to facilitate a feeling of connection. In a relational model of group work, the leader is careful to understand each interaction, each dynamic in the group, as a means for maintaining connection or as a strategy developed to remain out of connection. As in interpersonal therapy groups, the leader encourages the members to be aware of their availability in the here-and-now relationships of the group by understanding and empathizing with their experiences of the past. But it is the yearning for connection, rather than an innate need for separation or individuation, that fuels their development *both* in the here and now *and* in the past. The leader of a relational therapy group sets the stage for safety by providing a respectful, validating, and empathic relational space, rather than a critical or analytic atmosphere, no matter how " constructive" or essential the interpretation. Empathy is the primary emotional tool which a group therapist employs in understanding, validating, and being present with each member's experience. However, it is always the group member who is the "expert" and who decides whether an interpretation or an idea fits her experience. In this context, a member is empowered to risk vulnerability and feels safe enough to be moved and to move others in the group.

We have lived in and live in many relational spaces, often simultaneously and sometimes contemporaneously. Creating a group is a process of creating a new relational space, a safe relational context, that for many people, even quite successful ones, is a unique relational space. How does a group leader create safety? It is essential that the relational group therapist is present in an emotionally available and empathic way; she must complete the circle of connection. The leader must establish the norms of mutuality, attend to the group process, and minimize the power differential. Further, she must safeguard the relational environment and enlist members' collaboration in its creation. For example, the group therapist sets the tone with which to discuss feelings of anger or dissatisfaction with the group. Members are encouraged to discuss these feelings without judgments or harsh criticisms. In contrast to a model of a silent group leader, a relational one counters feelings of humiliation, endangerment, or criticism for the sake of safety.

The group becomes a here-and-now relational space where transferential relations of the past or devaluing relational spaces of the present can be safely and respectfully revealed in an atmosphere of emotional connection and healed in the dynamic process of ongoing mutual and empathic relationship. The goal of relational group work is to create a place where people experience a new possibility for connection, face inevitable disconnection, and strive for reconnection. This is the new and powerful experience that can occur. The group leader enhances communication by understanding the strategies that each member has developed to stay out of connection and by empathizing with the need for those strategies. She begins to visualize and articulate relational dilemmas or patterns for staying out of connection in the group. In a validating environment, the group can empower its members to utilize the strategies less and less. As one member described her experience, the group allowed her to "open up to the affirmations that had always been, the world, but that she hadn't been able to hear." At the same time, she began to "tune out the disaffirmations" to which she had been exquisitely attuned.

Some clients like to think of a group as a relational laboratory where one examines old assumptions and experiences a new possibility of relationship, where vulnerability can be tolerated because of the experience of safety. Van der Kolk (1993) describes his amazement at women's ability to remain open to relationships in therapy groups even in the face of histories of tremendous trauma. Despite each person's strategies of disconnection, it is women's relational capacity to also remain vulnerable (Gilligan, Rogers, & Tolman, 1991; Jordan, 1992; Miller, 1976) that is the heart of effective group work.

There are many aspects of relationship that need to be kept in awareness simultaneously: the transferences, the countertransference, and the real here-and-now relationship. The transferences certainly include all the connections and learned strategies for disconnections to all the relational figures of the past. In her book *Trauma and Recovery*, Herman (1992) describes a therapeutic context where the perpetrators of abuse are in the room. My experience is that in a group, everyone is in the room—all the important relationships are represented, some more vividly or audibly than others. I first realized this when I was leading inpatient groups that included women who had multiple personalities. We, as a group, would wonder how many people were in the room. But the reality is that there are always many relationships representing the connections and disconnections in the members' relational past. And the beauty of a group is that sometimes these transferences overlap with one another; that is, one women's transference toward another member is complemented by that member's matching transference. For example, Joan may be angry because Kathy's silence reminds Joan of her emotionally absent mother, while Kathy is terrified of Joan's direct expression of anger reminiscent of Kathy's volatile sister. Though this is a challenging situation in a group, it also provides an opportunity for both women to observe their reactions to familiar situations and see the impact of their actions. There is truly the possibility of movement. In the safety of a genuine relational context, representatives of old relational images can be expressed in the transference. Creating an environment that allows vulnerability in a group format involves the complexity of creating safety for all participants. The group therapist in understanding each member's transference can help the group understand what transferential "locking of horns" might be impeding movement in the real here-and-now relationship.

Because of the group format, the presence of so many memories in a room, and the similarity of a group to a family, many of the transferences evident in a group involve sibling issues in the family of origin, as well as issues with authority or getting enough from the family. Sibling issues can be quite profound, particularly when there is sibling rivalry or guilt because of the disadvantage of another sibling. There are often many strategies for disconnection around this material.

Certainly, it is important to understand our countertransferences as therapists. The relational view of countertransference (Miller & Stiver, 1991; Steiner-Adair, 1991; Surrey, 1991) includes anything which helps or hurts a therapist's ability to maintain a real connection with a client—to be truly present and truly aware. Stiver (1992) encourages us to examine our own paradox, our own ways of staying out of connection, and the impact on our work as therapists. I believe we do this by creating effective group networks to support our work and examine our own paradox in supervision groups and consultation groups. Understanding our strategies for disconnection allows us to resonate more effectively with—and ultimately to be more empathic with—the group process.

This brings us to issues of the therapist's disclosure around difficult group process material. This is a particularly important question for the therapist, for example, around recent unresolved grief or loss. It is a challenge to stay connected to a group that is dealing with intense feelings about loss without using our own strategies of disconnection. These strategies can interfere with our ability to remain connected and resonant with the group process. Since the anticipation of loss or rejection is always present in a group in some form or other, it is important to develop some authentic way of remaining connected with the group. One approach is to say "I can imagine what if feels like" or "I know what it feels like" without actually talking about your own experiences in the group. This authentic approach is usually honest and empathic enough to maintain the therapist's connection with the group. Because of the complexity of all the members' transferences, therapist disclosure of painful material needs to be approached with caution.

Another important countertransference issue involves not letting our biases, no matter how well meaning, interfere with the group treatment or influence our ability to allow each woman to find her own voice, her own experience, and her own feelings. The difficulties are demonstrated in the work that group therapists do with abused clients, whether the abuse is physical, sexual, or psychological. Group therapists need to provide members with a safe context to determine and acknowledge their own feelings. The therapist must be open to the level of positive feelings, as well as negative ones, that a client has toward an offender. The therapist cannot allow her own abuse or her own rage and feelings of helplessness at the amount of violence perpetrated against women to interfere with her openness to the member's full range of feelings. At the same time, therapists need to hold in highest regard the physical and psychological safety of the members.

To summarize, connection involves the development of the real here-and-now relationship in an authentic, mutually validating, and empathic manner. It is this relationship that provides the hope for defusing devaluing transferential relationships from the past and the creation of growth-enhancing ones in the future. Whenever the therapist or client experiences a break in connection, it is important to raise the question: What is interfering with my/our capacity to remain in relationship? If the therapist cannot create a space for movement, the question can be raised with the group. Why is everyone having a hard time connecting? Why are people keeping their emotional selves out of the experience? The leader needs to return to the paradox. Members who feel vulnerable in the face of their tremendous yearnings to connect will utilize their strategies for disconnection. The work of the group involves understanding how each person's strategies contribute to the group process, especially during a group impasse. The group consists of different people with different vulnerabilities and consequently different strategies for disconnection. It is difficult but tremendously powerful work to begin to untangle the fears and strategies that each member has developed to protect herself from feelings of isolation. Again, ironically, in talking about the disconnection, the group can get back on track and experience reconnection.

Resonance

The power of experiencing one's pain within a healing connection stems from the ability of an individual to resonate with another. Resonance, which appears in the literature on the Stone Center relational model, Gilligan and colleagues' work (1991), and studies on groups (Alonso & Swiller, 1993), implies one person responding to another person. It manifests itself in group work in two ways: The first is the ability of one member to simply resonate with another's experience in the group and experience some vicarious relief because of that resonance. The member need not discuss the issue in the group, but the experience moves her that much closer to knowing and sharing her own truth without necessarily responding or articulating it. The second way resonance manifests itself in a group involves the ability of members to resonate with each other's issues and thereby recall or reconnect with their own issues. This is an important element of group process in all groups but is dramatically obvious in groups with women who have trauma histories. Often, when one woman talks about painful material, other women dissociate. It is a very powerful aspect of group work that, if acknowledged, can help women move into connection. It can also cause problems if women become overwhelmed or flooded. The leader needs to modulate this resonance by helping each member develop skills to manage and contain intense feelings.

Empathy is a sophisticated and powerful tool that has its roots in the capacity for resonance. Jordan (1984, 1987, 1989, 1990) has done extensive work describing the cognitive and affective components of empathy in the relational model and empathy's role in the therapeutic relationship. In particular, she has described the various experiences of empathy that allows for a person's development in relationship. People experience empathy from others in the safety of connection. They are empowered to experience empathy with themselves (self-empathy), and they continue to develop the capacity to experience empathy with others. These three experiences revitalize empathic possibility and allow for relational movement in groups.

Given the proper conditions in a group (a safe, validating environment of connection), empathy becomes an essential element of communication and healing. It is often a woman's first full experience of others' empathy, of being heard and moving others in a dramatic way. This experience of empathy allows the member to reexperience her own feelings without immediately resorting to strategies for disconnection, even from herself. In experiencing these feelings within a safe group context the member develops the healing ability of self-empathy. In an earlier paper, Fedele and Harrington (1990) presented clinical material regarding the development of self-empathy in groups. The group environment also allows each member to fully develop her capacity to empathize with others. Although women have always had the ability to empathize, we need relational settings that validate this capacity because many popular theories about relationships cast this capacity in a negative light and cause women to blame themselves: "codependency," "masochism," or "love addiction" (Jones & Schecter, 1992). The ultimate relational goal of group work is the development of mutual empathy in growth-fostering relationships.

The use of countertransferential material as a window into the client's experience is addressed in relational writings (Miller & Stiver, 1991). The experience of countertransference in a group is another example of resonance as a therapeutic tool. In a group, the therapist's own strategies for staying out of connection, particularly if they are not her characteristic strategies, can indicate some group collusion to stay away from painful material. Extensive feelings of disconnection and isolation evident in the room are a good indication that the whole group is reacting and protecting their vulnerability. In group literature, this is termed a group-as-a-whole response. A leader might realize her own disconnection and share her own subjective experience of the moment in a way that discloses her present feeling. If this is empathically attuned to the other members' experience, someone often resonates with the expression and discusses her own disconnection, which, of course, leads to connection.

A respect for the group's ability to resonate with, and possibly to access, material from the leader's unconscious is also important. For example, members might notice if a leader is tired or sick, or a leader reacts when listening to sadistic or hostile feelings. Is there a way the leader tunes out (or uses her own strategies for disconnection) that communicates her feelings? Are these feelings in the group? Can the leader reflect them in an authentic way? Resonance is an important tool that fosters connection. And empathy, a more sophisticated and complex resonance, is the necessary catalyst that makes reconnection a possibility.

In summary, this chapter has included discussions on three relational concepts that are the important threads of group work: paradox, connection, and resonance. There are many paradoxes in group work. Three are highlighted: (1) sharing feelings of disconnections helps one become reconnected; (2) discussing diversity leads to connection; and (3) dealing with conflict can lead to connection. True, growth-enhancing connections in the safe relational space of groups are an integral part of the healing experience. The transference, countertransference, and here-and-now experiences are all important aspects of connection.

Resonance and its more sophisticated counterpart, empathy, are central in the process of healing in group work.

A CLINICAL ILLUSTRATION: CONFLICT IN CONNECTION

This and the next section consist of two ongoing examples of group process. The descriptions of group members are disguised composites. The first example is about *conflict in connection* and involves two women in a women's group composed of eight women. This is a common group dynamic and the descriptions represent many different members who experience differences in groups. One married woman, who will be called Sue here, joined the group because of intense feelings in relationships, which she wanted to modulate. She felt that she overwhelmed people easily. Her family of origin was a large chaotic Catholic family of 10; her mother had been diagnosed with a major mental illness and, in the best of times, would be silent. Her father was emotionally and sometimes physically unavailable to the children. He would put them in an orphanage when he couldn't take care of them. As you can see, there was a great deal of loss and grieving about what had been missing in the family. Sue had worked on all of these issues and had reached a good amount of satisfaction in her own life—a marriage and a successful professional career. As an adult, however, she saw a tremendous amount of dysfunction in her family members because they had developed dangerous strategies to deal with their feelings. Yet, she wanted to maintain some semblance of connection to them. She was the one that tried to help them deal with their feelings, and she would usually be disappointed. In the group, Sue would always look deep into the heart of feelings and try always to help people grapple with them.

Another member, who will be called Sally, tended to be quiet and frightened of interaction. She had also worked extensively in individual and group therapy on issues with her family around abuse, as well as the death of her mother at an early age. She joined this group because of her progress in dealing with her sadness and because of her wish for movement to the next step: to develop more relationships. Her family history was different from Sue's, although some similar issues were present. Her WASP family had been punitive toward her whenever she had expressed feelings of grief or dissatisfaction. One of her older sisters had been spared this criticism because she followed the family dogma: "Look good and keep silent." As a group member, Sally took a while getting used to the group. Her adjustment was so difficult that at times she would disconnect from the material, especially when it was about relationships that she felt, although difficult for others, were impossible for her.

As you can well imagine, the dynamics between the two were intense at various points in the 1½ years they were both in the group. Over and over again Sue would want the group to grapple with intense feelings and feel angry at what she perceived as Sally's silence, avoidance of feelings, and judgment. This was reminiscent of her mother's silence or criticism and her father's absence. Of course, this took a while to be expressed. Sally, on the other hand, would retreat because she was angry at Sue for being like her sister, getting all the attention and being what she considered the "group favorite." She would disconnect in the hopes that she wouldn't have to share her feelings. She literally would hold onto her seat in the hopes that nothing bad would happen and that she wouldn't be attacked for her feelings.

In each case, the group, by encouragement to express feelings, by empathy, and by a sense of being moved by both of them, would move the pair closer and closer to recognizing both their experiences—fostering connection by empathy with divergent experiences. The emotional awareness that both women could safely reveal their feelings in this different relational space slowly produced movement in relationship. Sue and Sally found that they could both get nurturance and empathy with their experience.

At the 1-year anniversary of the group, Sue brought in roses for all the members as a way to celebrate the importance of the group. She picked roses specifically because, though they are beautiful, they have thorns. To Sue, this represented the difficulty of the work in the group. The next week, Sally, when asked to share her feelings, carefully talked about how hard it was to have Sue bring in flowers: "It hasn't been a bed of roses to me." She was able to say that she knew that wasn't the true message but it was her feeling, her reaction. Being able to speak it and be accepted without judgment was crucial. In an exit interview from the group, Sue acknowledged the group's help in teaching her to value differences in experience. She had begun to understand how to be in conflict without getting out of connection. For her, it involved the issue of acceptance versus judgment—both being judged by others and judging others. Her efforts to get at intense feelings that were often overwhelming to other members was a strategy for disconnection, because she would quickly judge those members as inadequate to deal with her feelings. She was replicating her experience with her family members who truly were unable to deal with her feelings in any way. By explaining her feelings and her judgments, the group could begin to experience empathy for her feelings and remain in connection without utilizing their own strategies of disconnection. Sue and the other members began to experience mutual empathy in a conflict situation. This allowed her to enlarge her relational opportunities and develop more flexible relational possibilities.

ANOTHER CLINICAL ILLUSTRATION: LOSS AND DEPRIVATION

The second clinical example focuses on the experiences of loss and deprivation and their expression in the group. Since connection is the primary focus in our relational space, loss is an extremely difficult issue and permeates all aspects of change in a group. Group members often experience loss in reaction to the comings and goings in the group: the addition of new members, the absence of members, and the leave-taking of old members. Although there are many significant problems in groups, such as powerlessness and feelings of inauthenticity, loss and its resulting sadness are often the most powerful issues. The cycle of connections, disconnections, and reconnections is disrupted and sometimes drastically changed by loss.

Comings and goings both signify change and the potential for loss. I would venture to say that every therapy group session has some aspect of loss in it: losing time; losing dreams; losing childhood; losing members; losing a leader or co-leader; losing important relationships; losing feelings of acceptance and belonging; divorce, grief, depression. These are all frequent themes in women's groups. Memories of being left, of being put up for adoption, of being abused. One of the most salient factors in groups is sadness that underlies feelings of abandonment and isolation. Many members share the experience of feeling different, alone, and isolated—"the feeling of being the last kid chosen for the softball team."

A new person coming into the group engenders fear that the new person can change the relationships in the group in a negative way, fear that a new person would disrupt permanently the safe relational space and create an old transferential relational space. The loss of a member feeds the fantasies that the group will no longer be able to create a mutually empathic and empowering space. At the same time, experiencing a different kind of coming or going in a safe and validating space can break new relational ground, as these quotes from group members illustrate: "The memories of connection in sadness can soothe your pain in the present"; "People leaving catalyzes a process, it makes things happen; we get to a deeper level and talk about important things"; "I want to learn to say good-bye with the graciousness of a woman rather than the desperation of a child." They are all comments on the importance of experiencing a different approach to change and to loss.

The following is a series of group events that demonstrate how the creation of a safe relational space was crucial in catalyzing relational movement around deprivation and loss. The group had experienced a great deal of transition since a number of members had come to the group and a number had gone. These changes had been an integral part of the group discussion. During one particular session, the group was having a conversation about the experience of not having their feelings recognized and of "not having enough." One of the members talked about the group's experience as an indication "that I have never been heard in my whole life before." The members in this group discussed ways that each of them felt they did not have enough.

Trudy, the mother of three and herself a student, said she always felt that there wouldn't be enough. She keeps her refrigerator full of food, even though her children are away from home. Someone commented that they had seen a house while house hunting where someone had stored many gallons of cooking oil, a very neat stash; Trudy said that she had 15 gallons of oil on hand. She then began to talk about always needing more food to assure herself she wouldn't go hungry. She talked about her fears, then told of walking out of Europe as a child during the war. She had to live at a refugee camp for 10 years—the real fear of starvation was vivid—and had been diagnosed as malnourished at the time. It is important to note that in a pregroup interview she had said that she couldn't share these war memories in a group. She had been unable to share them with her mother and father, for it was "unspeakable." But she had been moved by the group process and, in turn, shared a poignant story that moved everyone.

A few weeks later, on her 20th wedding anniversary, Trudy came to the group with a bunch of papers. She announced that, because of the occasion, she had brought each of the members a present—a poem. This ritual of bringing presents on special occasions was begun by another member in the group. As a rule, these small gifts are not discouraged or interpreted. Trudy, all the while keeping her head in the papers, told of how she had forgotten them at school and then had asked to use my copy machine but it had cut off the copies in the wrong places. She wanted to fix the copies and give us the poem at the end of the group. I clearly remember sitting in my chair and, in what might be described as the moment when a therapist's training flashes before her eyes, thought of all the things I could say. What was her resistance? First she left the poems at school; now she is not paying attention to the group. Is she resistant to the group? Or, even, why is she not connecting to the group? And, of course, what is she trying to avoid by bringing presents? Or, the most insidious, why was she criticizing me as inadequate as a leader because my copy machine didn't work?

Luckily, I disregarded these old teachings and simply respected her decisions. I kept quiet, she finished quickly, and the group went on to talk about group transitions. I read the poem that night and discovered that it was a poem she had written.

The poem was about Trudy's hordes of oil. It mentions her and friends exchanging such revelations so, as you can see, the group is in the poem. In the description of the group, there is implied safety, validation, mutual empathy, and empowerment. The group process, however, had centered on the many transitions and losses in the group over the past few months. In the experience of connection within the group around feelings of never having enough, Trudy can connect with that part of her that holds painful memories of deprivation. She can speak the "unspeakable" and unburden herself of a painful secret. The sense of community is quite dramatic since there are actually two groups at work here. Trudy is also a member of a poetry group that gives interactive feedback on writing. This vignette demonstrates the power of issues of deprivation and loss to dominate our view of the world for a long time. Further, it confirms the healing climate of therapy groups and gives evidence of the enormous contribution of creativity as a transformative process. It is the ultimate paradox to create a meaningful and powerful work of art from the experience of extreme deprivation and sadness.

REFERENCES

Alonso, A., & Swiller, H. L. (1993). *Group therapy in clinical practice.* Washington, DC: American Psychiatric Press.

Bergman, S. J., & Surrey, J. L. (1992). The woman–man relationship: Impasses and possibilities. *Work in Progress, No. 55.* Wellesley, MA: Stone Center Working Paper Series.

Bergman, S. J., & Surrey, J. L. (1994). Couples therapy: A relational approach. *Work in Progress, No. 66.* Wellesley, MA: Stone Center Working Papers Series.

Boyd-Franklin, N. (1987). Group therapy for black women. *American Journal of Orthopsychiatry, 33*(3), 365–385.

Boyd-Franklin, N. (1991). Recurrent themes in the treatment of African-American women in group psychotherapy. *Women and Therapy, 11*(2), 25–40.

Brody, C. M. (1987). *Women's therapy groups: Paradigms of feminist treatment.* New York: Springer.

Burden, D. S., & Gottlieb, N. (1987). Women's socialization and feminist groups. In C. M. Brody (Ed.), *Women's therapy groups: Paradigms of feminist treatment* (pp. 24–39). New York: Springer.

Butler, S., & Wintram, C. (1991). *Feminist groupwork*. London: Sage.

Doherty, P., & Enders, P. L. (1993). Women in group psychotherapy. In A. Alonso & H. I. Swiller (Eds.), *Group therapy in clinical practice* (pp. 371–391). Washington, DC: American Psychiatric Press.

Dowd, S., & Forstein, M. (1993, November 6). *Gay and lesbian dialogues: Functions of an outlaw identity*. Paper presented at the Harvard Medical School Conference on Men and Women: A Clinical Dialogue, Cambridge, MA.

Ehrlich, E., Flexner, S. B., Carruth, G., & Hawkins, J. (1980). *Oxford American dictionary*. New York: Oxford University Press.

Fedele, N. M. (1993, February 26). *Relationships in therapy: Connection, paradox and resonance*. Paper presented at Grand Rounds, Charles River Hospital, Wellesley, MA.

Fedele, N. M., & Harrington, E. A. (1990). Women's groups: How connections heal. *Work in Progress, No. 47*. Wellesley, MA: Stone Center Working Paper Series.

Gilligan, C. (1982). *In a different voice: Psychological theory and women's development*. Cambridge, MA: Harvard University Press.

Gilligan, C. (1990). Joining the resistance: Psychology, politics, girls and women. *Michigan Quarterly Review, 29*(4), 501–536.

Gilligan, C., Lyons, N., & Hammer, T. (1990). *Making connections*. Cambridge, MA: Harvard University Press.

Gilligan, C., Rogers, A., & Tolman, D. L. (1991). *Women, girls and psychotherapy: Reframing resistance*. New York: Haworth Press.

Grunebaum, H., & Solomon, L. (1982). Toward a theory of peer relationships: II. On the stages of social development and their relationship to group therapy. *International Journal of Group Psychotherapy, 32*(3), 283–307.

Herman, J. L. (1992). *Trauma and recovery*. New York: Basic Books.

Johnson, M. (1987). Feminist therapy in groups: A decade of change. In C. M. Brody (Ed.), *Women's therapy groups: Paradigms of feminist treatment* (pp. 13–23). New York: Springer.

Jones, A., & Schecter, S. (1992). *When love goes wrong*. New York: HarperCollins.

Jordan, J. V. (1984). Empathy and self boundaries. *Work in Progress, No. 16.* Wellesley, MA: Stone Center Working Paper Series.

Jordan, J. V. (1987). Clarity in connection: Empathic knowing, desire and sexuality. *Work in Progress, No. 29*. Wellesley, MA: Stone Center Working Paper Series.

Jordan, J. V. (1989). Relational development: Therapeutic implications of empathy and shame. *Work in Progress, No. 39*. Wellesley, MA: Stone Center Working Paper Series.

Jordan, J. V. (1990). Courage in connection: Conflict, compassion and creativity. *Work in Progress, No. 45*. Wellesley, MA: Stone Center Working Paper Series.

Jordan, J. V. (1992). Relational resilience. *Work in Progress, No. 57*. Wellesley, MA: Stone Center Working Paper Series.

Jordan, J. V. (1993). Challenges to connection. *Work in Progress, No. 60*. Wellesley, MA: Stone Center Working Paper Series.

Jordan, J. V., Surrey, J. L., & Kaplan, A. G. (1983). Women and empathy. *Work in Progress, No. 2*. Wellesley, MA: Stone Center Working Paper Series.

Krugman, S., & Osherson, S. (1993). Men in group therapy. In A. Alonso &

H. I. Swiller (Eds.), *Group therapy in clinical practice* (pp. 393–420). Washington, DC: American Psychiatric Press.

Lazerson, J. S. (1991). Feminism and group psychotherapy: An ethical responsibility. *International Journal for Group Psychotherapy, 42*(4), 523–546.

Lerner, H. (1988). *Women and therapy*. New York: Harper & Row.

Miller, J. B. (1976). *Toward a new psychology of women*. Boston: Beacon Press.

Miller, J. B. (1983). The necessity of conflict. In J. H. Robbins & R. J. Siegal (Eds.), *Women changing therapy* [Special issue]. *Women and Therapy: A Feminist Quarterly, 2*(2), 3–9.

Miller, J. B. (1986). What do we mean by relationships? *Work in Progress, No. 22*. Wellesley, MA: Stone Center Working Paper Series.

Miller, J. B. (1987). *Toward a new psychology of women* (2nd ed.). Boston: Beacon Press.

Miller. J. B. (1988). Connections, disconnections and violations. *Work in Progress, No. 33*. Wellesley, MA: Stone Center Working Paper Series.

Miller, J. B., & Stiver, I. (1991). A relational reframing of therapy. *Work in Progress, No. 52*. Wellesley, MA: Stone Center Working Paper Series.

Miller, J. B., & Stiver, I. (1994). Movement in therapy: Honoring the "strategies of disconnection." *Work in Progress, No. 66*. Wellesley, MA: Stone Center Working Paper Series.

Mirkin, M. P. (1991). Female adolescence revisited: Understanding girls in their sociocultural context. In M. P. Mirkin (Ed.), *Women in context: Toward a feminist reconstruction of psychotherapy* (pp. 77–95). New York: Guilford Press.

Pines, M., & Hutchinson, S. (1993). Group analysis. In A. Alonso & H. I. Swiller (Eds.), *Group therapy in clinical practice* (pp. 29–47). Washington, DC: American Psychiatric Press.

Solomon, L., & Grunebaum, H. (1982). Stages in social development: Friendship and peer relations. *Hillside Journal of Clinical Psychiatry, 4*(1), 95–126.

Steiner-Adair, C. (1991). New maps of development, new models of therapy: The psychology of women and treatment of eating disorders. In C. L. Johnson (Ed.), *Psychodynamic treatment of anorexia nervosa and bulimia*. New York: Guilford Press.

Stiver, I. P. (1990a). Dysfunctional families and wounded relationships—Part I. *Work in Progress, No. 41*. Wellesley, MA: Stone Center Working Paper Series.

Stiver, I. P. (1990b). Dysfunctional families and wounded relationships—Part II. *Work in Progress, No. 44*. Wellesley, MA: Stone Center Working Paper Series.

Stiver, I. P. (1992). A relational approach to therapeutic impasses. *Work in Progress, No. 58*. Wellesley, MA: Stone Center Working Paper Series.

Surrey, J. L. (1987). Relationship and empowerment. *Work in Progress, No. 30*. Wellesley, MA: Stone Center Working Paper Series.

Surrey, J. L. (1991). What do we mean by mutuality in therapy? In J. V. Jordan, A. G. Kaplan, J. B. Miller, I. P. Stiver, & J. L. Surrey, "Some misconceptions and reconceptions of a relational approach." *Work in Progress, No. 49*. Wellesley, MA: Stone Center Working Paper Series.

Surrey, J. L., Kaplan, A. G., & Jordan, J. V. (1990). Empathy revisited. *Work in Progress, No. 40*. Wellesley, MA: Stone Center Working Paper Series.

Swift, C. (1987). Women and violence: Breaking the connection. *Work in Progress, No. 27*. Wellesley, MA: Stone Center Working Paper Series.

Swift, C. (1988). Surviving: Women's strength through connection. In M. B. Straus (Ed.), *Abuse and victimization across the lifespan* (pp. 153–169). Baltimore: Johns Hopkins University Press.

Trotman, F. K., & Gallagher, A. H. (1987). Group therapy with black women. In C. M. Brody (Ed.), *Women's therapy groups: Paradigms of feminist treatment* (pp. 13–23). New York: Springer.

van der Kolk, B. (1993). Viewpoint. *Northeastern Society for Group Psychotherapy Newsletter, 16*(1), 1–3.

Yalom, I. (1970). *The theory and practice of group psychotherapy*. New York: Basic Books.

Yalom, I. (1983). *Inpatient group psychotherapy*. New York: Basic Books.

This chapter was originally presented at a Stone Center Colloquium on December 1, 1993. © 1994 by Nikki Fedele.

11

Mothers and Sons
Raising Relational Boys

CATE DOOLEY *and* NIKKI M. FEDELE

> Achilles, mightiest of the Greeks, hero of the Iliad, was
> nearly immortal. According to myth, his mother, Thetis,
> dipped him into the river Styx. The sacred waters of this
> river that led to Hades, the world of the dead, rendered
> whomever they touched impervious to harm. But Thetis,
> good mother that she was, worried about the dangers of
> the river, and so she held onto Achilles by his heel. As the
> story goes, because of that one holding spot, Achilles
> remained mortal and vulnerable to harm. Thetis would
> be blamed forever after for her son's fatal flaw, his
> Achilles' heel.

T he holding place of vulnerability was not, as the myth would
have us believe, a fatal liability to Achilles. It was the thing that kept
him *human and real*. In fact, we consider it *Thetis's finest gift* to her son.

Every mother of a son hopes to prepare him for life's "battles"
while also preserving his emotional–relational side. Because mothers
value connection, they want to "hold on," to keep open that place of
vulnerability. But faced with cultural pressures that suggest restraint
and withdrawal, rather than comfort and nurture, many mothers feel

conflicted about their desire to stay connected to their sons. Traditional wisdom cautions that holding on will be damaging and create psychological problems for sons. Faced with this dilemma, mothers often yield to cultural pressures and disconnect from their young sons because they think it's the right thing to do.

Our work with mothers of sons is based on relational–cultural theory (RCT), a view of development for women and men that grew out of Jean Baker Miller's 1976 book, *Toward a New Psychology of Women* (2nd ed., 1987). In her book, Miller introduces a new view of women and their development. After many years of listening to and studying women, she concludes that relationship and affiliation are essential to healthy development. She has noted the pejorative attitudes about women and their roles, embedded in the fabric of Western culture, and states that these cultural views diminish women's self-worth.

We highlight the mother–son relationship because we feel that this same devalued view of women affects the mother–son relationship. The culture tells mothers to disconnect from their sons. A closeness with mom has frequently been misunderstood and pathologized. The mother–son connection is ridiculed ("Go run to mama"; "Crybaby"), cautioned against ("You better let him go"; "Push him out to the world"), prohibited ("Don't coddle him"; "No more hugs and kisses"), and maligned ("She's turned him into a mama's boy"; "He's tied to her apron strings"). We feel that this disparaging attitude and the resulting early call for separation from mother isolates boys from relationship.

In this chapter we are referring to the dominant cultural model for boys in the United States. We recognize that there are many diverse variations of this model dependent upon race, ethnicity, religion, sexual orientation, family structure, socioeconomic class, and other factors. We focus on the mainstream model supported by media images and messages because of the strong negative influence it has on boys' development. We feel that all mothers, regardless of diverse circumstances, are impacted in their relationship with their sons by this culturally prescribed paradigm of disconnection.

Infant studies show that physical and psychological development is dependent upon a good mother–infant connection. Without such a connection, we see a developmental "failure to thrive" in babies. Ed Tronick of the Brazelton Touchpoints Project (1998) notes that infant development occurs only within relationship. This is also Jean Baker Miller's belief about our lifelong experience. In her 1976 book she states that "all growth and learning takes place within the *context* of relationship." While the relational presence of mother is essential for babies to thrive early on, it continues to be essential for boys' emotional and relational growth.

Jean Baker Miller and Irene P. Stiver (1997) speak of the need for relationship and connection as a *human need* in their book *The Healing Connection*. They see this as a universal need, best met through the development of mutually empathic and mutually empowering relationships. But young boys, if deprived of sufficient opportunities to learn how to make real connections, try to meet these needs in superficial and manipulative ways. They are taught in the dominant "boy culture" to fulfill their desires and get ahead, even at the expense of others. In acting this way, boys and men are simply following established rules of the culture for males. A false bravado model not only deprives boys early on of parental empathy but also infuses them with a sense of esteem and power devoid of internal resonance. As a result, mutually satisfying connection with others becomes impossible. In our clinical practice, men tell stories of "working the room" in executive meetings, assured that they will ultimately sway others and (right or wrong) get what they want. These men complain, however, that they feel no internal gratification in these interactions. All this attention and power fail to gratify, and in fact leave them feeling empty and even more alone. We see in their experience how learned behaviors make it impossible for many men to connect authentically, leaving them with a debilitating sense of internal isolation.

This problematic developmental course may account for what appears to be a predominance of men who are self-absorbed and cut off from relationship. Perhaps, if we understand more deeply the impact of culture on boys' and men's development, we can bring a compassionate and understanding perspective to our male children, partners, friends, and clients as they sort through these difficult, deeply embedded relational patterns. Perhaps, if we create more empathic possibilities, these new experiences can prevent in boys, and heal in men, the wounds of this early disconnection.

A MOTHER'S PROSPECTIVE VIEW

We have found, in our work with more than 3,000 mothers of sons, that in spite of the cultural message, many mothers follow their inclination and stay in relationship with their sons. Tentatively questioning established norms, these mothers keep a place of emotionality open in their sons through continued connection. Yet, at the same time, they worry that they will affect their sons' development in negative ways. Mothers who resist the cultural call to disconnection are in need of validation and support. These courageous mothers are, potentially, the real experts in boys' development. Keeping a strong connection is the way to teach sons how to navigate the many and complex nuances of relationship. We believe that it is within the mother–son context that relational learning occurs and the groundwork is established for future relationships. Olga Silverstein (1994), in her book *The Courage to Raise Good Men,* demonstrated that the root of sons' difficulties as adults is linked to distance and disconnection in the mother–son relationship. Our workshops with mothers and adult sons, as well as our clinical work with men and couples, tell us that boys with a secure maternal connection develop stronger interpersonal skills and enjoy healthier relationships as adults.

Although RCT originally developed as a way to understand women's psychology, the capacity to create and sustain growth-fostering relationships is equally crucial for boys and men. Traditional views of boys' and men's development are embedded in men's experiences and men's fears. Men who have grown up in this culture often feel that the old model is best for their sons. Even men who want to change things may worry about these new directions for boys. Fathers can be pulled unwittingly into a retrospective analysis of present-day issues because of old fears based on their own experience. Because becoming a man is closely linked with traditional ideas about being one's own man (individuation), being dominant, and not being a "girl," evolving their thinking into the realm of emotional and relational development about boys can create worry for some men. Some men may be fearful of turning boys into girls. Women, on the other hand, not having grown up in boy culture, may have a clearer lens in viewing the currently evolving possibilities for boys and men. Most mothers *do* keep connection with sons, and sons *are* more aware of the benefits and possibilities open to them in relationship. These newly evolved attitudes and behaviors are actually already much more a part of everyday life for boys than are reflected in the media. Just as Jean Baker Miller (1976) insisted that we must listen to women to hear about their experiences, we must listen to mothers of sons to formulate a *prospective view* of the possibility of relationship for boys. It is our opinion that listening to mothers of sons will inform us about current realities and possibilities for boys.

At a recent lecture about middle school children, a mother asked the speaker how to talk to her 12-year-old son. The psychologist answered, "There's bad news and there's good news. The bad news is that you won't be able to get him to talk. The good news is that it won't last long, just a few years." Most of the mothers gathered at the back of the lecture hall disagreed with this notion. Even though it was difficult, they had managed to stay connected with their sons. As the "keepers of the connections" in our culture, women know about relationship. Mothers hold the hope for change in their sons' relational growth.

New developmental attitudes and directions for boys can change development in many positive ways. Changing cultural expectations to include relational development for boys can change outcomes for both boys *and girls.* Valuing relational skills and emotional awareness in boys will increase respect for girls in our culture. By creating a new vision for boys, we modify the course of development for both genders. Both girls and boys are born with the capacity to have responsible and collaborative relationships. It is the work of parents to provide a safe context for boys, as well as girls, through the development of family, community, and social values that support relationship.

BOY CULTURE: WHAT IS IT? HOW DOES IT AFFECT BOYS?

Invisible forces in the dominant culture take hold in the form of the implicitly communicated expectations of boy behavior we call "boy culture" (Figure 11.1). Images of male dominance are projected by the media and modeled daily by older peers in countless ways. These expectations are not consciously taught nor supported in most of our homes, schools, or communities. Rather, they are the insidious behavioral messages boys in our culture receive regarding boy behavior. These occur in the form of put-downs and intimidating threats in every day interactions on the playground and in the halls of our schools. When we do nothing to intervene, thinking "boys will be boys," we implicitly give our approval to and help normalize behaviors that are disconnecting and domineering, which may later lead to what has become a pervasive societal problem of violence.

- Closeness with mom is for sissies/babies
- Feelings are for wimps and girls (except anger)
- Be first, be in limelight
- Don't back down
- Banter/bravado
- "Power over" model
- Pride in noncompliance and disrespect
- Desensitization to violence
- Code of silence

FIGURE 11.1. Boy culture: Implicit cultural expectations (Dooley & Fedele, 1997).

When we name and question the impact of boy culture we are not critical of boys and men, but rather of the gender straitjacket imposed on boys by the culture. Boy culture focuses on who's in the limelight. It says "be first, win." It is built on a competitive, "power over" model in which there are winners and there are losers. Boy culture encourages young men and boys to take pride in expressions of noncompliance and disrespect, to act out, and to pretend not to care about their failings.

Teachers rate boys as problems in the classroom 90% over girls (Boston Public Schools, 1997; Lewis, Lovely, & Yaeger, 1989). Research shows that as the number of *boy* siblings in a family increases, so does the incidence of acting out, school truancy, and social delinquency (Jones, Offord, & Abrams, 1980). The fact that this is not the case with the increase of girl siblings may speak to the powerful influence of boy culture within families. Behaviors such as bullying, teasing, stealing, noncompliance, swearing, and teacher disrespect have become serious problems, even at the elementary school level. Children, largely boys aged 5–10 years, are imitating offensive interpersonal behaviors portrayed by the media and observed in older peers.

Boy culture also says that if you retreat, if you shrink from competing, you risk being labeled "wimp," "chicken," "sissy," "scaredy cat," "baby," or even, "girl":

A group of first-grade boys respond to a simple question posed by their teacher by rising up out of their seats and onto their toes, hands waving high, whispering "me first, pick me." They are so eager to be first, all their energy goes into this quest. When called on they have forgotten the question and have nothing to say.

A third-grade boy creeps along a high wall egged on by his peers. He is terrified, but continues on for fear of being called a "wimp" or "scaredy cat."

A fifth-grade boy proudly boasts to his friends that he chased another boy down, took his prized art project, and made him cry.

A seventh grader jokingly brags about not studying and takes pride in his prediction of a poor grade on a math test scheduled for that day.

One 8-year-old explained, "If my friends ever found out that I come home from school and go through my backpack with my mom and show her everything I did in school that day, they'd really make fun of me and call me a baby."

- **STAGE I: YOUNG BOYS (3–7 yrs.)**
  CULTURAL MESSAGE: Disconnect from mom and vulnerable emotions. Superhero influence: physical power and aggressive/violent play. Fewer empathic responses. Failure to thrive emotionally.
  RELATIONAL GOAL: Keep a strong, empathic connection. Teach and model emotions and relational skills. Differentiate emotions. Avoid normalizing gender stereotypes. Help initiate friendships. Keep boys and girls together; mix gender roles in play.

- **STAGE II: MIDDLE YEARS (8–13 yrs.)**
  CULTURAL MESSAGE: Bullies, banter, and bravado. Loss of "relational voice." Influence of peers and "boy culture." Daredevil and "bad boy" behavior. Desensitized to violence. Code of silence.
  RELATIONAL GOAL: Interactive, fun-filled, authentic relationships. Friendship skills. Expect and model receptivity and responsiveness to others. Limits with contingencies and reparation.

- **STAGE III: TEENAGE YEARS (14–18 yrs.)**
  CULTURAL MESSAGE: Locker room culture. Peer pressure. Physical and sexual dominance. "Shut down" emotionally; turn to drugs, alcohol, and sex. Drive/act recklessly.
  RELATIONAL GOAL: Keep a strong connection! Move toward greater mutual understanding. Talk out instead of act out feelings. Help navigate complexities of relationships and guide through conflicts. Clear expectations regarding drugs, alcohol, and sex.

- **STAGE IV: COLLEGE/ADULT**
  CULTURAL MESSAGE: Disconnection and distance from mother.
  RELATIONAL GOAL: Mutual responsibility for growth in the relationship. Work toward a positive, authentic connection that is mutual.

FIGURE 11.2. Breaking through the cultural straitjacket (Dooley & Fedele, 1997).

Our culture's established standard of individuation and independence moves both girls and boys away from relationship. But for boys, this push is especially difficult because it happens at a very young age and within one of their most intimate of relationships, their relationship with their mothers. This move toward independence and away from mom occurs at a time in development for boys when they are still thinking in concrete ways (Piaget & Inhelder, 1969). Boys' concrete view of the loss of mom at age 5 is that they have lost relationship and are on their own emotionally. Carol G. Gilligan (1996) and others link the increase in attention deficit disorder (ADD) to this early separation from mother. Diagnostic ADD rates are higher than ever and occur predominantly in boys. Boys' loss creates sadness and anxiety, which may manifest as hyperactivity and inattention. Maybe the first diagnostic criteria to look for in these hyperactive boys should be symptoms of what we call CDD, or *connection deficit disorder!*

The development of learning and behavioral problems in young boys has become alarmingly common. Boys learn that it is "cool" to be distant, inauthentic, and disconnected. They lose their *relational* voice, the voice that reflects authentic feelings and affiliative needs. What replaces real interaction is banter and bravado. Caught up in the expectations of boy culture, imitating behaviors seen in older peers and siblings, boys often become alienated from their own inner world. When boys disconnect from their mothers, they lose access to the relational way of being with others that mothers represent. They may lose the ability to be responsive and receptive (Miller, 1986, 1988).

Stephen J. Bergman (1991) has coined the phrase "relational dread" as a phenomenon in boys and men that grows out of early emotional disconnection from mom. Boys lose their place within the relational context. Eventually, when faced with emotion and relationship, they freeze. They become immobilized. Isolated in their disconnection from mother, they don't know what to do or how to be in relationship. Bergman aptly describes this experience of dread and the resulting avoidance of connection that has become an intrinsic part of traditional developmental models for boys. Girls and women don't always see this dread because men cover it up with avoidance, denial, and bravado (I. P. Stiver, personal communication, November 25, 1998). Its impact, however, is great. This is part of what makes mutually empathic interactions with and between boys and men so difficult.

When mothers move away from young sons and push them toward independence, boys are denied empathic resonance (Stiver, 1986). Without a safe relational context provided by mother, a boy feels alone. He is too young to protest. He knows no alternative. He thinks that disconnection is what is supposed to happen. Nevertheless, he still longs for connection—quite rightly. But now he feels shame and confusion about his inner longings. To deal with his pain and confusion, he shuts down emotionally. He hasn't yet learned to differentiate and name feelings. Confused, he suffers alone, in silence. The cost of this break in relationship from mother is significant for boys' evolving relationships with others. They deal with this inner confusion and pain by shutting down access to their emotional world and to relationship. When this happens, relational and emotional development slows down.

From this point on, there are fewer empathic possibilities for boys than for girls. This early loss of parental empathy creates a void in the area of responsiveness to and identification of emerging feelings. Judith V. Jordan (1989) notes that a lack of empathic responding will result in a feeling of personal shame. In the absence of empathy, this inner place of vulnerability and feelings fills with shame. Boys learn early that emotional needs, longings, feelings, or dependencies are shameful. They then have a more difficult time developing a healthy sense of self-empathy. Shame and shaming become the consequence of this empathy void. Emotional needs and longings often become covered up in boys through angry expressions and aggressive behaviors. Eventually, through continued exposure to boy culture, put-downs, and "power over" behavior, boys seem to lose their capacity for empathy toward others.

There is a further twist. We all yearn for a sense of connection; yet, the inevitable disconnections that happen in relationships can be painful and threatening. Everyone experiences this flow of connection/ disconnection in life. Because of these repeated interpersonal disconnections, we often pull back from relationship while we yearn for connection. Miller and Stiver (1997) write about this as the "paradox of relationship." Boys feel this paradox at a young age; they learn early not to fully represent themselves in relational encounters. Shamed for expressions of emotion, they begin to keep important parts of themselves hidden from others. They do this by developing a repertoire of behaviors for staying out of relationship. Miller and Stiver call these "strategies of disconnection." These strategies keep boys from experiencing the shaming and putdowns of boy culture at the cost of keeping them out of real connection with others. Some examples include silence, smart remarks that discourage conversation, elaborate demonstrations of disinterest, sarcastic humor, and the exchange of glances between boys that convey disrespect for the speaker. Beneath the bravado and banter, boys are hungry for connection and emotional expression. This is the paradox of relationship for them.

Carol Gilligan (1996) describes adolescent girls as sacrificing relationship for the sake of relationships. Boys sacrifice authentic emotional connection with others for the sake of inclusion within boy culture. This accommodation helps them avoid being teased and shamed, gains them the approval of peers, and creates superficial connection at the expense of real relationship.

Bullying, competitive banter, and bravado, these are the hurtful, "power over" interactions that pervade boy culture. At the same time, boys learn about the code of silence built into these interactions. You cannot "tell" on others even if you know their behavior is damaging and wrong. Boys learn early in life that to survive with peers they have to endure harsh, mean, even hurtful verbal and physical behavior. The dominant culture expects boys to be tough and shames them when they aren't. They can't let on when they've been hurt or humiliated. If they break the "code of silence," they risk humiliation, peer isolation, and further harassment. Boys plead with their mothers not to intervene.

They would rather submit to the bullying than be shamed for turning to someone for help:

> Walking home from school, a group of 9-year-old boys stop at the ballpark to hit a few fly balls. Waiting his turn, Max stands behind the backstop, his fingers curled around the metal links. Whack! One of the boys smashes the bat against the backstop and hits Max's finger. Max screams and crumples to the ground in tears, clutching his hand. The group of boys stares at him. Then one says, "Oh, c'mon. I don't see anything wrong. It's not bleeding. You're faking." "What a wimp!" yells another. "Poor baby hurt his finger?" chimes in Andrew, Max's best friend. Bewildered, Max gets up, trying without much success to hold back the tears. His finger throbs. "Maybe you should go over and play with those girls," taunts Andrew, shaking his head in disgust as he and the others walk off together, leaving Max behind. Max arrives home upset. His mother sees his tears and swollen finger turning black and blue. She offers ice, but it's not the finger that hurts most. She tries to comfort Max and asks what happened. "Nothing, Mom, it's okay," insists Max as he retreats to his room in shame.

Mothering can be seen as a political act. It is a form of the political resistance that Brown and Gilligan (1992) so eloquently describes for women—they need to speak their truth. In this case it is the truth about boys' code of silence.

The experience of being shamed by the culture, by peers, or by parents because of vulnerable feelings can have a significant impact. In response to the recent episodes of violence in young adolescent boys (Jonesboro, Arkansas; Paducah, Kentucky; Pearl, Mississippi) we, as a nation, are examining the roots of this behavior. James Gilligan (1996), in his recent book on violence in men, cites the experience of intense shame as an important dynamic in the histories of violent men. Shaming men and boys for exhibiting vulnerable feelings may contribute to their risk of engaging in violent behavior. Shame may be a precursor to the expression of anger, 6 an acceptable feeling for men and boys that may lead to aggression.

A liability built into boy culture is the expectation of repeated exposure to violent play, movies, and video games. Boys eventually become desensitized to violence. To avoid being teased or shamed, they stifle their natural emotional reactions of fear and vulnerability. Gradually, with daily exposure and practice, boys lose access to their real feelings and normal reactions to violence. Before long they can watch violence, abuse, and horror on the screen, in video games, even in peer interactions without flinching!

THE EBB AND FLOW OF RELATIONSHIP

Connection occurs when we experience a sense of mutual engagement, empathy, authenticity, and empowerment within the context of relationship. We have the mutual feeling of knowing and being with the other, immersed in their experience along with our own. Such connections provide a continual source of growth for the individual and the relationship. This form of connection has startlingly positive effects which Jean Baker Miller (1986) calls "the five good things": zest (vitality); a more accurate picture of oneself and others; an increased sense of self-worth; an increased desire and ability to act; and a desire for more connection. When we are in a disconnection, the opposite happens. We feel cut off from the person, experience the pain of not being understood and not understanding the other, and feel confusion about what is happening. The five outcomes of disconnection are decreased energy, confusion and lack of clarity, decreased self-worth, inability to act, and turning away from relationship.

Relationships are not static. Figure 11.3 illustrates the natural

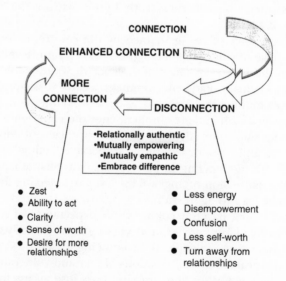

FIGURE 11.3. The ebb and flow of relationship connection (Dooley & Fedele, 1997).

movement of all relationships. The cycle of connection–disconnection–
new connection demonstrates how working through disconnections
can enhance relationships. Understanding this is the key to mutually
satisfying relationships. The inevitable disconnections become the signal that work needs to be done in the relationship. When we don't
acknowledge this and when we don't try to find a solution together, distance replaces closeness. The relationship suffers. The connection
becomes derailed in the confusion and ambiguity of the disregarded issue. On the other hand, when disconnections are addressed, they can
become opportunities to work together toward mutual understanding
and solutions (Bergman & Surrey, 1992).

Reconnection can be quick and easy, or it can take time, effort,
and creativity. This is the strengthening work of relationship. When we
find the way back, it is not just a reconnection but a strengthened, enhanced, growthful leap for the relationship. Even when sons seem to be
disinterested and uninvolved in this process, a mother's efforts are extremely important. This is how we continue to build relationships with
sons.

This creative work will differ depending upon the unique characteristics of each family: family structure, values, importance of the issue
at hand, temperament, culture, ethnicity, religion, and race. This work
provides opportunities to widen the lens for sons. For example, in dealing with a power issue, white mothers can talk with their sons about
how various power differentials create disconnection. By raising awareness of the dominant culture's racist views and how they affect relationships, mothers can help boys begin to see and deal with issues of privilege and power early in life. Discussions about social esteem (Jenkins,
1993) can help boys understand how their view of themselves and others is affected by (often negative) stereotypes and attitudes deeply embedded in our culture.

The mother–son relationship is a safe place for boys to learn how
to work through disconnection. Boys can learn to view disconnections
as cues in their relationships—not to let go, but rather to find creative
ways to reconnect. Mothers can then support, guide, and reassure their
sons through small and large conflicts in their relationships. Often
these conflicts happen first with mom, then with other family members, and eventually in peer and adult relationships outside the home.
The following example illustrates how a mother's emotional connectedness to her son enhanced his relational and emotional development.

> When 13-year-old Andy got home from school he learned that the
> dog belonging to his best friend, Sam, had been killed by a car. His
> own dog had died the same way just a year ago. Andy, in hearing

the news, froze. His body stiffened; his face registered fear. What could he possibly say or do to help his friend at this point? He had no words. He was confused, overwhelmed, and inundated with feelings about his own dog's death. He knew the horrible loss he experienced a year ago was what Sam was feeling now, but he felt immobilized by his own grief and discomfort. How could he possibly approach Sam in this vulnerable state? And what about Sam? Wouldn't he be embarrassed by his own sadness?

His mom put her arm around him and said, "You know how sad Sam must be. Remember how sad we all were when Trumpet died? Sam could really use a friend right now, especially one who knows exactly how he must be feeling." Andy panicked. "No, Mom, I can't. I don't know what to say. I'd sound really stupid," he said.

"You know it's a really important part of a friendship to go to your friend's side when something bad happens. He needs you now," said his mother. Andy couldn't move. He couldn't go to Sam's. He couldn't call. He was angry with his mother for her suggestion. He started walking out of the room, but his mother said, "Wait, let's do this together. We can write it out and then call him." Andy stiffened further, insisting he couldn't even think, saying, "I'm stupid. I don't know what to say."

His mother wrote the words out for him, encouraging him all the way. "Look, Andy, all you have to say is 'Sam, I'm sorry. I just heard about your dog. I'm so sorry. I know how you must feel. You know Trumpet died last year the same way and it crushed me. I'm really sorry.' " Andy backed away from the phone, but his mother dialed and handed it to him. As the phone rang, he mouthed "No" to his mother while dangling the receiver her way. Finally, the answering machine picked up. With a sigh of relief, Andy read the message.

Later his mom was worried about how these two teenagers could make a face-to-face connection. So she offered to let Andy have a beanie baby she had just bought for his younger brother. "You could give this to Sam in memory of Rumpus because it looks just like him," she said. Andy was insulted: "Wow! Step back, Mom! A *beanie baby*? Give me a break!" At this point his mom dropped the idea.

The next day, Sam came over to find Andy, who wasn't home yet. He repeated over and over to Andy's mom, "Tell Andy that it was so cool he called me. No one else did. Tell him I said thanks. Tell him I came over. Tell him to come over to my house when he gets home. Tell him that was really great to call." When Andy returned, his mother told him Sam had been there. Andy stiffened in fear. When his mother related how appreciative Sam was for the call, Andy's whole body relaxed. His eyes brightened, he had a burst of energy, and he was out the door to Sam's. His mom was relieved, and then a few minutes later she heard him come back into the house. As he ran up the stairs he smiled and sheepishly asked if he could give the beanie baby to Sam. On his way out the door his mom gave him a quick hug and told him what a great job he'd done. He smiled as he pulled away saying, "That's because I've got a *buena madre!* [good mother]"

Andy moved from alienation to emotional involvement. He moved from disconnection to not only reconnection but even better connection with his mom and his friend. When he first heard the news, Andy disconnected and became immobilized. He exhibited all five outcomes of disconnection: lack of clarity or confusion ("I don't know what to say"); decreased desire and ability to act ("I can't"); decreased self-worth ("I'll sound stupid"); turning away from relationship (walking away); and decreased energy. With empathy, support, and mutual involvement from his mom, he was able to make the move back into relationship with his friend and with his mom. By the end of the story we see how the individuals and both relationships benefit from the move back into connection.

Andy exhibited all of the five good outcomes: he was motivated to act and did (went to his friend, came back for the beanie baby); he felt better about himself (smiling, joking); he had a more accurate picture of himself and others ("*buena madre*"); he had a desire for more connection (with his mom and Sam); and he had more energy (went to his friend, energized in his interaction with his mom). Andy learned something important about relationship and loss. His relationship with Sam will deepen because the two shared a new awareness of themselves in relation to each other's grief. Furthermore, his relationship with his mother is enhanced as he more fully appreciates her efforts to help him with the difficult work of relationship.

PARENTING-IN-CONNECTION

Embracing the natural ebb and flow of relationship is the basis for a model of child raising we refer to as *parenting-in-connection*. The goals are to enhance connection and to circumvent distance and separation. As noted above, disconnections are *opportunities* to deepen and strengthen the relationship. Thus, the inevitable disconnections of parenthood become a signal that work is needed in the relationship. Mothers can teach sons, by example, to move toward reconnection rather than becoming derailed by disconnection. A mother's knowledge and ability can facilitate this learning process for a son and enrich the mother–son connection.

In a 2-year longitudinal study of 12,000 teenagers from across the country, researchers found that a close relationship with a parent is the best predictor of a teenager's health and the strongest deterrent to high-risk behaviors. The study published by the *Journal of the American Medical Association* was apart of a $24 million project funded by the National Institute of Child Health and Human Development and other agencies (Resnick et al., 1997). A strong emotional connection with at least one parent or significant adult figure reduces the odds that an adolescent will suffer from emotional stress, have suicidal thoughts or behavior, engage in violence, or use substances (tobacco, alcohol, or marijuana). Feeling that at least one adult knew them and treated them fairly buffered the teens against every health risk except pregnancy. This finding held up regardless of family income, race, education, specific amount of time spent with a child, whether a child lives with one or two parents or in an alternative family structure, and whether one or both parents work. The evidence is overwhelming. Good relationships help create resilience to dangerous acting-out behaviors in our children.

As parents and educators, we share the painful dilemma of having important family and community values that conflict with the realities of peer culture for boys. Together, mothers and sons can develop new ways of approaching these dilemmas. We help mothers introduce the notion of reparation when dealing with interpersonal violations and injuries. There is a growing need to set limits on emotionally, socially, and physically hurtful behavior toward others. But setting limits for the sake of limits doesn't work. Punishment without a relational context only further alienates boys. They take pride in getting busted. Acting out and noncompliance earns them points with peers. Naming the behavior that we want changed, providing alternatives to the traditional boy culture strategies, and encouraging interpersonal reparation are all essential parts of setting limits with boys. They often love structure and tend to go along with a clearly outlined and defined model that they *and their friends* are expected to follow. "If you build it, they will come!" Boys need adults to point out that the behavior is hurtful, offer better alternatives, and provide concrete consequences for relational injuries.

We are suggesting a simple yet powerful change in boys' development: move the emphasis of the mother–son relationship away from separation and isolation toward connection. When we do that, we have a chance to help sons with healthy emotional development daily in dozens of small but significant ways. We just might change the course of their lives by teaching them, through these everyday interactions, how to develop mutually empathic, mutually empowering relationships.

In reviewing boys' relational growth, we identified four stages in the development of mother–son relationships. Each developmental period has cultural expectations, which influence the mother–son relationship, creating conflicts and dilemmas. We have set relational goals for each stage and defined ways mothers can counter these cultural influences and keep sons on the path of relational development. Each stage is outlined in terms of age, imposed cultural pressures, problems created, and specific methods for meeting relational goals.

1. *The early years (3–7 years)*: The cultural message is the invincibility of the *superhero*. Little boys are besieged by superhero figures that imply that becoming a man depends on independence, strength, stoicism and total invulnerability, and the defeat of all others. The relational goal is laying the groundwork for relationship by naming, demonstrating, and validating relational abilities.

2. *The middle years (8–13 years)*: The cultural message involves banter, bullies, and bravado. Middle school boys are indoctrinated with the competitive ethic of winning at all costs and exploiting power over others. The relational goal is setting limits and offering alternatives by guiding sons toward interactive, fun-filled, authentic relationships.

3. *The teenage years (14–18 years)*: The cultural message is to shut down authentic feelings and interactions and engage in the "locker room" culture of social, physical, and sexual dominance. The focus is on dominance, not real relationship. The relational goal is maintaining relationships as multidimensional and encouraging mutual dialogue. It also involves viewing conflict and difference as opportunities to stay in connection and learn more about each other.

4. *College/adult*: The cultural message is disconnection and separation from mother. Adult sons worry about being too "attached." The expectation to disconnect can feel like disinterest and distance to their mothers. The relational goal is to encourage a mutually responsive, mutually empowering mother–son relationship.

Parenting-in-connection provides a new way of understanding and responding to disconnections. It can be teaching a 2-year-old to share, helping a 9-year-old to deal with the hurt and unfairness of being bullied, empathizing with a teenager's pain in being rejected by a girl, or sorting through the many decisions of adulthood together.

THE EARLY YEARS

One mom recalls how her son, Aaron, went from being the "best boy" in preschool to becoming that "wild boy" in kindergarten. "The kids he sat with on the first day of kindergarten were rambunctious, wild boys," she recalls. He sat at the same table day after day and very soon "he became a wild boy."

Before entering a traditional school setting, Aaron was an empathic little boy who asked his preschool teacher, "Are your feelings hurt?" when another child snapped at her. He was always the first to step forward and offer a welcome when a new child entered the class. With the move to kindergarten, Aaron entered a larger, traditional setting, which reflected more mainstream boy culture expectations. His new teacher seemed to assume that all boys were rowdy, and she didn't really know Aaron. Feeling isolated and disconnected, he sought to establish connection by mimicking the boys at his table. He became loud and boisterous, winning acceptance by succumbing to pressures to join in with "wild boy" behavior.

In the parenting-in-connection model, the early years (Figure 11.4) are the time to lay the groundwork for relational mothering. Noting how essential mutual respect, honesty, empathy, and listening are to every interaction can do this. Mothers can show sons how to put these skills into action, verbally and nonverbally. Mothers often direct boys outside or into the basement to watch a video when company arrives because their aggressive energy feels too incongruent to the occasion. Why not, instead, teach boys to stop, look at, shake hands with, respond to, and initiate conversation with guests that we welcome into our homes. Keeping boys in the picture offers an opportunity for practicing interpersonal skills. Over time, these relational skills will become second nature to boys and possibly replace the high-activity behaviors they seem to use to cover their anxiety.

Boys need to be told and shown how to interact in situations that extend beyond family and friends. Mothers can be clear about expecting receptivity and responsiveness to others in the home and community. Early childhood is the time to inculcate values like these. It is also the time to note the importance of being honest in communications with others and of respecting others' feelings, even though we might feel differently. These are the show-and-tell years, a time when children are open to guidance and learning that the culture doesn't offer and even opposes.

Our culture convinces boys early on that invincibility and imperviousness are hallmarks of strength. Little boys are fascinated by stories

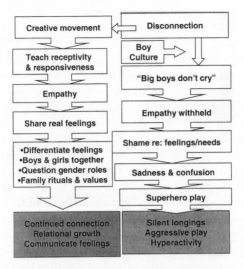

Stage: Early Childhood (3–7 yrs.)

Cultural Issues: Disconnect from mother and vulnerable emotions, superhero influence, aggressive/violent play

Problems Created by Cultural Stereotypes:
1. When boys disconnect from mom they lose access to emotion and relationship.
2. They lose the place for differentiating feelings and practicing relationship skills.
3. The loss impacts both: Mom feels sad; son confused, can't name his emotions.
4. Premature independence creates a connection deficit that looks like ADD.
5. With loss of mom, boys connect with "boy culture."
6. Desensitization: Exposure to aggression and violence in media and superhero play.
7. Adults begin to withhold empathy; "don't cry," "you're ok," "be a big boy."
8. He loses self-directed empathy, shaming his feelings instead: "Only babies cry."
9. He conceals/loses access to his vulnerable feelings; feels shame.
10. He begins to lose his natural empathic responsiveness to others.
11. Peer interactions become more aggressive/less empathic.

Relational Strategies:
1. Show and tell: Relational expectations and values
2. Keep the connection; relational "chats" at bedtime, in car, at meals, etc.
3. Develop family rituals that structure and model relational skills and emotionality
4. Show rudiments of verbal/nonverbal receptivity and responsiveness to others.
5. Continue to respond to boys with empathy. Teach/show them "how to."
6. Praise relational behavior/emotional expression. Help differentiate emotions.
7. Reframe concepts of strength, courage, and bravery relationally.
8. Name the relational part of every activity
9. Encourage boy/girl friendships. Discourage "boys will be boys" type behavior.
10. Add a repair piece to "time-out."

FIGURE 11.4. Choice of the early years: Boys stay connected to mom or connect to superheroes (Fedele & Dooley, 1998).

about Superman, and they love to play superheroes. They learn that they have to be able to fix everything and protect everyone from evil forces. There is little room for expression of their vulnerable, dependent side. This inner part of boys can be quickly buried beneath shame if parents let the message of the culture take hold at this age.

Superman is powerful and invincible. But, as the story goes, his survival and strength depend upon his being apart from any trace of his "mother" planet, Krypton. Like Achilles, the underlying mythology presents the allure of invincibility and the dangers of the mother connection for sons. And the price for these illusions of strength for boys is the loss of access to feelings and authenticity in relationships.

In these early years, children are beginning to practice skills of empathy. Being responsive to family members' feelings and expressive of his own can give a little boy the opportunity to learn about mutually empathic relationships. Highlighting and validating the relational part of an activity, not just the activity itself, is another lesson for the early years:

> Maria takes her 7-year-old son cross-country skiing for the first time. When they come to a hill, John has a rough time. His mom braces him from behind to keep him from backsliding. Resting against her, he looks up and says, "You must really hate skiing with me. I'm terrible and you're awesome." "Oh, no," says Maria, "I love this. I love being with you and helping you. That's what's important to me." "Really?" says John, smiling broadly.

Another simple way to create a space for relationship at this early age is to make a daily chat a part of a boy's routine. Mothers can designate a time for a private chat. This can be done in the car on the way to an activity. It can be done at bedtime as a way of wrapping up the day. It can be combined with a game or other joint activity. A mother needn't pressure a son to speak, but rather should let him know that he has the opportunity. As the chat becomes ritualized, this will be a special time together. This sets a relational frame within which he can learn that it's safe to talk about *anything*.

Parenting-in-connection in the early years is a matter of teamwork. Instead of sending a little boy out to master a two-wheeler without any preparation, mother and son start by peddling a bicycle-built-for-two. Mom is there to help her young son navigate life's inevitable bumps and twists. Working through difficult feelings and problems with his mom not only teaches the boy relational skills but also nourishes and enriches his self-worth and their relationship. These lessons and experiences with his mother give him the confidence to remain in touch with his inner world as he ventures into the greater world beyond family.

THE MIDDLE YEARS

At this age we see the "playground" influence of teasing and bullying (Figure 11.5). This behavior can be both emotionally and physically hurtful. Boy culture behavior says: "I'm tough"; "It doesn't bother me"; "You can't hurt me"; "I don't care." As noted above, when we stop responding to boys from an empathic, compassionate perspective, we give them the message that they should be tough and independent, both emotionally and behaviorally.

In the Max story told earlier, the mother went to her son's room and sat with him. Her acknowledgment of and compassion for his pain offered both validation and comfort to Max. Left on his own to deal with this experience, Max would learn to avoid the shame he felt by denying his feelings of physical and emotional pain. Mothers sometimes worry about embarrassing sons further by acknowledging and responding to their vulnerable emotions. Yet, it is this very naming of and feeling compassion for hurt feelings that offers empathic responding where they otherwise feel shame. This interaction teaches boys alternatives to avoiding shame by denying feelings.

We encourage mothers to jump into their sons' world and react authentically to what they see and feel. Naming their emotional reaction and eliciting their sons' view of the situation creates a dialogue. Mothers and sons can then further this process by sharing differences and exchanging values. While this process doesn't always give immediate answers, being together in a real way can create the connection necessary for them to work toward possible solutions.

A couple of years ago, a weekly yearlong values class became the setting for teaching relational skills to ten 9-year-old boys. Previous teachers warned about the impossible task of working with this group of boys, stating: "Every one of these boys meets criteria for attention-deficit/hyperactivity disorder (ADHD). They are impossible to work with in a classroom setting. Let them go outside to run off their energy. This group desperately needs girls to tone it down." Similarly, the boys greeted the new teacher with "We are powerful! No one can control us! We rule! You have to let us go outside and run around."

The teacher spent the first month reinforcing good relational behavior with pennies and letting the boys trade these for candy at

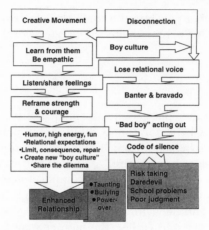

Stage: Middle Childhood (8–14 yrs.)

Cultural Issues: Disconnect from vulnerable feelings, loss of relational voice, boy culture, teasing/bullying

Problems Created by Cultural Stereotypes:
1. Loss of *relational voice*. Vulnerability, sadness, desire for connection, and honest expression in relationship fade.
2. Inauthentic interaction with peers; denial of feelings.
3. Boy culture bravado takes over.
4. Loss of empathic connection; fear of honest connection.
5. Further desensitization to violence (through video games, movies, TV, Internet access)
6. Daredevil tactics with peers; poor judgment regarding risks.
7. Behavior/discipline problems in elementary school.
8. Noncompliance/disrespect leads to poor performance.
9. "Bad boy" behavior further alienates/isolates boys.
10. Discipline/limit setting with no compassion/connection.
11. Alienation from mother.
12. Girls adopt "boy culture" as power model, "Anything you can do, we can do."

Relational Strategies:
1. Expand relational expectations; teach receptivity and responsiveness to others.
2. Mutual responsibility for relationships; guide with role-play and scripts.
3. Reframe strength and courage in relational terms.
4. Continue relational "chats" and rituals.
5. Sit with his feelings/talk about your feelings; help him differentiate emotions.
6. Define dilemma: home and school; father tells his story.
7. Jump in/join his world; create your own "boy culture" with relational values.
8. Enjoy activities because "we're doing it together."
9. Talk together about "boy culture" and alternatives; define family values.
10. Continue to keep boys and girls together in friendships.
11. Set limits with clear consequences, especially regarding relationships; institute "relational violation" with reparation.
12. Use humor. Have FUN.

FIGURE 11.5. Boy culture: Implicit cultural expectations (Dooley & Fedele, 1997).

the end of class. She walked around the classroom dropping pennies into paper cups whenever someone was *not* participating in disruptive behavior. She was eventually able to reinforce the new relational behavior as it appeared. Slowly the boys, through the introduction of a new model of interacting, started to engage with one another in a real way. The class brainstormed ideas about old and new models of relationship for boys. As they shared their experience in the old model, they were able to share feelings of isolation and an awareness of how unfair the old model is to boys. One child likened the expectations of boy culture to racism: "It's like racism—you can't even have a friend who's a girl without being called her boyfriend or a wimp for hanging around with her!"

This class created its own new culture and value system for boys. Instead of running wild, they talked about relationship. They interacted honestly and respectfully with one another. They even learned to meditate to the resonance of a meditation bell!

In the same classroom, Stein and Sjostrom's "Bullyproof" curriculum (1996) introduced language and concepts for participation with peers outside the group. The boys brought in examples of boy culture from their school life and talked about the dilemma of doing the right thing in the face of peer pressure to do the opposite. Stein and Sjostrom's "web of courage" exercise renamed being honest and supportive with friends as bravery and strength. There are countless ways we can praise and build confidence in boys for going against the cultural model. One boy's brave act was calling his friend on the phone. He expressed his hurt feelings to this friend who had joined with other boys mocking him on the way home from school. The boys seemed relieved to tell their real stories and talk about feelings in a place that was relationally safe. When we create new models with new values, boys can grow in new ways.

Boys at this age respond well to structure. Mothers can name the relational violations they see, stop the hurtful interactive behaviors, and provide meaningful concrete consequences. We teach the notion of relational reparation to boys. When a behavior is hurtful to the person and the relationship, we call it a *relational violation*. Reparation, through some concrete form of giving to the relationship, is required to move back into connection. Boys are responsive to structured ways of coming back into connection. Making reparation to a younger brother who's been hurt can mean engaging him in his favorite game and having fun together. This can be a quick 15-minute interaction between siblings during which all other freedoms are on hold. Reparation fits with a boy's desire to fix things. The shift is important: move the focus from fixing concrete things to repairing relationship.

Mothers can draw on established family relational rituals to open dialogue and process feelings and interactions with sons. Mothers can share the stories of their lives and welcome their sons' stories. Children are particularly interested in their parents' stories of childhood. A mother might tell her sons how she struggled at their age. She might encourage their daily stories. She might show interest in their day-to-day struggles with peers and praise their creative attempts to deal with these obstacles. When mothers do these things, they can enhance their sons' relational skills that are otherwise ignored or even put down by peers and the culture at large. By joining with their sons, mothers can widen their sons' views of new possibilities and change.

THE TEEN YEARS

As boys enter the teen years, the cultural message is to get as far as possible from their vulnerable emotions (Figure 11.6). The "power over" model of boyhood is transformed into a model of dominance in adolescence. Social, physical, and sexual dominance replaces authentic interactions. Because they are disengaged from their feelings and are disconnected from their parents, adolescent boys tend to act out rather than talk out their problems and conflicts. This leaves them at risk for forming insecure or abusive relationships. They may experiment with drugs, alcohol, and other risk-taking behaviors. Peer competition and pressure often motivate premature sexual intimacies. This type of quick intimacy is devoid of relational depth; it can lead to frequent shifts in their choice of sexual partners.

Confusion about who they are and what they feel extends to their future and their goals. Often this can translate into underachievement in school and a feeling of general discontent with their lives. This path for boys leads to further disconnection and alienation from relationship. They learn to become relationally silent.

Mothers of teenagers often interpret their sons' silence as rejection or as a desire for independence. They retreat from their sons' distance. They are fearful that if they pursue connection they will be ignored or will increase the animosity they already feel from their sons. They are also afraid of being intrusive. They think they should respect their sons' need for distance.

A group of 15-year-old boys responded to the question: "What are the important mother–son issues for you?" One boy went on and on saying, "She should stay out of my room, leave me alone, stop telling me to do my homework and to clean up my room." This

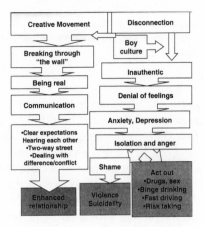

Stage: Adolescence

Cultural Issues: Locker room bravado, peer pressure, physical and sexual dominance, experimentation (drugs, alcohol, sex)

Problems Created by Cultural Stereotypes:
1. Have only a vague awareness of feelings, except anger.
2. Desensitized to violence (through movies, video games, etc.).
3. Act out, rather than talk out, problems and conflicts.
4. Shut out from communication within the family.
5. Physical and sexual dominance; power over gets magnified in cliques, turf, sex.
6. Underachievement; confusion about future goals.
7. May use drugs/alcohol to reduce interpersonal anxiety.
8. Group/peer pressure to drive recklessly, drink, act out, be sexually active, etc.
9. Code of silence.
10. Date rape, teen pregnancy, frequently shifting sexual intimacies, AIDS.

Relational Strategies:
1. Participate in son's world; make him the expert; raise issues and ask questions.
2. Continue relational "talk time." Together, find ways to communicate, be together, and enjoy each other.
3. Expect to talk out rather than act out his/your feelings.
4. Mutual empathy/responsibility for relationship. It takes two!
5. Value conflict as an opportunity for greater connection.
6. Guide him in negotiating friendships at new level; honing of relational skills.
7. Continue to set limits with consequences; expect reparation for disruptions.
8. Friendship with girls is prerequisite to sexual intimacy.
9. Plan/navigate through transitions; brainstorm.
10. Predict feelings ahead and ways to deal with these.
11. Sit with his confusion about feelings; help him name and process emotions.
12. Clear expectations about drugs, alcohol, sex; teach him how to deal with peer pressure.
13. Accept his humor/use your own to make connections.

FIGURE 11.6. The choice of adolescence: Boys tune in or tune out (Dooley & Fedele, 1998).

same boy when questioned further about whether his mother ever tried to talk with him about important things, responded, "Yeah, but she gives up too easily."

In our work we encourage mothers to work hard at keeping the connection with their sons. Adolescence is a developmental time when sons need their mothers to hold onto the relationship. Even when it seems to mothers that they are "talking to a wall," these efforts mean something to boys and can become the early threads of connection. A mother can raise issues and questions and let her son know what she thinks and feels. As boys mature, mothers can expect increased mutual responsibility for the work of their relationship. Mothers need to remain authentic while interacting with their sons. For example, voicing frustration because she is doing all the work of the relationship and wanting more effort on his part can spark a son's awareness and make connection start to happen. Even if interactions seem to be conflicts and disagreements, the dialogue itself moves the relationship out of silence and distance into connection. Mothers need to make explicit the work of relationship so that boys learn what to do. Boys need guidance and real-life examples.

At the same time that the relationship with mother becomes more balanced relationally, it can also become more balanced regarding the concrete work of family life. Mothers sometimes hold onto the role of provider and caretaker in a concrete way because that's all they have with their sons. As roles and responsibilities evolve, boys feel better about themselves and their growing mutuality with mom. They learn how to be in relationship in a real way. A mother can share her feelings and perspective while remaining receptive to her son's effort to communicate his viewpoint. Receptivity to a son's initiative is essential, whatever form this may take. Sometimes just being together in silence can create enough connection for sons to share a little bit more of who they are. As the relationship evolves, boys will begin to include mothers in discussions regarding dilemmas they face in the world and with peers. Learning to communicate with parental support gives boys the skills they need to deal with complex and difficult situations in life. As mentioned earlier, when there is a strong connection with at least one parent, teens don't need to turn to drugs, alcohol, or other forms of distraction and acting out.

As boys start to deal with bodily changes and emerging sexuality, mothers can provide a safe place to learn about both physical and interpersonal changes in relation to girls. Mothers can keep the dialogue open by being responsive to questions, initiating concerns, and even sharing their own story. When it comes to teaching and guiding sons

1. Keep boys and girls together. Encourage, reinforce, expect friendships.
2. Avoid normalizing "boys will be boys" and stereotyped girl behaviors.
3. Value relational skills in girls and foster relational skills in boys.
4. Keep the language of emotion across and within gender groups.
5. Recognize "dangerous edges" for boys and girls:
   - "Rough-and-tumble play is on a dangerous edge for boys (they can't say when it hurts).
   - "Dieting and external body focus is on an edge for girls.
6. Provide adult intervention. Raise expectations for boys regarding peer interactions: name, intervene, and structure alternatives.
7. Focus on girls' internal strengths (aptitudes, creativity) rather than externals.
8. Name emotional and relational interactions with peers as courageous.
9. Structure alternative models taught within peer groups in a sanctioned setting, like the school, by respected adults in authority (teachers).
10. Introduce structured programs in the home, community, school: relational rituals, antibullying programs, gender dialogue, cross- and same-gender peer mentoring, violence prevention, role modeling, peaceable school, co-researchers, reframe bravery and courage, highlight relational leadership.
11. Reinforce, name, notice, and acknowledge new behaviors when you see them.
12. Set limits with contingencies on relational violations.
13. Keep "opening doors" with boys (getting through defenses) until you get to their authentic emotional and relational voice.
14. Assist and model for girls how to lead with relational skills in the face of "power-over" behaviors (putdowns, jokes, mocking, etc.) from boys.
15. Provide media literacy education for students: How does it influence and maintain gender roles?
16. Structure leadership opportunities and positions for girls.
17. Teach relational leadership style to boys.
18. Resist stereotypic gender role expectations. Enlist our higher cognitive functions to evolve beyond old models.
19. Question, educate, reframe stereotypic interactions as they occur or are observed through media examples.
   - "Increase boys' and girls' psychological mindedness in understanding where cultural models come from and how to step aside from these.
   - "Social/political action raises consciousness toward evolutionary change.

FIGURE 11.7. Breaking through the gender straitjacket (Dooley, 1999).

through the emotional developmental topography of intimacy, mothers (as well as fathers) can be good resources! Today's teens have few guidelines or structures in place to set the pace of intimacy for them. Dating standards have changed; there are no rules. Teens "hook up" at parties. "Going out" and "hooking up" are loosely defined descriptions of boy–girl partnering that can mean anything from talking on the phone regularly to having some form of sex together. This "no rules" situation creates problems especially for boys. Our culture shames boys for their lack of knowledge about sexual intimacy and for exhibiting any reluctance to initiate it. Boys feel they should know what's going on, be in charge, and take the lead sexually. When sons appear to not want to talk about sexuality, it can be due to their shame of not knowing enough about intimacy. If mothers can voice their own feelings about this difficult topic, sons can begin to overcome their shame and feel safe enough to talk. Mothers need to hold this connection with their sons, creating possibilities for dialogue about relationships, intimacy, and sexuality.

THE ADULT YEARS

Adulthood is composed of many developmental stages for men. During this time, an adult son's energy may be directed toward developing an intimate relationship; similarly, a son may need to invest time and energy in a demanding work schedule, or he may choose to have children. All of these features influence the mother–son relationship. Furthermore, there are many diverse configurations of the adult, mother–son relationship: mothers of single sons, married sons, sons with children, gay sons, divorced/separated sons, to name a few. Essentially, as an adult, the son is developing more interpersonal commitments and career opportunities at a time when his mother may be doing the opposite: he is less available, and she is often more available. This juxtaposition of the two can create misunderstandings and hurt feelings if not addressed by mother and son.

The challenge for mothers is to understand their sons' expanding relationships and relational responsibilities while voicing an interest in being included in some way. It is our hope to reframe the relational goal of men's development to discover renewed connection with their mothers as they enter into mutually supportive adult to adult–child interactions.

Many mothers of sons feel isolated and alienated. At one of our first workshops, 40 of the 100 participants were mothers of adult sons. There was uniform concern about remaining in connection with sons while they attended college, during their marriages, and throughout their adult lives. We began a session of the workshop by saying the refrain: "A daughter is a daughter for the rest of your life; a son is a son . . . " and everyone in unison joined in spontaneously " . . . 'til he takes a wife." The cultural message of disconnection at this stage is the culmination of years of distance between mothers and sons (Figure 11.8). The cultural stereotypes are always of the intrusive or meddling mother or mother-in-law. There are numerous negative images in the media of close mother–son relationships. The cultural mandate of disconnection we've talked about is fiercely reinforced through exaggerated stereotypes, which mockingly refer to adult men who are close to their mothers as "mama's boys":

> At age 37 a young man was reflecting on the anger and distance he had felt toward his mother since adolescence. At this stage in his life he wanted to establish a better relationship with her.
>
> In answer to the question, "What was your early relationship like?" he suddenly recalled, "I remember the wonderful feeling of her sitting on my bed talking with me before I fell asleep every night. Then one night she didn't come in. I called to her, but she said she couldn't come in any more. She never told me why and she never came in again."

A mixture of pain and shame was evident in the telling of his story. Sharing his past experience seemed to bring him greater understanding of his feelings. This clarity motivated him to discuss the incident from the past with his mother.

One way of connecting with an adult son is to revisit past interactions and talk about how cultural pressures affected your mother–son relationship. Many mothers who disconnected did so because the culture told them to, not because they wanted distance from their sons. In opening a dialogue, both mother and son can share their perspectives and their feelings about these experiences. Processing old interactions in an effort to understand each other's point of view creates connection. This can be the beginning of the mutual effort and understanding that is needed in order to heal past hurts and misunderstandings.

One mother of an adult son told us that she had been having concerns about the distance in her relationships with her grown son. When she told him she was attending a "Mothers and Sons Conference," he suggested that they have lunch afterward to talk about it. It seemed that letting him know about her interest in the conference opened a door for them and had an immediate effect on their relationships. Talking openly and clarifying feelings can help reestablish the connection and decrease the misunderstandings caused by silence.

Mothers and adult sons need to respect and embrace each other's relational efforts across differences in needs, perspectives, and situations. Mothers can value attempts at connection by their sons, even when they feel as if they need more. Being authentic about one's feelings but responsive to the others' needs and circumstances is the challenge of the adult years. At this point, the relationship is the mutual responsibility of both mother and son. Being aware of conflicting needs and discussing the natural dilemmas they create can result in an atmosphere of greater acceptance.

Finally, and most important, mothers need a strong support network of other mothers and other family members to help them deal with their evolving relational needs. Many mothers of adult sons have voiced the need to talk together about these issues. Joining with others in similar life circumstances can be healing and can help create the kind of connection that is often lacking. This network of connections can empower mothers to find positive solutions to dilemmas with sons.

SUMMARY

This chapter reviews traditional and relational models of boys' development and the impact of these models on the mother–son relationship. It explores the important developmental issues of empathy, self-esteem, and shame in the context of gender, specifically for boys. Traditional theory calls for separation and distance from the mother at a very early point in a boy's development (age 3–5). We define problems and outline developmental issues and dilemmas faced by boys and mothers of sons because of this cultural injunction to disconnect. We examine a prospective view of the capacity for relational development in boys. Then we present a model of parenting-in-connection based on RCT, highlighting relationship as central to psychological health. Furthermore, we define the dominant boy culture and examine its impact on boys' development and the mother–son relationship. Finally, four stages in boys' relational development are detailed, including in each stage an examination of the impact of culture, relational goals, and methods mothers can use to reach these goals. Examples from workshops and clinical work are used to demonstrate this model.

REFERENCES

Bergman, S. J. (1991). Men's psychological development: A relational perspective. *Work in Progress, No. 48.* Wellesley, MA: Stone Center Working Paper Series.
Bergman, S. J., & Surrey, J. L. (1992). Couples therapy: A relational approach. *Work in Progress, No. 66.* Wellesley, MA: Stone Center Working Paper Series.
Boston Public Schools. (1997). [Survey of classroom behavioral problems by gender.] Unpublished raw data.
Brazelton Touchpoints Project. (1998). *Touchpoints project manual.* Boston: Child Development Unit, Children's Hospital.
Brown, L. M., & Gilligan, C. (1992). *Meeting at the crossroads.* New York: Ballantine.
Federal Bureau of Investigation. (1987). *Uniform crime reports for the U.S.* Washington, DC: U. S. Department of Justice.

Gilligan, C. (1996). The centrality of relationships in human development: A puzzle, some evidence, and a theory. *Psychoanalytic Review, 82*, 801–827.

Gilligan, J. (1996). *Violence.* New York: Vintage.

Jenkins, Y. M. (1993). Diversity and social esteem. In J. L. Chin, V. De La Cancela, & Y. Jenkins (Eds.), *Diversity in psychotherapy: The politics of race, ethnicity, and gender.* Westport, CT: Praeger.

Jones, M. B., Offord, D. R., & Abrams, N. (1980). Brothers, sisters and antisocial behavior. *British Journal of Psychiatry, 136*, 139–145.

Jordan, J. V. (1989). Relational development: Therapeutic implications of empathy and shame. *Work in Progress, No. 39*. Wellesley, MA: Stone Center Working Paper Series.

Jordan, J. V. (Ed.). (1997). *Women's growth in diversity: More writings from the Stone Center.* New York: Guilford Press.

Lewis, D. O., Lovely, R., & Yeager, C. (1989). Toward a theory of the genesis of violence: A follow up study of delinquents. *Journal of the American Academy of Child and Adolescent Psychiatry, 28*: 431–436.

Miller, J. B. (1976). *Toward a new psychology of women.* Boston: Beacon Press.

Miller, J. B. (1986). What do we mean by relationships? *Work in Progress, No. 22.* Wellesley, MA: Stone Center Working Paper Series.

Miller, J. B. (1987). *Toward a new psychology of women* (2nd ed.). Boston: Beacon Press.

Miller, J. B. (1988). Connections, disconnections and violations. *Work in Progress, No. 33.* Wellesley, MA: Stone Center Working Paper Series.

Miller, J. B., & Stiver, I. P. (1997). *The healing connection.* Boston: Beacon Press.

Piaget, J., & Inhelder, B. (1969). *The psychology of the child.* New York: Basic Books.

Resnick, M. D., Bearman, P. S., Blum, R. W., Bauman, K. E., Harris, K. M., Jones, J., Tabor, J., Beuhring, T., Sieving, R. E., Shew, M., Ireland, M., Bearinger, L. H., & Udry, J. R. (1997). Protecting adolescents from harm: Findings from the national longitudinal study on adolescent health. *Journal of the American Medical Association, 278*(10), 823–832.

Silverstein, O. (1994). *The courage to raise good men.* New York: Penguin.

Stein, N., & Sjostrom, L. (1996). *Bullyproof: A teacher's guide on teasing and bullying for use with fourth and fifth grade students.* Wellesley, MA, and Washington, DC: Wellesley College Center for Research on Women and the NEA Professional Library.

Stiver, I. P. (1986). Beyond the Oedipus complex: Mothers and daughters. *Work in Progress, No. 26.* Wellesley, MA: Stone Center Working Paper Series.

12

Applications of the Relational Model to Time-Limited Therapy

JUDITH V. JORDAN, MARYELLEN HANDEL,
MARGARITA ALVAREZ, *and* ROBIN COOK-NOBLES

AS RELATIONAL APPROACH TO SHORT-TERM THERAPY

Judith V. Jordan

Although managed care has recently made short-term therapy the therapy of choice for most clients, the practice of time-limited therapy did not begin with managed care and it is not synonymous with managed care. A study done in 1984 indicated that patients remained in therapy an average of 6–12 sessions, regardless of the setting, the diagnosis, and the motivation ("Mental Health," 1995). In other words, most patients who come into therapy are in short-term therapy either by design or by chance. While there has not been a great deal of research comparing the merits of short-term versus long-term therapy, there has been much debate about the relative merits of both. The same *Consumer Reports* article indicated that the longer the course of therapy, the more improvement occurred. But proponents of time-limited therapy also point out that there have been excesses in the application of long-term therapy. And we are all challenged by the current economic pressures to come up with ways of providing some kind of short-term, limited therapy that is effective and has integrity. We also, however, need to carefully research who can benefit from time-limited therapy and who will not; then, professionals will need to educate both themselves and insurance companies about these differences. The idea of managed care originally was intended to provide better treatment for more people; problems arise when the profit motive enters the picture and when nonclinicians are shaping clinical policy. The joint contributions presented in this chapter explore several different views and applications of time-limited therapy.

Most time-limited therapies hold in common a need to focus on specific objectives. Therapists practicing short-term therapy tend to take an active role in collaboratively building the therapeutic alliance, in defining problems, in setting goals, in making shifts in behavior, and in trying to stabilize these shifts. Historically, short-term therapy had its inception when Eric Lindemann, who was treating survivors of the Coconut Grove fire in Boston in 1942, found that in such a crisis situation patients improved greatly after 6 weeks of intervention (Sifneos, 1979). Two of Lindemann's residents, Peter E. Sifneos and Habib Davanloo, went on to develop something called *anxiety-provoking therapy*, one of the primary models of short-term therapy practiced in this country (Davanloo, 1980; Sifneos, 1979). This model can be a rather confrontational, stress-filled therapeutic regimen, and this approach is not considered appropriate for many clients. James Mann (1973), who emphasized working with grief and loss, suggested 12 sessions as optimal. In his work, too, there is an emphasis on facing, bearing, and resolving longstanding conflicts. Malan (1979), another leader in short-term therapy, believes that character can be changed in 30 sessions or less if the therapist brings pressure to bear on the experience of affect. And Davenloo's (1980) therapy, called *short-term dynamic psychotherapy*, depends on the provocation of anxiety and challenging defenses. Each of these mainstream models of short-term therapy place heavy emphasis on challenging the client's defenses, producing anxiety, and moving toward separation. There's also a focus on termination from the very onset of the treatment.

Recently, two clinicians have suggested some modifications of the prevailing emphasis on separation and confrontation in short-term therapy. Leigh McCollough Vaillant (1997) frames her work as *anxiety-regulating* therapy (in contrast to *anxiety-producing therapy*). She emphasizes the importance of connection rather than what she calls "collision" in therapy. Her approach departs dramatically from the confrontational style of many of her predecessors. In addition, Susan Edbril (1994), reflecting on what may be a gender bias in short-term therapy, points out that most time-limited therapies are based on male models of health, which stress the importance of separation. Edbril suggests, instead, that in short-term therapies we need to address the importance of continuity of connection. Both of these women are calling for a different kind of time-limited therapy, and both point to the centrality of connection and relationship in the therapeutic process.

Some of the central points that we might look at in thinking about a *relational model of time-limited therapy* are as follows: an emphasis on connection rather than separation; spacing of sessions to promote the development of relationship; promotion of *relational awareness*; and an emphasis on resources of connection. Spacing of sessions should be planned in terms of building a comfortable working relationship between the therapist and the client. That may involve utilizing several closely spaced, consecutive sessions at the beginning of therapy to build a sense of connection. After two to four of these weekly sessions, sessions can be spaced farther apart. Rather than calling this time-limited therapy, we might think of it as intermittent therapy that stresses continuity of therapy over time.

To help build *relational awareness* (Jordan, 1995), the therapist and client will pay attention to the relational patterns and images that emerge in the therapy relationship itself, as well as in the current relationships in the client's life. Homework assignments that guide the client to attend to relational patterns would complement the work done in sessions. Focusing on two or three *core relational issues*, patterns of connection and disconnection in and out of the therapy sessions, would provide a powerful focus for the work. In assisting people to change *their relational images* (Miller & Stiver, 1997), we work on developing moment-by-moment awareness of the longing for connection as well as the movement toward disconnection, which arises from the terror of connection. The more painful or violating relationships have been for people, the more they will have developed strategies for disconnection in order to maintain a sense of personal safety and integrity. These strategies of disconnection must be honored, and the therapist must acknowledge the underlying longing to connect (Jordan, Kaplan, Miller, Stiver, & Surrey, 1991).

Developing a person's awareness about her/his *resources for connection* is also important. Thus, the therapist will help the client look at her/his patterns of *relational resilience* (Jordan, 1992). As part of this work, the therapist helps the client identify her/his wants and needs, and helps find ways to express these needs so that people other than the therapist can be responsive to them. Furthermore, recognition of nonmutual or hurtful relational patterns is encouraged so that the client can appropriately protect her/himself and make decisions about engagement in relationships. The therapist tries to help the client alter what might be called maladaptive perceptions of self and other, and helps alter relational expectations. In time-limited therapy, this is done in a focused way. A *relational awareness handbook* (Jordan, 1995) assists the clinician and client in tracing relational patterns.

In addition, two group formats have been developed. One, originally called a *self-in-relation group* (C. Dooley, C. Kaufmann, & J. L. Surrey, personal communication), is a psychoeducational group meant to be conducted over 8–12 sessions. It introduces participants to some of the core concepts of the Stone Center model. A relational practice manual is currently being written for application to a wide array of group and institutional settings (Jordan & Dooley, in press). Another format called *relational awareness groups* (Jordan, 1995) also includes psychoeducational/conceptual material, a special relational check-in process, ongoing development of awareness of patterns of disconnection and connection, and awareness of relational vulnerabilities and strengths. Relational awareness groups can be tailored to time-limited interventions (8–12 sessions) or can be more open ended. These groups have been very effective in helping people look at the ways in which they get into relationships that are maladaptive or destructive for them; but they also help people begin to develop and explore constructive relational resources and begin to alter existing relational patterns. Both these group models have been used in various settings, including a women's prison with inmates and guards, a psychiatric inpatient setting, a partial hospital setting, trauma programs, programs for chronically disabled psychiatric patients, a women's housing project, a group of 10-year-old boys, and staff groups in various institutional settings.

Unlike most of the traditional session-limited therapies that emphasize termination from the moment the person walks in the door, a relational approach maintains an "open door policy" and stresses the continuity of relationship, even when therapy sessions are not taking place. The therapist and client do a piece of work together, but it should be clear to the client from the outset that the therapist will be available for future work. This is not a therapy that prescribes a "stand on your own two feet" or a "Lone Ranger" ethic. Very often people can do a piece of therapy and then come back, possibly 6 months or a year later or longer, and do another piece of therapy. The relationship that has been built in this initial phase continues in the absence of meetings; it offers the possibility of reconnection when more work is needed. Furthermore, growth-fostering relationships outside of the therapy relationship are encouraged and other relational resources are emphasized and explored.

In summary, a relational approach to session-limited therapy stresses connection not separation, support not confrontation, relational awareness in addition to symptom reduction, and the building of relational strengths and networks that provide support and encouragement for the client when the therapist and client are not having frequent regular meetings. A relational approach also maintains that it is essential to differentiate when a client can make use of such limited therapeutic contact and when more intensive or long-term work is indicated. And it is imperative that clinicians, not cost-cutting administrators, be in charge of clinical decision making. Furthermore, clinicians have a responsibility to work on an organizational and legislative level to try to get better care for all clients.

THE MANAGED CARE MODEL

Maryellen Handel

Many relational therapists feel that managed care, with its inherent time limitations, is a barrier to building connections and therefore to the healing process. I would like to suggest that a short-term model and the relational model need not be mutually exclusive. I propose that these two approaches can, under optimal circumstances, work hand in hand, and in addition can provide an opportunity to empower women as they actively participate in the therapeutic process.

In this section, I make several assumptions at the outset: (1) that the therapist and client are able to make workable connections with the managed care company; (2) that the managed care company is respectful of the clinician's recommendations; and (3) that the patient has the psychological resources to utilize the model that we are presenting.

It is important to acknowledge the difficulties that disconnections with managed care companies create for therapists and their clients. For instance, communications from managed care companies to carry out treatment for clients in short time frames may lead to disconnections between therapists, clients, and the managed care company. In the service of clients, who depend on managed care company payments, however, it is important to succeed in building good connections with the managed care companies, and thus be to able to carry out the work. For many people, this is their only chance for any therapy at all. Despite the barriers that are present when working with managed care, I have found that the model for treatment presented here can work and can enhance women's growth and connection.

This section begins by delineating the basic tenets of this short-term model, then connects these to the relational model as described by Jordan above, and then proposes ways in which this combined model can empower women. Clinical material is used to illustrate the approach.

The Ideal Model of Managed Care

Most clinicians are aware only of the problems and barriers that sometimes exist when working with managed care companies. Yet, there is a positive theoretical basis in the *ideal* model of managed care delivery. The three basic tenets of this ideal model are easy access, quality maintenance, and cost effectiveness. The concept of easy access ensures that there should be no barriers to care for those who need it. Ideally, networks are established to provide clients with services that are geared to their clinical, cultural, and geographic needs. Quality maintenance ensures that the treatments used are effective and delivered by qualified clinicians. Finally, cost effectiveness ensures that treatment should be provided at the appropriate intensity or "level of care."

A fourth concept of managed care is "customer focus." This assumes that the client is an active participant in the healing process and in the selection of the clinician who can provide the care. It is a collaborative model and the power disparity of the medical model (i.e., "You are sick and if you do as I say you will be well") is altered.

The managed care model envisages a client/customer at the center with the therapist serving the client's needs according to the client's values, according to the client's customs, and according to the client's level of comfort. Connection is very important throughout this type of work. One must connect rapidly and work in a focused way in fewer sessions. So, how does the managed care construct fit with the relational model?

Weaving Together the Relational and the Managed Care Time-Limited Model

The work itself, in the context that has been described above, can dovetail with the relational model. The therapist works with the client's strengths and works to ensure connections that are collaborative. In the evaluation, as it focuses both on strengths and problematic areas, the therapist and client select two or three focal relational issues. Together the client and therapist can look at patterns of connection and disconnection. They can collaboratively look at the resources for connection and also look within the therapeutic relationship for the issues of connection and disconnection. In addition, the assessment must conclude that the client is a good candidate for this type of short-term empowering treatment plan.

The next step is to plan, with the client, how this therapy is going to take place. In other words, with these resources and in a limited number of sessions, how are the therapist and client together going to help strengthen this client's abilities to make and sustain connections to meet her/his current needs. As mentioned above, one can begin with several sessions close together to support the therapeutic connection. The client and therapist may decide to spread the sessions further apart after the initial connection has been established. For example, the client may say, "I want these sessions to last for 6 months; so, I'd like to come once a month because I anticipate a problem in September and maybe in October. That is usually a tough time of year for me, so I think I would like to spread these sessions out."

The therapist can also empower the client by encouraging her/him to seek connections within her/his own communities. These connections are important as they can build lifelong bridges and connecting networks that the client can access over an unlimited period of time. The client can be encouraged to seek out support groups, relaxation classes, exercise venues, and the like, on her/his own; therapy encourages and helps repair the client's ability to make connections outside of the therapeutic alliance.

As stated above, the assessment must evaluate the client's resources for connection. Focusing on these attributes empowers the client, helps her/him to establish connections, and reinforces her/his ability to bring strengths to the healing process. It is important to use this collaborative, connected approach in the assessment process. I usually continue the assessment for two sessions. For example, after assessing the connections and disconnections (assessment of strengths and delineation of problem areas) during the first session, I may use the Beck Depression Scale to help quantify the level of depression if that is an area of concern. Then, I attempt to build a connection with the client, helping to empower her/him through education to understand symptoms within the context of connections and disconnections. Knowledge and increased clarity regarding the client's subjective discomfort can begin to build strength for the healing process and, in addition, fosters the sense of connection and working relationship with the therapist.

An Example

The client, whom I'll call Mary, was referred by her primary care physician. I work with the client in a two-session evaluation. Mary, as customer, presents her problems requesting that I help her to solve them. She says, "I am anxious and I don't know why. I am not sleeping well. I'm angry and irritable at work. These symptoms have come on in the last month, and it is very unlike me." We work together to look at past issues, particularly connections and disconnections. We learn that the client was adopted and never thought about looking for her birth mother. She and her husband have been unable to conceive a child and are in the process of a fertility workup. The client had an abortion when she and her husband were engaged. As she talks, it emerges that this past loss, connected now with the infertility issues, is particularly painful.

The client is not at all connected to her siblings, both the biological and adoptive ones. Her husband and his family are from another culture (they are new immigrants), and she often feels disconnected from them. The client works at night and the husband works during the day—more disconnections.

We establish goals for treatment together. The client says, "I don't want to feel the way I am feeling. I want things to change." We select three issues to work on over time. During the eight sessions, the client (1) grieves the abortion; (2) sets out her own plans for getting involved with an adoptive children's group; and (3) works to connect to her own creative energy through craft projects. As a creative project (her "psychological baby"), she starts making flower arrangements, which gives her a good deal of satisfaction. During the therapeutic work, she is able to see that her depression is related to issues of connection and disconnection, and that she has the skills and the resources to find ways to reconnect to the things that are important to her and to grieve the losses that she has had.

Empowerment

Despite the fact that the managed care model as outlined above has often not been implemented in a way that is faithful to its theoretical construct, it still can work to empower women. For example, the therapist can encourage the client to be active and collaborative in deciding what she needs and how that can be accomplished.

The empowering aspects of managed care and the relational model assume that the client can evaluate the treatment session by session. As a matter of course, I now ask clients at the conclusion of every session, "How was the session today?" If they reply, "It was good," I continue, "Can you tell me what made it good for you today?" and "Which parts of the session didn't work; which parts were particularly helpful?"

This ongoing evaluation and responsiveness on the part of the therapist is very powerful and serves to enhance both the relational and managed care models. First of all, by carrying out this dialogue at every session you are encouraging the connection with the therapist in a collaborative way. You are also helping the sessions to be efficient and focused as you are getting feedback that can help both participants to steer the work toward the most healing and connecting areas. It assumes a mutual respect that is essential in making connections.

Conclusion

In my experience, the managed care model of time-limited therapy can be viewed as fostering connection, empowerment, and a sense of worth and initiative. Both the managed care model and the relational model ideally value the client as a person whose strengths in connection can be known and brought explicitly to the healing process.

RELATIONAL TIME-LIMITED PSYCHOTHERAPY: DEVELOPMENTAL AND CROSS-CULTURAL CONSIDERATIONS

Margarita Alvarez

Although time-limited psychotherapy is not a panacea for the solution of all types of psychological problems, it can be effective as an approach when addressing dilemmas that are developmental (i.e., entering into adolescence; graduating from school; moving away from home) and/or transitional in nature (i.e., adjusting to the pressures of a new job; losing a significant support system). Time-limited psychotherapy is helpful with people who are internally resourceful, with flexible meaning-making systems, and with accessible supportive networks. Additionally, this approach might be particularly useful if congruent with the person's worldview and meanings regarding her/his presenting dilemmas, previous help-seeking experiences, and view of helping professionals.

Developmentally related difficulties can be addressed in a time-limited fashion if the focus centers on normative versus pathological processes. Shifting expectations connected to changing roles, contexts, and relationships can be confusing and disorienting. Connecting empathically to clients' grief associated with separating from loved ones, or to their anxiety related to the unknown, as well as with their confusion when experiencing conflicting role expectations, can facilitate reframing these processes as normative. Having a resource-oriented perspective opens up the possibility of exploring options and coping strategies. Shifting from a problem or deficit perspective to a positive meaning-making framework can be liberating and growth promoting (Jordan, 1989; Miller & Stiver, 1995).

A time-limited approach may assuage feelings of incompetence or family disloyalty if the person's culture and worldview are congruent with solving problems on their own and/or within their family or extended network of close friends. Similarly, people concerned with becoming dependent on a therapist benefit from approaches that frame the focus of intervention in a short-term fashion.

This approach can also address therapeutic needs in an efficient fashion if the person seeking help prioritizes her/his needs and commits to working on them expediently because of constraints around money, time availability, and/or energy. Additionally, persons with vulnerable coping skills may fear in-depth exploration of events and affect that may tax their functioning and interfere with meeting commitments. In these situations, a time-limited approach that focuses on facilitating problem-solving strategies for their most pressing concerns while respecting defenses might be more appropriate. Considering that psychotherapy has a culture of its own (Rendon, 1996), it can be argued that people not "acculturated" to its benefits, or perhaps with a history of negative experiences with mental health professionals, can shy away from the notion of lengthy treatments, but be more open to a time-limited approach. For many people, shame, despair, and lack of hope are deterrents to engaging in therapy, even more so when they feel they have to bare their souls to a stranger. A time-limited and nonhierarchical therapeutic stance, where the client and therapist together share responsibility in elucidating and working toward mutually agreed goals, can help restore a sense of empowerment and control for the client (Jordan, 1986, 1989). Lengthy treatments may signify for some people that their problems are too serious and severe, further contributing to a sense of despair and hopelessness. One wonders if this factor contributes to the high rate of attrition in outpatient psychotherapy.

In short, time-limited and "present-oriented" approaches can be effective and appropriate for individuals with pragmatic and "present-oriented" styles; for those dealing with life transitions, including sudden losses and dislocations; for younger populations dealing with developmental shifts and family changes; and even for people with time and financial limitations or with more chronic but stable problems. However, these are assumptions that would need to be verified with each particular individual requesting help.

In the next subsection, I discuss some difficulties embedded in developmental and life cycle transitions that often present in clinical practice through the manifestation of "symptoms," where a time-limited approach can be effective.

Developmental and Life Cycle Shifts: From "Symptom" to Context

People usually tend to seek psychotherapeutic services when experiencing internal distress or a disconnection from parts of themselves during times of significant changes, disruptions, or discontinuities in their lives. Growing up, changing physically, adjusting to shifting gender roles, accommodating to shifting internal and/or contrasting external expectations, moving away, leaving behind significant emotional attachments and familiar social contexts that nourished and validated primary identifications, or finding different ways of being in the world are all examples of normative experiences that can challenge a person's sense of self and continuity. Developmental discontinuities can also be experienced, for example, in children transitioning from elementary to middle school. Moving from a structured, familiar, and supportive setting to one which is less familiar, protected, and nurturing, and where autonomy and emotional independence are emphasized, can derail a youngster's sense of belonging if peer relationships cannot be established soon and a sense of being an outsider prevails. Similarly, the experience of becoming uprooted in order to pursue a new career or job, or to follow a loved one into another culture, faith, lifestyle, or tradition, contributes to an internal sense of disruption due to crossing into new territories (Espin, 1994) where internal maps available to making sense of oneself, others, and the world become incongruent or irrelevant. Discontinuities in the validation received in relationships with significant others as well as in the "average expectable environment" (Hartmann, 1950/1964; cited by Akhtar, 1994) can be emotionally disorganizing and contribute to the appearance of emotional, physical, and/or social difficulties.

Lack of external support or tolerance for the manifestations of emotional pain associated with these developmental transitions can influence the appearance of emotional disconnections with oneself and others, contributing to the appearance of symptoms (Miller, 1988). While these can be transient, they can also become chronic and debilitating forces in a person's life if the emotional reactions to the losses experienced are lived in isolation and/or experienced as illegitimate (Miller, 1987).

All these issues can be addressed effectively in a relational, empathic, and validating manner (Miller & Stiver, 1991), especially when symptoms are understood in light of the person's experiences in context. As Judy described before, the therapist needs to be actively engaged in helping the client access her/ his resources for connection. As therapists, we also need to provide information that will enhance the person's access to external resources. A relational time-limited therapy that resonates to the person's culture would attempt to—

- Enhance awareness of internal and external resources in light of changes and shifts
- Increase clarity regarding previous functioning
- Increase understanding of a symptom's metalanguage as she/ he enters a new context with different rules
- Facilitate relational images that provide comfort and holding while expanding other images that may help in the shifts and transition

If these goals are met, clients will be more likely to get back on their developmental path and fulfill their optimal potential while adjusting to new shifts and demands.

Non-Normative Transitions

A relational, time-limited approach can also be effective when dealing with the effects of disruptions in peoples' lives that transcend normative life cycle transitions. For example, natural disasters, wars, forced migrations, and immigration contribute to significant emotional, identity, and relational disruptions in peoples' lives due to geographic dislocations and loss of significant relational contexts that previously sustained their cultural identity (Alvarez, 1995). When people are moving to different places or social contexts because of traumatic circumstances, various forces will inevitably influence how such people will function, adjust to changes, and view themselves. The culture of the new place shapes how one experiences and interprets one's experiences through the lens of different ways of being, relating, communicating, and so on. The status of outsider, minority, ethnically different, or marginalized because of language, race, and class will cast new

meanings on previously held identities (Akhtar, 1994). All of these processes influence the emergence of self-doubt and of a devaluing of
one's known way of being and interpreting the world. Different behavioral patterns will be tried in order to adjust to new role prescriptions
and to new identities, chosen or imposed. If one experiences these processes in isolation, the loss of significant relationships and attachment
figures will further contribute to patterns of grief and mourning.
Symptoms will most likely emerge if the new culture does not resonate
to the emotional expression of these losses (Alvarez, 1995).

Coping Styles as Mobilizers or Inhibitors

Clinical data indicate that people's coping strategies become paralyzed
or mobilized around times of anticipated and/or of actual change.
However, people get stuck when old coping strategies (which were once
functional) become reactivated despite their lack of effectiveness in
solving the new challenges at hand.

Old coping patterns become reactivated because people tend to re-
sort to what they know best. It is difficult to let go of what is familiar if
there is nothing to replace it. Furthermore, if maintaining old coping
patterns preserves a connection with significant others, places, and
times, it makes sense that giving them up may trigger a fear of losing a
sense of who one is. Loyalty conflicts can also crystallize apparently
dysfunctional coping strategies when a person carries an "unsettled account in the family" (Boszormenyi- Nagy & Spark, 1984), usually mobilized by guilt and anxiety. Anniversaries commemorating the loss of
significant loved ones tend to reactivate unresolved grief reactions or
symptomatic behaviors that serve to connect with the lost loved ones.

Other problems that emerge during developmental and life cycle
transitions may relate to peoples' fears of the unknown. Becoming paralyzed or reactivating old coping patterns are ways of responding to the
anxiety elicited by the uncertainties about the future or unfamiliarity
with the demands at hand. The new maps for interpreting the new territories may not readily describe behavioral patterns that can be easily
emulated in order to function effectively according to the norms of the
new place. However, other difficulties may arise from the person's interpretation or meaning-making of these events.

Conclusion

In summary, a relational and culturally informed time-limited approach can foster clients' optimal functioning and adjustment to con-

flicting and shifting demands in times of normative and non-normative transitions. The therapist's nonpathologizing stance can facilitate the client's access to internal and external resources in a growth-promoting and cost-effective fashion. This approach can be effective with developmentally and culturally diverse populations.

SHORT-TERM THERAPY IN A COLLEGE COUNSELING SERVICE
Robin Cook-Nobles

In transitioning from a long-term to a short-term model of psychotherapy, it is important to have a theoretical frame. Theory provides guidance and direction to the work. The focus of this section is our work at the Stone Center Counseling Service and how we work relationally with students within a limited time frame. We primarily provide short-term counseling, which typically ranges from six to eight sessions. However, there is flexibility around the actual number of sessions per student, which is tailored to the student's individual need(s) and circumstance.

Clients do not exist in isolation but in relation to the world and their immediate environment. It is important to acknowledge this larger context. Some important questions to consider are whether the environment is supportive and whether other people are available to help provide a supportive network that will complement the work of the therapy. The environment at Wellesley College is supportive. There are a number of resources on campus that can be tapped into to empower the client and the therapy.

Time-limited treatment meets a practical need. It allows us to provide a service while remaining available to the student body at large. Thus, there is no need to maintain a waiting list; we can accommodate a student in crisis, and most students are seen within a week. Students are therefore able to get the services they need within a relatively short time period.

The short-term work that we provide is relational. We focus on the connection, working collaboratively, and empowering the client to connect and work with other resources in the community. This is contrary to the belief that short-term work is all about separation and termination. I therefore suggest that you consider the larger context in your clinical work. Identify other supports that can be tapped into that can empower the clinical work. It could be the community at large, the family, or grassroots groups.

Practical Considerations

We provide periodic counseling. If a student comes to the Counseling Service and has a good experience, then she knows that the Counseling Service remains available to her and that she can return for support. The mere presence of the Counseling Service on campus provides a holding environment for the student, whether or not she is availing herself of the services at a particular time. She may come back with a related problem or a completely different problem in the future. Thus at the end of brief therapy, the relationship has changed but has not abruptly ended. The student can remain in relation to the Counseling Service and/or the therapist even when she is no longer an active client of the Counseling Service. It therefore provides continuity for students. It increases the connection and lessens the disruptions and disconnections.

By engaging in short-term work, the client is learning new coping skills and different ways of managing her behavior. The role of the therapist broadens to that of an educator whose goal is to teach the client new and different ways of managing and coping, which she can internalize and use when other similar situations arise in the future. These new skills may also be transferable to other problems or situations that arise. The client also has the option of coming back later and reengaging in treatment with the same or a different therapist. Thus, one of the important goals of the treatment is for the client to have a positive clinical experience so that she will feel free to reengage in treatment in the future should the need arise.

In assessing the appropriateness of short-term therapy, one has to assess the client's resources. Margarita Alvarez has already mentioned resilience. It is important to assess the client's survival skills, ego, strength, coping mechanisms, and relational resources. Some important questions to consider are the following: what has the client gone through before, and how did she manage; what made a difference for her at that time; and what shifted things for her? The financial resources of the client can be addressed as well. Such questions help the client become cognizant of her resources and what may have been useful (or not so useful) in the past in getting her through a difficult period. By helping the client identify what worked then, she can begin to explore what might work now.

As previously mentioned, it is important to look at the client's social supports. We have found that students who are connected to other people tend to do much better than students who are isolated. The therapist helps the client to identify her social supports and encourages her to use them. Sometimes, when a support network is lacking, the goal of the therapy is to help the student build a network or expand her social group. Sometimes the focus of the therapy is to help the client develop more mutual supports in which there is balance in the relationship and/or to help the client to learn to relate to people differently.

Short-term therapy does not work for everyone. It is important for clinicians to assess the type of intervention needed and to take into account the needs and wishes of the client. One client might need to be seen for the duration of the academic year; another might need a limited amount of sessions spaced out over a semester or academic year. She might need a referral to a private clinician in the community for ongoing psychotherapy, or a referral to an agency or hospital might be appropriate. Sometimes a combination of the available services is indicated. It is important to be open to a number of treatment options and to collaborate with the client in making treatment recommendations.

In providing a thorough assessment, it is important to look at the other stresses that are impacting the client. An academic environment can be quite challenging, and other life stresses, such as family history, background, and/or ongoing family problems, may be interacting with academic demands. Given the amount of stress and the degree of distress that the client is experiencing, the therapist may choose not to delve deeply into the presenting concerns nor attempt to uncover underlying issues. The focus of the clinical work might be to hold, support, contain, and stabilize the client. After the academic year/semester is over, the student may then decide to look more closely at the underlying issues and engage in more intensive psychotherapy.

Clinical Considerations

The appropriateness of short-term therapy may be determined by the presenting concern or the manner in which the client presents or tells her story. For example, a student may present with homesickness, which typically is seen as a reasonable presenting concern for short-term work. However, her presentation may raise concern as to whether there are major loss issues, which may contraindicate putting a time limit on the treatment. For example, the client may talk on and on and have a hard time ending the session. She may experience the limited number of sessions as an initial rejection and may flee from the treatment rather than connect with the therapist. The homesickness may be the immediate presenting concern, but the long-term issues of loss may be the underlying issue that needs to be the focus of treatment.

Another example of the presenting problem having implications for the treatment modality is the client with a trauma background. One might automatically assume that long-term work is indicated. This is not necessarily the case. If a person is struggling with issues of trauma but has a lot of other factors impinging upon them at a particular time, long-term intensive treatment might be contraindicated. Instead, it might be more appropriate to focus on safety and stabilization, rather than on the long-term issues. Providing a supportive, safe holding environment might be the focus of the treatment. Thus, even though the presenting concern is important in determining the appropriateness of short-term work, other factors also need to be considered.

Margarita Alvarez already has discussed the attitudes toward therapy and cultural factors that impinge upon the therapy. I want to reiterate their importance and add that therapy is a culture. People from a certain culture, background, and experience created therapy. As culture shifts and changes, and as people have different cultural experiences, therapists need to remain flexible and open. The rules and techniques of therapy are neither sacred nor static. In some cultures it is appropriate to accept gifts. In some situations the boundaries around the therapy hour and place have to be more flexible (for instance, home visits for those unlikely to come to our offices). In connecting with clients from varied cultures, it is important to acknowledge the culture out of which the therapy grew. We should also acknowledge aspects of the training that are helpful to maintain and those which might need to be modified.

Process

Last, it is important to focus on the process. The primary therapeutic ingredient is the relationship and the working alliance between the therapist and the client. Within this relationally focused context, there are three phases of treatment (i.e., assessment, treatment, and what has been called termination). During the assessment phase, the relationship is central and two primary processes are in operation. The therapist and client are establishing a connection and simultaneously identifying the problem, establishing the goals of the treatment, and devising a contract or plan of how to work together.

In addition, in short-term work the therapist needs to be active. One cannot let the work unfold as is the case with time-unlimited therapy. Within the first two or three sessions a decision has to be made as to whether the therapist and client will continue to work together. The time frame has to be decided upon as well. If the problem cannot be addressed fully within the agreed upon time frame, then a smaller piece (focus) of the larger problem might be addressed. Or the client might feel that she needs support over an extended period of time and decide to take a referral for long-term treatment. The focus could also be an extended assessment, in which the client gains greater understanding of the problem and what is needed therapeutically. In sum, during the assessment phase of treatment, the therapist and the client decide on a focus and contract for treatment.

The treatment phase follows, in which the client and therapist work together to help resolve the primary concern (focus) and to meet the established goals. The client identifies patterns of behavior that might be counterproductive or destructive, relationships that might be problematic, and so on, develops new ways of coping, and/or makes significant life changes.

During the final phase there is a review and an evaluation of the work, as well as an identification of next steps. Closure on the treatment is gained while also identifying other areas of concern and future treatment options. The therapist and the client clarify options for support in the future, including counselor availability. The relationship remains central throughout the treatment and models mutuality, which might well transfer into other relationships.

The therapist makes creative use of the limited number of sessions. Therapeutic time includes the traditional 50-minute sessions, half-hour check-in or follow-up sessions, and 15-minute telephone calls. Together client and therapist devise a contract or plan that spells out the ways in which the time will be used. The relationship remains key throughout the treatment. It establishes the working alliance, maintains trust and commitment to the treatment, and provides holding and support during time of crisis.

Summary

In sum, short-term therapy is a different way of working, both qualitatively and quantitatively. We believe that it is most effective when the focus is on the relationship, connection, and continuity. The therapy is active and has a specific focus, and the client is empowered as an active participant in the treatment. The client has both a voice and a choice. This empowerment of the client is important when working across cultures and with disenfranchised groups of our society. Also, short-term therapy can assist the new client in understanding the therapeutic process and how to make use of therapy. Furthermore, in relationally focused brief treatment, termination is not as final. The connection is central, and the therapeutic door remains open. The client can therefore return without the stigma that she has failed.

REFERENCES

Akhtar, S. (1994). A third individuation: Immigration, identity, and the psycho-analytic process. *Journal of the American Psychoanalytic Association, 43,* 1051–1084.

Alvarez, M. (1995). The experience of migration: A relational approach in therapy. *Work in Progress, No. 71.* Wellesley, MA: Stone Center Working Paper Series.

Boszormenyi-Nagy, I., & Spark, G. M. (1984). *Invisible loyalties.* New York: Brunner/Mazel.

Davanloo, H. (Ed.). (1980). *Short-term dynamic psychotherapy.* New York: Aronson.

Edbril, S. (1994). Gender bias in short-term therapy: Toward a new model for working with women patients in managed care settings. *Psychotherapy, 31*(4), 601–609.

Espin, O. M. (1994). Crossing borders and boundaries: The life narratives of immigrant lesbians. *The Society for the Psychological Study of Lesbian and Gay Issues: Division 44 Newsletter, 10,* 18–27.

Hartmann, H. (1964). Comments of the psychoanalytic theory of the ego. In *Essays on ego psychology* (pp. 113–141). New York: International University Press.

Jordan, J. V. (1986). The meaning of mutuality. *Work in Progress, No. 23.* Wellesley, MA: Stone Center Working Paper Series.

Jordan, J. V. (1989). Relational development: Therapeutic implications of empathy and shame. *Work in Progress, No. 39.* Wellesley, MA: Stone Center Working Paper Series.

Jordan, J. V. (1992). Relational resilience. *Work in Progress, No. 57.* Wellesley, MA: Stone Center Working Paper Series.

Jordan, J. V. (1995). Relational awareness: Transforming disconnection. *Work in Progress, No. 76.* Wellesley, MA: Stone Center Working Paper Series.

Jordan, J. V., & Dooley, C. (in press). Relational practice in Action: A group manual. *Work in Progress Project Report, No. 6.* Wellesley, MA: Stone Center Working Paper Series.

Jordan, J. V., Kaplan, A. G., Miller, J. B., Stiver, I. P., & Surrey, J. L. (1991). *Women's growth in connection: Writings from the Stone Center.* New York: Guilford Press.

Malan, D. M. (1979). *Individual psychotherapy and the science of psychodynamics.* London: Butterworth.

Mann, J. (1973). *Time-limited psychotherapy.* Cambridge, MA: Harvard University Press.

Mental health: Does therapy help? (1995, November). *Consumer Reports,* pp. 734–739.

Miller, J. B. (1987). *Toward a new psychology of women* (2nd ed.). Boston: Beacon Press.

Miller, J. B. (1988). Connections, disconnections, and violations. *Work in Progress, No. 33.* Wellesley, MA: Stone Center Working Paper Series.

Miller, J. B., & Stiver, I. P. (1991). A relational reframing of therapy. *Work in Progress, No. 52.* Wellesley, MA: Stone Center Working Paper Series.

Miller, J. B., & Stiver, I. P. (1995). Relational images and their meanings in psychotherapy. *Work in Progress, No. 74.* Wellesley, MA: Stone Center Working Paper Series.

Miller, J. B., & Stiver, I. P. (1997). *The healing connection.* Boston: Beacon Press.

Rendon, M. (1996). Psychoanalysis in an historic-economic perspective. In R. P. Foster, M. Moskowitz, & R. A. Javier (Eds.), *Reaching across boundaries of culture and class: Widening the scope of psychotherapy.* Northvale, NJ: Aronson.

Sifneos, P. E. (1979). *Short-term dynamic psychotherapy: Evaluation and technique.* New York: Plenum Press.

Vaillant, L. M. (1997). *Changing character: Short-term anxiety-regulating psychotherapy for restructuring defenses, affects, and attachment.* New York: Basic Books.

This chapter was originally presented at a Stone Center Colloquium on February 7, 1996.
© 2000 by Judith V. Jordan, Maryellen Handel, Margarita Alvarez, and Robin Cook-Nobles.

13

Relational Theory in the Workplace

JOYCE K. FLETCHER

*T*his chapter will overview the findings of a research project[1] that used a relational model of growth and development (Jordan, Kaplan, Miller, Stiver, & Surrey, 1991) to explore women's experience in the workplace. As Jean Baker Miller noted in *Toward a New Psychology of Women* (1987), work organizations are likely to be hostile environments in which to seek growth-in-connection. This is true because organizations, like most of society's structures, are based on masculine models of growth that are antithetical to connection, models that privilege separation and independence rather than interdependence and collectivity. The study overviewed here started from the premise that if women truly were operating from a different belief system about what

[1]This project was part of a larger study on gender equity that was funded by the Ford Foundation through Grant No. 910-1036. Before I began this independent part of the study, I had been on site for nearly 2 years as a member of a larger research team that included Lotte Bailyn, Deborah Kolb, Susan Eaton, Maureen Harvey, Robin Johnson, Leslie Perlow, and the consultant to the project, Rhona Rapoport.

leads to growth and effectiveness, this belief system would be evident in the way they worked, even though organizations might not support or encourage this way of working and might even, in their practices and reward systems, actually discourage it. So one goal of the study was to observe women as they worked to see if there was any evidence of work practice that reflected a relational belief system about what leads to growth, organizational effectiveness, and success. The intent was not only to describe the behavior but also to link it to a motivational belief system, a way of thinking that might challenge—and offer an alternative to—masculine norms about how organizations need to be structured in order to be successful.

The second goal of the study was to explore the gender/power implications of relational ways of working. That is, rather than simply describe a different way of working, the study sought to explore what effects this way of working might be having on women and their ability to get ahead in organizations. If, as Jean Baker Miller (1987) suggests, women are expected to shoulder relational work invisibly in personal relationships so that the "myth of independence" remains unchallenged, might this also be happening in organizations? If women were doing "invisible work" in organizations, what effect was this having on them and their career progress? So, the goal of the study was twofold: the first was to make visible, give language to, and build theory about relational activity as practiced in organizations; the second was to explore the power implications of the findings through understanding what happens to people, particularly women, who work this way.

METHOD

The research design reflects the exploratory nature of the research questions. Qualitative data were gathered using a method of structured observation, as well as individual and group interviews, to capture the everyday work experience of six female design engineers. Structured observation is a data-gathering process characterized by the systematic unselective recording of events in their natural setting (Jacques, 1992; Mintzberg, 1973; Weick, 1968). The advantage of this method over more common self-report diary techniques is that it generates data about how people *actually* work as distinct from how they *talk* about how they work. However, in order to explore issues of gender and power, it was also important to understand how the engineers and others in the work environment talked and thought about their work, the language they used to describe it, and the sense they made of it and its effect on their tasks. In order to collect both types of data I devised a protocol in which I shadowed each engineer for a full day, closely observing and recording her behavior and interactions not only with people but with all aspects of the environment. The day after the shadowing I held a long interview with each engineer; I walked her through the day's events asking for comments and explanations of what I had observed. I also interviewed other members of the work site and held a focus group of all the participants in which I fed back some of my early findings and gathered further input and reactions from them.

FINDINGS

Part I: Relational Practice

Analysis of the shadowing data revealed four types of relational practice:

1. *Preserving:* This is behavior associated with tasks. It includes relational activities intended to preserve the life and well-being of the project.
2. *Mutual empowering:* This is behavior associated with enabling others' achievement and contribution to the project.
3. *Achieving:* This is behavior that uses relational skills to increase one's own effectiveness and professional growth.
4. *"Creating team":* This behavior has to do with teamwork. It includes activities intended to create an atmosphere of collegiality, where the positive outcomes of group life—things like collaboration, trust, mutual respect—can occur.

Tables 13.1–13.4 detail the many specific behaviors associated with each type of relational practice, the skills and belief system underlying the practice, and its intended effect on the project. To capture the essence of relational practice in the engineers' own words, selected examples of each type are presented below.

Preserving

This practice had to do with preserving the life and well-being of the project. It included things such as taking responsibility for the whole and doing whatever needed to be done to keep the project connected to the people and resources it needed to survive. People who acted this way had an attitude of "doing whatever it takes" or "if I don't do it, nobody will." Sometimes preserving meant taking on jobs that were technically beneath them—like soldering a board themselves if a technician

were busy—and sometimes it meant going the extra mile by coming in
on a weekend to prevent what they considered "substandard" products
from going out the door. And sometimes it meant scanning the environment for information that needed to be passed on and then taking
the initiative to pass it along. For those who did it, this type of behavior
was considered an essential part of the job and they were hard on those
who refused to work this way. As one engineer put it:

> "What's wrong with picking up a soldering iron? Nothing. Your
> hands aren't going to fall off."

And another:

> "I just could not *believe* Marketing was going to let those prints go out
> the door—I mean, I showed them to Tony [the copy quality person]
> and he just shrugged like 'whatever' and I just said to myself 'no
> way' . . . so Sara and, I we came in on Saturday and redid them, be-
> cause, I mean, it had to be done."

Preserving also included activities that were meant to keep the
project connected to people it needed. For example, this engineer describes how she takes the initiative to make sure that people who supply
valuable resources to the project, but who have no reporting relationship to their team, feel appreciated and valuable:

> "[I]t's just that [I spoke up] because I was more sensitive to it than
> Ned [the manager]. I would—like, someone didn't feel that it was
> their job and I might have sensed that they were getting to the point
> that they were going to get hurt or feel that they were being taken
> advantage of. . . . Then I've put myself in that role and I've just said
> to Ned, 'Maybe we should send so-and-so a thank-you [note] or
> whatever."

Another type of preserving had to do with rescuing, or calling attention to problems. For example, one engineer identified a problem
she thought was serious. She convinced her boss and her boss's boss
that it was a problem, and she arranged for a meeting with another division. At the meeting she took a backseat, deferring to her boss and
letting him explain her data. Later, she describes this taking a backseat
as a conscious decision she made:

> "If we've got someone at a higher level like Mike who can communi-
> cate to them that it's a problem . . . (*pause*) . . . I mean if it was just
> me saying it . . . I mean, otherwise, they might not think it really is

... (*pause*) ... but I could tell. I thought it was a really good meeting because you don't see them that wound up about problems that often, you know? They would rather dust them under the rug and say look, if its just one occurrence."

In summary, the relational practice of preserving is rooted in a belief that being a good worker means taking responsibility for the whole. In many ways, preserving activities are similar to what Sara Ruddick (1989) calls "preservative love," one of the three practices underlying maternal thinking. Like a mother caring for a child, the engineers accept a responsibility for the life and well-being of the project—anything that threatens its health is deserving of time and attention. However, unlike the exclusivity of the mother–child relationship, the project has many "parents" and it is clear that these engineers expect others to assume this same sense of responsibility. It is apparent in the way they talk about their work that their definition of working effectively means not only attending to specific job duties but also connecting across functions, even if such connecting is beneath one in the hierarchy of job duties. Furthermore, there is an implied belief that good workers will have the skills needed to see things holistically and be able to operate in the context of implications and consequences rather than in an atmosphere of separation and specialization.

Another belief underlying this notion that everyone should put the needs of the project ahead of individual issues such as status, hierarchy, or self-promotion is the belief that such action will be seen as a sign of competence and commitment. In other words, the indirectness and apparent "invisibility" of these activities is assumed to be characteristic of their effectiveness, such that doing them invisibly and indirectly does not mean that they won't be recognized but rather, when recognized, will be even more highly valued because they were done without calling attention to them. Thus, the engineer who sacrifices an opportunity for self-promotion and defers to her boss in order to give the problem visibility describes her action with pride, as evidence of her competence—because of her action they are now "wound up" about the problem. This belief that indirectness adds value and that being quietly competent will be recognized is characteristic of relational practice.

The final dimension of the underlying belief system is evidenced by the engineers' willingness to put effort into maintaining relationships they deem critical to the project's health and vitality. Whether it means sending thank-you notes to show appreciation, sending a peacemaker to smooth ruffled feathers, or protecting the project from the consequences of severed relationships, these activities imply a belief

TABLE 13.1. Preserving

Relational practice	Underlying belief	Inputed skill	Intended effect
Shouldering "Do whatever it takes" Scanning Connecting Preventive connecting Maintenance connecting Rescuing	Work includes responsibility for the whole Interdependence is a natural state Relationships need to be in good working order for project to thrive/survive Indirectness adds value Competence will be recognized without self-promotion	Anticipating consequences Holistic thinking Ability/willingness to minimize status differences Sensitivity to emotional context Ability to strategize emotional response	Problem prevention Generalized responsibility for the whole Keep project connected to critical outside sources Protect project from outside threat

that keeping relationships in good working order is an important aspect of ensuring the life and well-being of the overall project. This way of working depends on a certain set of skills, including the ability to think contextually, the ability to anticipate consequences, and the ability to sense the emotional context of situations so one can recognize and take action when someone "might be feeling like they're getting taken advantage of" or is being seen as incompetent.

Mutual Empowering

The second type of relational practice, mutual empowering, includes behavior intended to enable others' achievement and contribution to the project. This practice is characterized by a willingness to put effort into what Cato Wadel (1979) calls "embedded outcomes." These are outcomes embedded in other people, such as increased competence, increased self-confidence, or increased knowledge. The most common empowering activity I observed was empathic teaching—a way of teaching that took the learner's intellectual or emotional reality into account and focused on the other (What does she/he need to hear?) rather than on self (What would I like to say?). As one engineer said when explaining why she talks someone through the whole process while she is fixing a computer file, "Look, the whole point is so they can do it without you next time, right?" Sometimes empathic teaching meant simpli-

fying the information intellectually, like giving an everyday example of
a statistical concept, and sometimes it meant modifying the emotional
context of a teaching interaction. As one engineer put it:

> "Well, the way I work with Frank is a little different. You have to be
> careful not to intimidate men. I wanted Frank to feel comfortable,
> so that's why I sat down next to him and worked through stuff with
> him. . . . It's just a style thing."

Making people feel comfortable about asking for help was a major
part of empathic teaching. Over and over I observed engineers prefac-
ing some information or instruction with comments like "Well, this
may be a silly way of doing this, but what I like to do is . . . " or "There
may be lots of ways to get around this but what works for me is. . . . "
They seemed to use these somewhat self-deprecating comments not
only to minimize status difference but also to communicate an openness to learning and to indicate that they, as teachers, were open to additional input in the interaction.

Another way of enabling others was by keeping them connected to
people, either acting as a go-between to smooth difficulties or stepping in
to handle difficult people for them. For example, one engineer took on
part of her boss's job by offering to take the responsibility for dealing
with a woman on the west coast who was difficult. As she said, "Carl was
getting really frustrated dealing with her, so I just said, 'Look, I'll do it.' "

In summary, mutual empowering activities are those that enable
others to produce, achieve, and accomplish work-related goals and objectives. Unlike the previous theme of preserving, which in many ways
is analogous to traditional dependency relationships based on a mother–
child model, this theme of empowering draws on a model of relational
interaction characterized by *interdependence* and more fluid power relations. It is behavior rooted in the belief not only that outcomes embedded in others are worth working for but that everyone needs and
should be able to expect this kind of help. As one engineer stated:

> "But everyone should feel like that. Because if everyone knew every-
> thing, we all wouldn't be here, you know? We all know something
> other people don't know, so it shouldn't be a big deal. . . . [P]eople
> should realize that . . . but some people don't though."

So mutual empowering is motivated by a different expectation
about enabling, one based on a concept of power and expertise that is
fluid and rooted in a belief that we are *all* dependent on others. Implicit in all of this is the expectation that parties operating in this more

TABLE 13.2. Mutual Empowering

Relational practice	Underlying belief	Imputed skill	Intended effect

Empathic teaching
Modifying information
  Responding to emotional
  Responding to intellectual
Protective connecting
Eliminating barriers
  Emotional barriers
  Practical barriers
	Interdependence is a natural state
	
	Expectation of reciprocity
	
	Expectation of mutuality
	
	Empowering is a skill, a source of self-esteem
	
	Achievement goal is to enhance interacting sense of self
	
	Definition of outcome includes outcomes embedded in people
	
	Growth, development, and achievement occur in context of connection
	
	Enabling requires attending to emotional context
	
	Enabling requires attending to practical context
		Ability to take on another's perspective
		
		Sensitivity to emotional context
		
		Ability/willingness to minimize status differences
			Embedded outcomes (skill, knowledge) in others
			
			Enhanced achievement of both parties
			
			Enhanced ongoing knowledge transfer
			
			Enhanced diffusion of ideas throughout organization
			
			New ideas, enhanced creativity

fluid environment, where power and/or expertise shift from one party to the other, will have two sets of skills. One is skill in empowering others (sharing—in some instances even customizing—one's own reality, skill, knowledge, etc. in ways that make them accessible to others) and the other is skill in *being* empowered (willingness to step away from the expert role and/or minimize status differences in order to learn from or be influenced by the other). In other words, it implies a belief that each party is dependent on the other to achieve a desired outcome and both parties will be motivated to engage in the interaction. This notion of mutuality differentiated this type of enabling from other, more traditional forms of helping. It was clear from the way engineers spoke about it that they weren't engaging in this kind of enabling out of some sense of altruism or selflessness. Rather, they got a positive sense of self-esteem and self-efficacy out of enabling others. In fact, it was part of what it means to be good at your job:

> "I know I'm doing a good job when people think of me when they have a problem. I've succeeded when people think of me as someone who is (1) competent and (2) someone who will help. Most people around here only care about the first thing—competence—they don't care if they are seen as approachable. I do."

Achieving

The third type of relational practice, achieving, uses relational skills to enhance one's own professional growth and achievement. It is a way of working rooted in the belief that I will be most effective as a worker if I am connected to others. So, much of the behavior had to do with maintaining connection and with creating good, solid working relationships with people. For example, one engineer went out of her way to track down someone whose feelings she had hurt; another made a point of following up with someone after a disagreement in a meeting. What was striking about these activities was the distress and sense of urgency

TABLE 13.3. Achieving

Relational practice	Underlying belief	Imputed skill	Intended effect
Reconnecting Reflecting Self-reflection Reflecting on emotional context Relational asking	Growth, development, and achievement occur in context of connection	Ability to admit mistakes	Enhanced achievement through relational asking
		Ability to recognize and acknowledge responsibility for breaks in relationship	Diffusion of ideas throughout organization through relational asking
	Authenticity is important to relationships		
	Severed relationships obstacle to future growth and achievement	Ability to respond to another's emotional state	Complex understanding of phenomena
		Ability to strategize an emotional response	New ideas, enhanced creativity
	Interdependence is a natural state		
	Expectation of reciprocity	Complicated thinking, (synergy of thinking, feeling, and acting)	
	Expectation of mutuality		
		Ability to call forth responsiveness	

to "make things right" that accompanied these reconnections. Theories of growth-in-connection suggest that this urgency to reconnect stems from a belief in the long-term potential of relationships that are in good working order. Thus, as this engineer indicates, the urgency and desire to maintain connection is not so much a fear of separation as it is an avoidance of conditions that might preclude future growth:

> "I get my point across, sometimes indirectly . . . the more it bothers me the more indirect I get. If I feel that confronting the issue may end the relationship, I won't confront it."

Her desire to maintain the connection is evident in the way she enacts a conscious, intentional strategy to speak more and more indirectly to minimize the negative impact of direct confrontation until finally, after making an assessment that the relationship is in jeopardy, she gives up. In effect, she decides not to pursue growth in the *current* connection but preserves the possibility of future growth by not severing ties completely.

At times the practice of achieving entailed paying attention to the emotional overlay of situations in order to understand what the most effective response would be. For example, one day we were sitting in the lab and another engineer came in and demanded, in an angry voice, to know what was going on. The engineer I was shadowing gave him some information about the problem she was working on and he turned and left. The next day when I asked her about it, she explained it this way:

> "Well, I told him about the problem because I think he feels a little territorial about it. He thinks of the lab as his area. Also, the meeting I have with him later is to get information from him that [our boss] wants me to document because she wants it documented in my style. Technically, this is his job, so I don't think he feels real comfortable with that, so he may be a little threatened and that may have something to do with his coming in here now and wanting to know."

Her ability to understand how he might be feeling prevents her from using the information as power or lording it over him. This not only keeps her relationship with him in good working order in the short term, it appears to be an intentional strategy to enhance her own effectiveness by increasing the chance that the meeting they have later on in the day will go smoothly.

This ability to use emotional data seemed to come so easily to these engineers that they were amazed when others didn't do it. One said:

> "These are smart people, they're engineers . . . and yet some of them don't seem to realize that they are never going to get that person to say what they need him to say because two hours earlier they made him look stupid in a meeting. They can't seem to figure out that the way to get someone to support you is not to call them stupid!"

Another type of achieving had to do with something I called "relational asking," or asking for help in a way that made it likely you'd *get* the help you needed, that is, in a way that called forth responsiveness in others. One engineer described it this way:

> "A lot of people around here will say something like: 'Katie, I'm in a position of leadership over you and you have to do this for me. Make these files.' And I tend to like to say, 'Katie, can you show me how to do one of these?' "

But it wasn't just the way of asking for help that was important, it was the kind of help sought. As another said, "I know people don't mind helping me, because they know I'll share it with others in my group, so its not like everyone will be coming to them." They contrasted this sort of "empowering helping" with people who asked for help in an exploitative way. As one says, "I'll show you what you don't know, but come on, everyone can make a file . . . I'm not going to do your *job* for you!"

In summary, the relational practice of achieving is based on a belief that not just personal, but professional growth is rooted in connection. It's a practice that depends on an acceptance of interdependence, where asking for help isn't a sign of weakness but an invitation to empower. Achieving behavior required an ability to use emotional data to understand a situation and strategize a response. It helped the engineers chose their battles and avoid unintentionally creating obstacles to their own effectiveness.

"Creating Team"

The relational practice of "creating team" had to do with working to create the background conditions in which group life can flourish. Working to create an environment in which the positive outcomes of relational interactions can be achieved—outcomes like cooperation, collaboration, trust, respect, and collective achievement—included two types of activities: creating conditions within the individual and creating conditions between individuals.

Creating conditions within individuals entailed all kinds of verbal and nonverbal interactions that acknowledged people and seemed to be intended to communicate a sense of "I hear you" or "I see you." It included things like nodding and smiling when others were talking, maintaining eye contact with speakers in meetings and chuckling at their jokes, or making encouraging comments like "right," "good point," or even just "uh-huh." It also included listening and responding to others feelings, preferences, or unique circumstances. As one engineer says:

> "The other thing is, because men joke around so much with each other, when a man does have something he wants to talk about he won't go to another man . . . he'll go to a woman. I've had men who I know don't even like me, use me to vent about really personal things. Like this one guy I know doesn't like me and I don't like him much, started to talk about the fertility problems he and his wife were having. I mean that's heavy stuff. And I've talked to several women who say that men come in and sit down and talk to them. You don't really have to say anything, just listen. They just want someone who will listen and not joke around about it. I feel bad when others are feeling bad or having a hard time, and I know its not going to kill me to spend some time with them. And also, who else are they going to go to? It doesn't cost me anything, really, just to listen. But sometimes it just feels like a big responsibility because even if you are not really in the mood, you have to do it. I mean, if they are coming to you it must be pretty bad, and where else can they go?"

One of the interesting things about this quote is how she responds empathically even though she is fully aware that "he doesn't like me and I don't like him much." So the response is not based on affection but is a conscious decision. Like the nodding and smiling, it seems to be rooted in a belief that people deserve to be acknowledged and to have their experience validated in some way and that they, as coworkers, have a responsibility to do this type of acknowledging for others. But it didn't seem to be just a personal responsibility as a human being. Rather, their actions appeared to be motivated by a desire to create a certain kind of environment in the workplace. As this engineer says:

> "What I think is—the more team-spirited people are more effective in what they're doing. And I equate being conscious of other peo-

TABLE 13.4. Creating Team

Relational practice	Underlying belief	Imputed skill	Intended effect
Creating conditions within individuals	Growth, development, and achievement occur in context of connection	Ability/willingness to affirm others with no loss to self-esteem	Create conditions within individuals that may lead to enhanced individual/team achievement
Responding/ respecting			
Empathic listening	Definition of outcome includes embedded outcomes	Empathic listening	
Responding to preferences			
Creating conditions between individuals	Outcomes of relational practice are valuable		Create conditions between individuals that may lead to new ideas or understandings through relational interactions
Smoothing			
Envisioning/creating	Value involvement over abstraction		
Reality of interdependence			
	Interdependence is a natural state		Enhance collaboration
			Enhance ongoing knowledge transfer

ple's feelings with working in a team spirit. I think people are much more effective this way."

Creating conditions between people had to do with creating an environment that would foster collaboration and cooperation. Sometimes this meant something as simple as creating the reality of interdependence by using collaborative rather than confrontational language in expressing ideas in a meeting. For example, saying things like "What I like about Dave's idea is . . . " and then going on to add to it. As one engineer notes:

> "I *like* to talk about things, explain why I think something, hear about what the other person thinks about something. But I know there are some people who like to operate in a state of conflict . . . with voices raised, like 'That's not a good idea,' instead of 'Why do you think that's a good idea?' "

In summary, "creating team" appears to be characterized by a certain set of beliefs and assumptions about group life. First, is the belief that individuals have a right to be "noticed" and that part of what it means to be a good coworker is to do the noticing. Second, is a belief that team spirit and achievement depend on paying attention to others' feelings and preferences and that the intangible outcomes that result from these efforts—outcomes embedded in other people and in social relations—are things worth working for. Third, it is a practice rooted in the assumption that a collective understanding of problems or situations, where other's ideas are fully explored and built upon, will enhance organizational effectiveness and lead to better decisions.

Summary

These four types of relational practice encompass a way of working that springs from a relational belief system, one characterized by a generalized responsibility for the whole and based on notions of connection, interdependence, mutuality, and reciprocity. It is a way of working that depends on the use of relational skills—things such as being sensitive to emotional contexts and others' emotional realities and the ability to think and act contextually. But the most important feature of relational practice, the feature that tied it most clearly to a relational model of growth and development, was that *its use was strategic*. The engineers in this study made a conscious decision to work this way because they believed that operating in a context of connection was more effective, better for the project, better for getting the job done.

This belief system—in which relational interactions are assumed to be sites of growth, achievement, and professional effectiveness—stands in sharp contrast to organizational norms and beliefs about competence, effectiveness, and organizational success. This brings us to Part II of the analysis: what happens to this relationally motivated behavior, and to the people who do it, when it is practiced in an environment that is hostile to its basic assumptions?

Part II: Gender, Power, and "Getting Disappeared"

As noted earlier, this project was part of a larger research project on gender equity. As part of that larger effort our team had done a cultural diagnosis of the work environment at this site. We found it to be a work environment similar to other environments in which design engineering is highly valued (McIlwee & Robinson, 1992). That is, we found that it is a workplace characterized by autonomy, self-promotion, and individual heroics, where time is a surrogate for commitment and competence is measured by short-term results. It is a workplace in which technical competence is highly valued and is seen as the route to organizational power and where self-promotion is essential to being seen as competent. Real work is defined as "solving problems," and engineers who moved on to supervisory positions even spoke of "no longer hav-

ing a job" because all they did now was help other people do their
work. It is a culture in which the definition of outcome is clear. Outcomes are tangible measurable and concrete. In fact, in this environment, if you can't quantify or measure something, it is assumed to not
exist.

So, what happens to relational practice when it is done in this
work culture? Well, it's not just that it is invisible or behind the scenes,
although it is that. What happens when relational practice is lifted
from its own belief system and brought into the organizational discourse on work is that the system *acts* on this behavior. It is not just invisible—it "gets disappeared." This happens because behavior based on
a model of growth-in-connection violates many of the assumptions underlying this culture, assumptions that reflect a different model of
growth, development, and achievement, one rooted not in connection
but in independence and individuation. By observing and listening
closely to how others responded to relational practice, how the engineers themselves talked about their behavior, and even how I as an observer sometimes misinterpreted their actions, I began to get a sense of
the ways in which relational practice "gets disappeared" in this setting.

Disappearing Preserving

The practice of preserving is rooted in a belief system that privileges
context and connection. However, in this engineering culture based
on individualism, hierarchy, and specialization, operating in a context of connection is literally non-sense. It is behavior that lies outside
the job description, and it tends to mystify the people who observe it.
So, for example, an engineer who attempts to pass information
across divisions by telling her manager that marketing will be sending out substandard prints is met by a shrug—that's not her job, don't
worry about it. Other attempts to call attention to things that could
cause future problems were met with the same type of response. After all, in a culture where you get ahead by solving high-visibility
problems, it is a waste of time to put effort into the routine, maintenance things. It tends to be seen as nit-picking or as an excessive de-
votion to detail. In fact, it can prevent problems and be of great
value to an organization.

And being quietly competent or sacrificing an opportunity for
self-promotion tends to be seen as not being competent at all. In fact, I
found that even I sometimes "disappeared" this relational competence
and misinterpreted what I observed. For example, when I observed the
event described earlier of an engineer who took a backseat in a meet-

ing and let her boss talk about her data, I at first coded this as evidence of her fear of power and success. I was making sense of her behavior as some sort of personal aberration, assuming that she was uncomfortable with self-promotion or with being seen as an expert. It wasn't until later, as she spoke of the incident with pride and explained to me that it was an intentional strategy on her part to give the problem increased visibility and make sure it was taken seriously, that I began to realize that her behavior at that meeting could be understood differently.

Others might see some aspects of preserving behavior, like sending thank-you notes, as "wives' work" (Huff, 1990) and attribute it to women's desire to humanize the workplace. The real point, however, is that these explanations are fundamentally different from viewing the behavior as work—intentional action meant to enhance effectiveness.

Disappearing Mutual Empowering

In a culture of self-promotion—where independence is prized and competition means beating the other guy out so you finish on top—helping others achieve doesn't make sense. In this culture, where secretaries and other support staff who get paid to help others are low in the hierarchy and have little opportunity for advancement, it makes sense that those who *voluntarily* enable others are considered either inherently nice or incredibly naive. They either don't know any better, or they don't understand the rules of the game. As one engineer says:

> "If you try to nurture around here, they just don't get it. They don't understand that is what you are doing. They see it as a weakness, and they use it against you. They don't see that you are doing it consciously . . . they think you have missed something or that they've gotten something over on you. So if you try to be nice, you end up doing other people's work."

What her experience makes clear is that here, in a work culture governed by "metrics," where all outcomes are tangible and measurable, it doesn't make sense to put effort into achieving outcomes embedded in others. In fact, there really is no organizationally acceptable language to describe the practice of embedding outcomes in others. The words she herself ends up using—nurturing, helping, being nice—tend to gender and de-skill the practice, making it seem more like a personal attribute than strategic action.

In this work setting, support activity in any form is routinely "disappeared" from the final product, reinforcing the myth of independence and individual heroics. This engineer is well aware of how this myth disappears enabling activity and wonders why they can't operate in an environment in which both enabling and *being* enabled are valued:

> "If we rewarded someone who said, 'You know that action item I got yesterday? I found this great source of information [within the company]. So and so's team did all this work, and here is some of the output,' and if [the boss] could say, 'That was good of you to not reinvent the wheel,' . . . you could actually get recognized for the *way* you got the job done rather than just getting it done. But just getting it done is what is important here . . . so you alone . . . *you're* the one who got it done . . . so you alone get the credit."

Disappearing Achieving

The relational practice of achieving "gets disappeared" in a similar fashion. Within organizational discourse, the world is divided into those with achievement needs and those with affiliation needs. In this framework, relational interactions are assumed to be motivated by strong affect and the desire—indeed, the *need*—to have those feelings reciprocated. The possibility of having achievement needs met through relational interactions isn't representable in this sense-making schema—it is non-sense. Thus, individuals who seek relational interactions as sites of growth and achievement in the workplace are destined to be understood as seeking something else, such as affect, and operating out of a "need to be liked." And in this engineering environment, a need to be liked is considered such a sign of personal deficiency that merely suggesting that certain people are motivated by this need is enough to taint them and their behavior as worthless, inappropriate, and a sign of incompetence. Again, as members of the system, engineers themselves are able to give voice to how any evidence of behavior motivated by a desire for growth-in-connection gets disappeared:

> "So if I do get into a situation that is confrontational, not angry necessarily, but even if we're just being very direct with each other and this person wants to do it one way and I want to do it another way, I'd be concentrating more on (*pause, then little laugh*) *winning* than on how they felt about it. I gave up a long time ago caring about how they felt about it, other than if how they feel about it is going to get in the way of getting it done. But if I don't perceive that their feel-

ings are going to get in the way, then I kind of don't notice anymore (*laugh*). So that's the only reason why I'm paying attention to their feelings. It isn't that I care that much about their feelings. It's because if they feel threatened enough, I won't make any progress and not because. . . . (*pause*) If I thought I'd win in spite of that, it wouldn't bother me at all. So it isn't that I'm terribly worried about whether the guys that I work with like me. I worry a lot about whether they respect me. *I don't really care if they like me or not.* (*emphasis added*) (*laugh*) . . . (*pause*). . . . I happen to think that usually those kind of end up going together, though. If you respect someone, you usually end up liking them, too . . . at the end of it all."

The contradictions and inconsistencies in this quote give a good sense of the disappearing dynamic that occurs when relational practice is brought into the organizational discourse on work. The language she has available to represent her experience is limited, and she is careful to distance herself from attributions of inappropriate behavior—she would be more concerned about winning, she wants me to know, than she would about someone's feelings. But then she gets all tangled up as she tries to describe her experience that these two things are not dichotomous. If feelings are going to get in the way of success, then of course she is concerned about them. If feelings weren't real, that is, if she accepted the conventional wisdom that feelings are irrelevant to organizational phenomenon, she wouldn't care about them at all because they wouldn't stand in the way of winning. But she wants to make it clear that the *reason* she is concerned about feelings isn't because she wants to be liked. She understands that this would be the "normal" attribution, and she wants to make sure I don't make it regarding her. So she falls back again into the dichotomy—she doesn't care if they like her as long as they respect her. Any language available to her to describe worrying about the effect of confrontation on the relationship, or to describe the possibility that behavior that gets you liked might make you more effective, would risk the attribution of "needing to be liked," an attribution that would taint her as incompetent. Not having the organizational language to describe such a possibility and still be considered competent, she chooses competence and unwittingly reinforces the dichotomy between the two. But after giving me the party line, she recognizes the inadequacy of what she has said in trying to capture her experience, so—after a slight pause and a little laugh—she undermines this dichotomous thinking: she happens to believe these two things go together, that being liked and being respected are not mutually exclusive.

Disappearing "Creating Team"

Many of these same dynamics operate to disappear the relational practice of "creating team." In an environment where a relational model of
growth and development is non-sense, it is difficult to articulate or understand a motivation to engage in activity to create a feeling of
"team." So, if one operates from a relational belief system and, for example, use language that invites collaborative discussion, rather than
being seen as effective, you are not seen at all. You and your ideas disappear. In the focus group, one engineer describes this disappearing so
vividly that the group laughs in recognition:

> "Sometimes you're in a meeting and somebody states an idea. If I
> stand up and I say, 'That's totally inappropriate, that's just plain stu-
> pid, this is what we should do,' or if I stand up and say, 'Well, that's a
> really good idea but how about if we look at it this way?,' the person
> who stood up and was abusive about it is the person that people are
> going to remember as having come up with that idea later, when it's
> time to evaluate people. Because even though it's a bad impression,
> you've made an impression. The other person, in being polite and a
> little self-effacing, has sort of melted into the background (*pause*).
> Sometimes, if you're nice you'll say something like 'Well, that's a re-
> ally good idea, but I looked at it this way and this is what I came up
> with.' And then [after you give your idea] they'll say, 'Well, anyways
> . . . ' (*general laughter*). And because you haven't like stomped on
> them, *you're not even in the room.*"

What she recognizes is that if there is only one right way, and discover-
ing it makes you the winner, then building on others' ideas is considered inappropriate or a sign that you have nothing new to add. Again,
the language available—nice, self-effacing—tends to devalue the approach she is trying to describe, making it more a sign of weakness
than strength. So this collaborative approach, like other things that create team—the affirming, the acknowledging, the listening, the smooth-
ing—is not seen as competency but as a personal attribute or a natural
expression of gender (women are naturally nicer, more polite, and
more self-effacing). As a result, team spirit is assumed to be something
that "just happens."

Summary of "Getting Disappeared"

This discussion suggests that there are three separate but synergistic
mechanisms operating on relational practice to disappear it as work

and construct it as something *other* than strategic action. The first mechanism is the attribution of "inappropriate." This occurs when relational practice is interpreted as a symptom of some sort of personal aberration, not appropriate to the workplace. This includes some positive attributions, such as being called "nice" or "thoughtful" as well as some more negative labels such as "naive" or being seen as someone who "doesn't know the rules of the game" or who has an emotional dependency or a strong "need to be liked."

The second mechanism through which relational practice gets disappeared is through the lack of language to describe it as work. The words the engineers have available to describe this kind of behavior ("helping," "nurturing," "nice," "polite") tend to associate it with the private sphere, with mothering and home. These words are not organizationally strong. At the same time, words that *could* describe it, words like "outcome" and "competence" are defined organizationally in ways that implicitly exclude the kind of behavior they are trying to describe. Like the engineer who said:

> "I've succeeded when people think of me as someone who is (1) competent and (2) someone who will help. Most people around here only care about the first thing—competence—they don't care if they are seen as approachable. I do."

It's clear here that what she is trying to do is describe an expanded definition of competence, one that includes a willingness and an ability to share and empower others. But there is no good language available to her to describe this kind of outcome—an outcome that would be embedded in another person—as evidence of competence. So she uses "approachability" and "help," words that are not nearly as organizationally strong and leave the definition of competence unchallenged. Ironically, her struggle actually ends up *reinforcing* the notion that enabling others is not part of competence but that it is something separate.

The third way in which relational practice gets disappeared has to do with the social construction of gender. It is different from the first two ways of getting disappeared because it has to do with how this way of working gets conflated with images of femininity and motherhood. Thus, the first two mechanisms of disappearing—being labeled inappropriate and not having the language to describe these things as work—would operate on *all* who worked this way, regardless of gender. But when women enact relational practice, something else happens. Because of gender roles, women are *expected* to act relationally, to be soft, feminine, helpful, good listeners. In fact they don't believe they have the option of acting any other way. As one engineer said, "I try swearing, but I feel so stupid!" Or another, describing what happens when she tries using confrontation to make a point:

> "People notice that you said it, and it definitely gets the point on the table. But it certainly isn't good for your long-term relationships with that person. Especially, I think, if it comes from a woman to a man. I think that another man could do that, could say the exact same words, the exact same tone, and after the meeting it would just be over . . . (*pause*) . . . I don't think it would be over if one of those players was a woman, even if it was over for the woman. I don't think it would be over for the man."

These gender expectations end up confusing the issue. It is difficult to articulate a relational way of working as an intentional choice when you sense that you don't *have* a choice. So the engineers get confused as they talk about this and they end up talking about it in contradictory ways, trying to capture the experience that they simultaneously resent being forced to use relational strategies *and* they believe it is actually more effective to work this way.

But even more problematic for women is that because they inhabit a female body, when they try to enact relational practice (work from a base of connection, mutuality, interdependence, and reciprocity), they often get misinterpreted as enacting mothering (selfless giving). That is, they get responded to as *women*, not as *workers*. So, if they try to limit helping (as one engineer said, "I'll help, but I'm not going to do your job for you,") or if they refuse to use collaborative language when their ideas are getting stepped on, they are labeled (jokingly) "Queen Bee" or "Tarantula Lady." Interestingly, these are names that label them not unhelpful but *unfeminine, poisonous, arrogant*. Getting called names for not being willing to help limitlessly, or for expecting reciprocity, over-whelms their belief in this as an alternative way of working. Because they recognize the career implications of being exploited or of being seen as naive, they end up cautioning themselves and others not to do too much relational work. As one said, "Although it might be good for the project, if you do it, you'll end up being a gopher your whole life."

The Disappearing Dynamic

These three mechanisms operate in concert, creating a self-sealing loop I call the "disappearing dynamic," pictured in Figure 13.1. The easiest way to read the loop is to start in the upper right of the circle. The loop gets engaged when women enact any one of the four types of

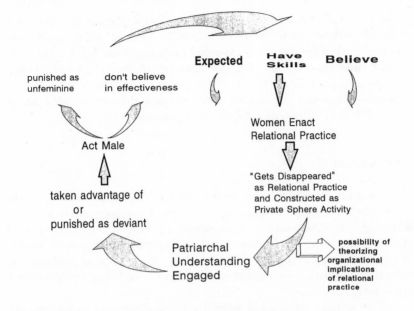

FIGURE 13.1. The disappearing dynamic.

relational practice. This practice gets disappeared as something new (an alternative way of working in the public sphere) and gets constructed as something familiar (private sphere activity, inappropriately applied to the public sphere). Two things happen at this point. First, the model of growth-in-connection and the intentionality motivating the behavior gets thrown out of the loop, truncating any possibility of analyzing this behavior as an alternative to organizational norms. And, second, the people who work this way are seen as acting inappropriately. *A patriarchal understanding* of the motivation underlying their behavior gets engaged and, at least for females, rather than being seen as good workers, they are seen as good women or good mothers. This tends to construct relational practice as an expression of woman's essential nature—not only does she like doing these things, she is *supposed* to do them. Again, this leads to two possible outcomes, both with negative career consequences. Either women get punished for being too feminine (she doesn't know how to play with the big boys, she's not aggressive enough) or she gets taken advantage of because she is seen as naive or exploitable. So, not wanting to be exploited, she tries to change her behavior and act more appropriately—Act Male—but that doesn't work either, because now she gets punished for being *unfemi-nine*. But also, her heart isn't in it because she really does not believe it is the most effective way of working. In addition, she has the relational skills to work in a way she does believe is more effective. So, for all these reasons—because she is expected to, because she has the skills to, and because she believes in it—she tries again. And the loop gets engaged once again. There are several important conclusions to be drawn from the loop and the way in which relational practice "gets disappeared" from organizational definitions of work.

CONCLUSION

The first implication of the loop is that relational practice gets absorbed by the system but challenges to ways of working—and ways of organizing that would support this way of working—"gets disappeared." So the main power implication is that the patriarchal nature of the status quo in organizations is not challenged. In fact, organizational norms of hierarchy, individualism, autonomy, and independence end up getting reinforced.

The second implication is that relational practice is undertheorized in the organizational literature. It is not theorized because, within the loop, it does not "exist" as an alternative strategy for organizational effectiveness. The result is that organizational understandings of the nature of work are both limited and one sided. For example, the understanding in the business literature about what it means to enable, what it means to collaborate, or what it means to work as a team is quite narrow, relying for the most part on private sphere models of relational interactions—like the mother–child relationship or the wife–husband relationship—rather than developing a new language or new models. Ironically, relational practice is exactly the kind of behavior "re-engineered" organizations *say* they need: holistic, team oriented, flatter, less hierarchical (Hammer & Champy, 1993; Senge, 1990). But, because of its association with the private sphere, when this type of behavior is enacted in organizations not only is it not rewarded, it is turned into a career liability.

The third implication is for women's mental health. Behaving in ways they believe exhibit competence, skill, and power but being branded naive, inadequate, or incompetent must be taking its toll on women's self-esteem. Certainly all the engineers I shadowed spent a lot of time reflecting on these issues. In fact, in my analysis I had a separate category labeled "Am I crazy?" to reflect the ambiguity and self-doubt they often expressed. The problem is that the loop constructs all these issues in terms of personal aberration. What gets lost is the fact that women's experience is being *systematically distorted* in order to protect the status quo from challenge. So, it is natural that women start to think of these issues as their problem and believe they have to solve it individually. And it is no wonder that lots of women—even those who have made it to the top—are leaving organizations to start their own small companies or are refusing promotions or refusing to compete for top positions. Again, conventional wisdom holds that these women are leaving because they can't hack it. Either career and work aren't important enough to them or they can't take the pressure. But interestingly, follow-up interviews with women who have left high-level jobs indicate that they *can* do these jobs, they've just decided they don't *want* to. Years of trying to change the system has taken its toll.

And for all the women who don't have the option of leaving, what does it mean for them? Well, it may mean they are ending up in a lot of psychologist's offices, feeling dispirited, lethargic, or incompetent and not really understanding why. If they are doing double duty at work—scrambling to be seen as competent in the current system and yet doing invisible relational work on the side in order to change the system or at least do their own job differently—it is easy to understand why they might be feeling dispirited.

We seem to be locked in a battle. Women need to change organizations, and organizations seem to be doing their best to change women. The real question is, what can be the next steps? Can we find the ways to convince organizations to recognize models of growth-in-connection?

DISCUSSION SUMMARY

After each colloquium presentation a discussion is held. Selected portions are summarized here. At this session, Maureen Harvey, Jean Baker Miller, Sung Lim Shin, Irene P. Stiver, Janet L. Surrey, and Maureen Walker joined Joyce K. Fletcher in leading the discussion.

QUESTION: In looking for evidence of relational practice, did you shadow any men?

FLETCHER: I did not include men in my data analysis. However, as I mentioned, this project was part of a larger study and as part of that study we did shadow a number of men. We did see in them some evidence of relational practice, particularly the helping and enabling type of behavior. Interestingly, the men who did do some of these things tended to be men of color who came from another culture, not the

United States. But I also want to add that the reason I did not analyze men had to do with the goal of the study. I was really trying to further our understanding of relational practice, not just as a way of working but as a way of *thinking*, one that is rooted in a belief that relational interactions are sites of growth, development, and professional achievement. So, to further the thinking required studying people who were likely to be operating from this model of growth and that meant studying women.

QUESTION: For the men that were shadowed, did the same thing happen to them? Did they "get disappeared"?

FLETCHER: Well, to a certain extent they did. That is, they weren't rewarded for their behavior and they often were seen as just being helpful or nice people. But they did not have the gender dynamic operating on them. In other words, they didn't get labeled as mothers and they didn't get punished or called names for not helping or listening or whatever. So it was a different experience for them.

QUESTION: Did you observe women mentoring each other? I have not seen a lot of mentoring of women by women. Instead, there seems to be a lot of backstabbing.

HARVEY: Well, I think that what you are seeing is that women get caught in the system. They get caught between what they have to do to succeed in this very masculine environment and the demands from other women for help. I've seen this played out in lots of senior women. There is sort of a love–hate relationship with the skills they have. They know they have the skills to enable others, but on the other hand they know if they do it they won't get rewarded for doing it and it might even hurt them because they won't be seen as tough enough or aggressive enough to do the job. It's really this whole disappearing dynamic. So, they are in a real bind and it's a real problem for them.

STIVER: Another thing is that often women are very isolated in these senior positions. They are disconnected from relationships with others, and it is in these instances of isolation that I think you see the kind of negative behavior—the backstabbing and so forth—that you alluded to. It seems to me that just the fact of being shadowed, of having someone listen to them, must have been an empowering experience for these women and maybe made them feel more able to claim this behavior. I guess that is really a question. If we really want to empower women to work the way they want to work, maybe it means we have to listen to them and be some sort of support, to provide that connection so they are not so isolated.

FLETCHER: I want to say one more thing about mentoring, and that is that I think the notion of mentoring we have is a very masculine notion, very hierarchical and one-directional. What I observed was a more generalized, more informal kind of mentoring. These engineers wanted *everyone* to succeed, and their everyday, ordinary interactions with people were geared to enable whomever they were with. It's different from formal mentoring where you are training and protecting a specific person. I also want to add to what Maureen said. I think we as women put extraordinary demands on women at higher levels, expecting them to be all things feminine and *also* to demonstrate all the masculine competencies that will advance them in the organizations. It's a lot.

SURREY: I also think that mentoring for men is somewhat different. What I've seen is that when men mentor, it's sometimes a narcissistic interaction. It's not so much a focus on the needs of the other as it is just feeling good about being in a superior position where you can pass on your knowledge and wisdom. So it's a different definition of what it means to enable someone else—you are doing it because you are getting credit for doing it.

WALKER: One of the things your question brings up is the need to acknowledge that being part of a socially devalued group does create a "dearth mentality." There is this feeling that there isn't enough to go around and if I have internalized what I need to get in order to succeed then I am going to do whatever it is I need to do in order to get it. So, for example, one of the things we see is that people in a socially devalued group go out of their way not to give special treatment to people who are like them and in many ways treat people who are *not* like them better. So that is one of the sticky questions we are going to have to deal with in all of this, the very human element of wanting to get ahead and doing whatever it takes to do it.

SHIN: I want to add that I think we can't ignore the issue of cultural differences. I think that in this culture it is not only women that have difficulty, it is people from different cultures as well. I am struck by the fact that some of the men who worked relationally came from other cultures. So I am struck by how *Western* male this focus on individualism and autonomy is. It is not just gender.

QUESTION: I love these findings. I've worked for years in organizations, and I would like to just scream for joy because some of these things are being named! I've worked where women after a number of years did turn the culture around from very hierarchical to more team focused where people can work together. And to answer where we go from here, we do need to start naming some of these things. Name it as a *nonhousehold* function to create the vision of what we are doing. Once we have the language, the real question is are we really ready to move toward a new model? I mean, is capitalism just inherently too competitive and are we really talking about a revolution here?

FLETCHER: Actually, I do think we are talking about revolution. And I think this challenge to hierarchy and competition is what makes this work "feminist."

HARVEY: I want to say something about naming. In the Stone Center Project at Digital Equipment Corporation (DEC) we were trying to name women's relational skills. It was the most difficult part of the project, and there were always things that stood in the way, that made it hard to really challenge the system. In some ways, we never seemed to get it right. The thing is, it's the most challenging part because it's the most threatening to the system.

QUESTION: I wanted to address the issue of organizational change. What I have noticed in years of working in organizations is that many men espouse the values of organizational change and talk as if they understand the intricacies of the process but they don't *actually* value these things. I am a consultant, and I have actually been forced to reduce my billable hours because the organization didn't believe that what I was doing was "real" work. So I am intrigued by the notion of language—that we need a language to talk about these things to get them valued. And what is frustrating me is that some of the language is out there . . . so much so that it has almost become a cliché to talk about teams and team building. But even though the language is there, there isn't a real understanding of what this type of work means and what it takes to really do it well.

WALKER: Well, I think naming is a very radical act. There is a huge investment in *not* naming or in using language to obscure reality. But if we start naming what it is that women do and naming it in strong language, that is radical because it is a direct challenge to the status quo. If we name these things as necessary, what we are doing is pointing to neediness in that segment of the population that doesn't have these skills. And there is nothing more shameful in this masculine hierarchical structure than to have a need!

MILLER: Just to add a little ray of hope. The Stone Center Project at DEC that Maureen Harvey mentioned *did* achieve some success in this regard. People did begin to name these things and make recommendations for how they could be valued and some real changes were made. So, it is possible to do this. And even though with downsizing, all the changes didn't last forever, they had a real impact on the people there.

QUESTION: I really would like some concrete suggestions. For years I have been consulting to a group of women, and when I try to name some of these things and talk about team building and process, I often get accused of being too touchy-feely.

STIVER: One of the things your comment points out is how hard it is to *own* this type of behavior. If we start to think of these things as strengths, that puts us in a very different relationship with the rest of society and in some sense it threatens the relationships we have. And so sometimes we as women tend to back away. So, it really points out how we need to support each other and help each other because it really is very scary to challenge society in this way.

MILLER: In terms of a specific suggestion, I think one important contribution this work makes is that we can name these strengths not just as process, as we in psychotherapy do, but as *practice*. And that is a big difference.

COMMENT: I want to make one comment about the way women are expected to listen to people's troubles at work, like the woman who had to listen to that man's fertility problems. It just strikes me that if men are in these really competitive positions, they absolutely need someone who will listen and relieve some of the pressure. But before they can go to someone they have to be absolutely certain that person will never be their boss or be in a position to compete with them. So they have to have some marginalized group they can dump this stuff on. But then the thing is, they have a tremendous motivation to make sure the marginalized group *stays* that way and is never in a position to use that information against them. So there is a way in which doing this kind of relational work really contributes to keeping you in a one-down position.

REFERENCES

Hammer, M., & Champy, J. (1993). *Reengineering the corporation.* New York: HarperBusiness.

Huff, A. (1990, May). *Wives–of the organization.* Paper presented at the Women & Work Conference, Arlington, TX.

Jacques, R. (1992). *Re-presenting the knowledge worker: A poststructuralist analysis of the new employed professional.* Unpublished doctoral dissertation, University of Massachusetts, Amherst.

Jordan, J. V., Kaplan, A. G., Miller, J. B., Stiver, I. P., & Surrey, J. L. (1991). *Women's growth in connection: Writings from the Stone Center.* New York: Guilford Press.

McIlwee, J., & Robinson, J. G. (1992). *Women in engineering.* Albany: State University of New York Press.

Miller, J. B. (1986). *Toward a new psychology of women* (2nd ed.). Boston: Beacon Press.

Mintzberg, H. (1973). *The nature of managerial work.* Englewood Cliffs, NJ: Prentice-Hall.

Ruddick, S. (1989). *Maternal thinking*. Boston: Beacon Press.

Senge, P. (1990). *The fifth discipline*. New York: Doubleday.

Wadel, C. (1979). The hidden work of everyday life. In S. Wallman (Ed.), *The social anthropology of work* (pp. 365–384). New York: Academic Press.

Weick, K. (1968). Systemic observational methods. In G. Lindzey & E. Aronson (Eds.), *Handbook of social psychology* (2nd ed.). Reading, MA: Addison-Wesley.

This chapter was originally presented at a Stone Center Colloquium on November 1, 1995. © 1996 by Joyce K. Fletcher.

Index

Page numbers followed by an *f* indicate figure; *t*, table.